The Doctor's Book of Natural Health Remedies

Unlock the Power of Alternative Healing and Find Your Path Back to Health

Peg Moline and the editors of **NaturalHealth**

Published in the United States of America by
Galvanized Books,
a division of Galvanized Brands, LLC, New York

Galvanized Books is a trademark of
Galvanized Brands, LLC

BOOK DESIGN BY GEORGE KARABOTSOS

SECTION OPENER ILLUSTRATIONS BY MARIE-ELAINE CUSSON

LINE DRAWING ILLUSTRATIONS BY MCKIBILLO

QIGONG POSE ON THE COVER PHOTOGRAPHED BY Z. WENDELL

Printed in the United States of America on acid-free paper.

ISBN 9780989594080

GALVANIZED

DEDICATION

This book would not be possible without the doctors who have been invaluable to us at *Natural Health* magazine over the years: the medical doctors, researchers, integrative physicians, acupuncturists, naturopaths, chiropractors, TCM practitioners, yoga therapists, homeopaths and more.

Specifically, thank you to: Andrew Weil, M.D., James Gordon, M.D., Mark Hyman, M.D., Joan Borysenko, Ph.D., Frank Lipman, M.D., Alice Domar, Ph.D., Christiane Northrup, M.D., John Douillard D.C., Dean Ornish, M.D., Neal Barnard, M.D., Judith Orloff, M.D., Elson Haas, M.D., Woodson C. Merrell, M.D., Judith Lasater, Ph.D., Mehmet Oz, M.D., and many, many others. I appreciate the generosity and patience you've shown my staff and writers as they wrestled this wealth of information into place.

The *Natural Health* staff! Couldn't have done this book without your excellence: Meghan Rabbit, Stephanie Birdsong, Jennifer Carofano, Yvonne Duran, Virginia Pelley, Cassie Tomlin, Maura Weber, Stacey Harper, Sharon Cohen, Beth Katz, Kate Wertheimer, Michele Hauf, Tracey Whitney, Nicole Dorsey, Maria Vega, Tara Thompson, Alexa Joy Sherman, Diana Gonzalez and all past designers and editors: copy, deputy and otherwise. Hillary Dowdle, thank you for your words, wisdom and guidance.

The writers, you know who you are. I'm especially appreciative of Kris Carr, Leslie Goldman, Kristina Grish, Lauren Piscopo, Ashley Koff, Susan Hayes, Dorothy Foltz-Gray, Linda Shelton and Teri Hanson.

And the team at Galvanized. Michael Freidson, thank you for your wise and witty editing, Lynette Combs, for your thorough research, George Karabotsos for your beautiful, clean design, Steve Perrine and David Zinczenko for the opportunity. Thanks!

Barbara Harris, you taught us how to be skeptical, report complicated health information responsibly and not jump on any bandwagons. It will serve me the rest of my life.

Ken Ng, you're the best ex a girl ever had—thanks for helping with kids and house so I could work and travel. And to my daughters, Lily and Maggie, love you so much. Thank you for bringing joy and meaning to my life.

—Peg Moline
former Editor-In-Chief, *Natural Health*

CONTENTS

PART 1

Find what ails you, and then find the remedy,
backed by the latest research.

PART 2

PART 3

PART 4

Introduction

You are the most important part of your health care system.

Gone are the days when you saw your family physician, filled a prescription and crossed your fingers—doctor knows best. Now the patient is part of the solution, with more choices than ever. Pick your health plan. Change your provider. Select your treatment. You've got hundreds of sources, thousands of cures and millions of opinions a click away.

What many of us are choosing—today more than ever—are natural remedies. And we're choosing them because they work.

In fact, natural remedies have been proven effective for thousands of years—herbal treatments, yoga, massage or simply restoring balance to one's diet. Many of the techniques detailed in this book, all backed by stunning new research, are literally ancient, and still being proven effective today. More than 80% of the world's population relies on herbs for health and healing. Americans are finally joining them en masse because we're sick and tired of our health care system, in addition to being sick and tired. Cue the Natural Health Care Boom.

One number says it all: $740. That's the average cost of going to the doctor for a common cold, before insurance deductions. Throw in prescription costs, time off work, and money spent on over-the-counter meds, and of course we're looking into more affordable alternative therapies. Our country's health bill is $2.7 trillion annually, and drugs account for 10%—how much of that bill are you paying? How much do you desperately need to save?

And more to the point, are you even happy with the expensive health care you're getting? Overworked and underpaid, many Western doctors simply don't have the time to spend with patients, churning them out faster than ever, according to recent studies. There are also more patients than ever, as the obesity epidemic and disease rates soar. And the Affordable Care Act may put even more responsibility into your hands, as well-meaning providers become overwhelmed by an increased caseload and more paperwork.

Additionally, the medications Western doctors prescribe, even the seemingly benign ones, give us pause, as we grow more skeptical of pharmaceutical companies. Most drug ads resemble an episode of *The Walking Dead,* since "side effects may include" diarrhea, hallucinations, ejaculation failure, severe depression. One drug, a popular hair-loss product, could cause grown men to lactate. Worse, doctors are over-prescribing these "cures"—one new study, in the peer-reviewed *JAMA Internal Medicine,* found docs doled out antibiotics to 60% of sore throat patients—when only about 10% can actually benefit. Another headline-making study found azithromycin—a catch-all antibiotic you've probably taken if you've had an earache or pneumonia—increases the chances of sudden death in adults. The scariest line from *The New York Times* article which detailed the findings: "Two related antibiotics... were already known to raise the risk of sudden death. But azithromycin was thought to be safer."

The American health system itself has become the leading cause of death in the United States, according to a riveting peer-reviewed piece of research by some of the nation's leading Ph.D.s and M.D.s, titled *Death by Medicine*. Each year in the United States, 783,936 people die from medical mistakes—many in hospitals—including adverse drug reactions (106,000), bedsores (115,000), unnecessary procedures (37,136) and just plain medical errors (98,000). No wonder so many are choosing alternative routes.

So, too, are many doctors and health researchers. By applying Western science to the study of alternative cures, *The Doctor's Book of Natural Health Remedies* is intended not to scare you, but to arm you, with the most authoritative information available about natural, beneficial treatments that may work separately or in tandem with your current care. The reasons for doing so are legion.

1. Natural health remedies are less invasive.

Not all solutions involve going under the knife. Acupuncture was shown, in a landmark 2012 study, to help relieve back pain and arthritis, and to improve symptoms of Parkinson's disease. Meditation, done right, can reduce your risk of a heart attack by 48%. And botanical remedies like milky oat seed can help those sick with stress, without the nasty side effects of a Prozac or Gaviscon.

2. Natural health remedies can be taken long-term.

Natural remedies can be continued for life, and also work to improve your general health while treating your illness—unlike prescription medications, which are targeted, generally used short-term and eventually stop working, sometimes causing your symptoms to return.

3. Natural health remedies are backed by science—now more than ever.

Although plenty of Western doctors still brand any nonconventional treatment as quackery, this is quietly changing. In 2013 the American Board of Physician Specialties, a national body that offers board certification, announced that it plans to start accrediting integrative doctors; and in 2012 the American Medical Association removed this line—"There is little evidence to confirm the safety or efficacy of most alternative therapies"—from its official policy.

4. Natural health remedies can perform as well as Western medicine—and even improve its effects.

For instance: A 2013 controlled study compared the effects of turmeric to the antidepressant fluoxetine (Prozac), on depression. After six weeks, researchers found that the turmeric worked just as well as the antidepressant. Ginkgo has also been studied extensively for its benefit in resolving erectile dysfunction; a 2013 review found that after taking it for six months, participants had a 50% improvement. And a University of Maryland study found that acupuncture significantly improved the odds of pregnancy for women undergoing in vitro fertilization. This book is filled with revelatory proof like this.

5. Natural health remedies are already working for your friends and family.

Nearly 40% of American adults use some form of complementary or alternative medicine (we'll call it CAM), according to a 2009 report from the National Institutes of Health (NIH) and its National Center for Complementary and Alternative Medicine (NCCAM). The NIH also reports that we spend more than $33 billion a year on alternative remedies and practitioners. To put that in context, the $11.9 billion spent on visits to CAM providers is about a quarter of what we spend on conventional doctor visits. (That there even is such a center run by the U.S. government proves how very seriously the establishment is investing in alternative therapies.)

6. Natural health remedies are easy to find and easy to use.

A niche market for hundreds of years, herbs, vitamins and alternative therapies are now trusted by your mom, your yogi, your girlfriend (maybe even your M.D., if you're lucky) and everyone's getting in on the action: local healers, farmers' markets and even those young, patchouli-smelling upstarts, Walmart and Mickey D's. Shops specializing in natural products used to stereotypically be a refuge for hippies, cultists and vegan masochists. "This stuff tastes awful," Woody Allen joked in *Sleeper.* "I could make a fortune selling it in my health food store."

Now, Whole Foods has gone from six stores in 1988 to 350 mega-marts today. Throughout the Southern U.S.—home to fried chicken and Busch beer—you'll find the farmers' market-like chain Sprouts; New York is home to growing chain Fairway (with 300 locations expected nationally); and Wild Oats, the organic pioneer based in Boulder, Colo., is also expected to expand, taking over the more traditional Fresh & Easy chain nationwide. Each of these mega-chains carries organic fruit and vegetables—and has an all-important herbs, supplements and vitamin aisle.

But the world of alternative medicine—especially those nutritional supplements, homeopathic remedies and herbal concoctions that are so widely available—can often be the most intimidating. Sales of herbal dietary supplements reached an estimated total of nearly $5.6 billion in the U.S., according to the nonprofit American Botanical Council. That's up 5.5% from the year before. And the NIH's NCCAM puts the total Americans spend on non-vitamin, non-mineral products such as omega-3 fish oil, glucosamine and echinacea at a whopping $14.8 billion. When there's that much money to be made, you can bet there's some snake oil mixed in with the fish oil.

Think of this book, then, as a decoder ring for these new stores—your authoritative guide on what to buy, how to use it and what should make you wary.

Mini-Glossary

"ALTERNATIVE" means used instead of conventional medicine.

"COMPLEMENTARY" and "integrative" medicine generally refer to non-mainstream therapies used with conventional medicine.

"BOTANICAL" means anything based on a whole plant. Herbalists believe whole plants are more effective than the isolated elements and synthetic ingredients used in drugs.

Overall Precautions

Most of the information about therapies, herbs and supplements you'll find on the following pages includes a section called "Precautions"; what you'll find below are general precautions you should take before trying any alternative or complementary treatment. And keep in mind that the information in this book is meant to guide you toward treatments you might not have considered. Always get medical advice from your doctor and/or a reputable source of medical information.

Tell your primary care doctor if you are using, or considering, any form of alternative or complementary treatment or herbs.

Tell your complementary practitioner about any treatments—conventional or nonconventional—drugs or herbs you are currently using.

If you are being treated for an illness, do not stop treatment without consulting your doctor, and do not stop any course of treatment that is working. Do not stop conventional treatment solely on the recommendation of an alternative practitioner.

Be extra careful if you're pregnant, nursing or trying to conceive; most herbs have not been tested on pregnant women or babies—and remember that whatever you ingest, your baby ingests. Most doctors will not recommend herbs or homeopathic remedies during pregnancy. Always consult with your caregiver before embarking on a nonconventional course of treatment.

Always check the credentials, professional alliances and education of a practitioner you are planning to see. Beware of any practitioner who will not see you for an informational appointment before signing you up for a course of treatment. In fact, beware of practitioners who insist on signing you up for a course of treatment.

Always ask how long treatment should be expected to last, and what the total cost will be.

Avoid any practitioner who makes you feel uncomfortable or pressured. Be wary of practitioners who seem to make excessive claims and guarantee a cure, especially if they stand to make a lot of money. Also be wary of a nonconventional practitioner who will not talk to your conventional doctor, especially if you are being treated for a serious illness.

Be sure to tell your doctor or practitioner if you have a sexually transmitted disease.

7. Finally, as we said at the beginning, natural remedies are less expensive.

Less expensive than a stay in the ER; less expensive than generic drugs; less expensive because they come from Mother Earth. This book has already paid for itself!

But wait....

You're skeptical—that's OK. You should be. For every zinc supplement proven to soothe colds, there are a dozen more "wonder cures" that may do more harm than good, sold by marketers preying on the vulnerable. (The word "quack" derives from a Dutch word meaning "hawker of salve"—this was back before there were infomercials and Nigerian spam.)

The concerns about herbal and alternative cures are reasonable. There's the paranoia: Are you getting ripped off? The placebo effect: Are the benefits psychological, rather than pharmacological? Wouldn't your sniffles have gone away over time, without that myrrh smoothie? The lack of FDA approval: Who's overseeing all this? What's next—Goldfish crackers advertising omega-3s? And, worst of all, irresponsible claims being made by advertisers and practitioners alike who, so confident in their remedies, may overstretch the truth and promise results you just aren't going to see.

Now's a good time to draw your attention to the box on page xi—"Overall Precautions." Our recommendation generally is to explore the world of natural healing in tandem with your doctor or physician, and to be conscious of dosages, claims and medical realities. There is no instant cure for the common cold—herbal or otherwise.

But it's also a good time to point out that many supplements—including most in this book—have research to back them up, with more studies being done every day. One of the benefits of growing consumer interest is that the more people who flock to alternative remedies, the more studies will arise. Remember, Louis Pasteur was once called a quack. So was Lovisa Åhrberg, the first female Swedish doctor. Are we at the beginning of what may be a major, holistic revolution?

The Beautiful Mind

Several elements unite the healing therapies we've included in this book: They involve lifestyle changes, particularly in diet, exercise and stress management. Self-help is a huge component in most. But believing in the power of your mind to heal your body is quite evident in all.

Study after study proves the power your mind has over your body. To us, one recent piece of evidence says it all: In 2008, U.S. Track & Field—and most visibly, officials of the New York City Marathon—banned the use of personal stereos during competition; iPods, MP3 players, anything with earbuds was disallowed, especially for anyone running a championship race. Why? Research has shown that runners experience less pain during training if they are listening to music. Psychologists believe music has a dissociative effect, diverting attention from fatigue and promoting a positive mood state.

In other words, music is considered a performance enhancer by USTF. The same effects have been shown in other sports, such as weight-lifting, and tennis players are famous for using music to calm pre-match jitters. What therapies such as biofeedback, yoga, ayurveda and even acupuncture teach you is how to harness that power to heal yourself and stay well.

Take a look at the facts here, talk to your doctor and decide for yourself what to trust.

The time for this is now. *Natural Health* has been the leading authority on natural remedies for two generations, making this book essential for anyone who wants to live a longer, healthier life. The work is honest. Balanced. Inspiring. And it is, most of all, authoritative.

How We Break It Down

With choice comes confusion. So we've organized the book based on how we think you'll want to use it, starting with...

Conditions

When your IBS flares during a big meeting, you probably don't immediately think of the cure. You think of the problem (and the laundry). So we've organized the ailments alphabetically by name, from Acne to Yeast Infections, with biggies like Cancer, Diabetes and Heart Disease in between. Throughout, you'll learn about causes, discover reduction techniques and get advice from the nation's leading experts.

Alternative Healing

The alt-docs, and why their remedies work. In this chapter, you'll find physical therapies (acupressure, chiropractic), sensual adventures (aromatherapy), psychological escapes (meditation) and a combination of all three (yoga). Yoga, for instance, continues to be the best therapy for low back pain, stress and fatigue; a 2011 study found that patients with moderate low back pain were significantly better, and using less pain meds, after 12 weeks of classes.

Herbs

This is what you've always wanted, if you've ever walked a garden and thought: aloe vera, black cohosh, feverfew, milk thistle—what the heck is milk thistle? (It's good for the liver—and a hangover. Oh, now you're interested.) These are cures straight from Mother Nature's garden, essential for every kitchen or medicine cabinet—including the 12 best herbs for women.

Supplements

CLA. CoQ10. L-glutamine. Your local vitamin store is an unsolvable alphabetical algorithm of supplements, with no one but the kid behind the counter to guide you. But in *The Doctor's Book of Natural Health Remedies*, you'll find an exhaustive, essential and scientific breakdown of supplements, and the complete evidence on what does, and does not, work.

The result is the most current, comprehensive guide to natural remedies available, at a time when you need it most. The best expert on your body is you, so stay informed. Use *The Doctor's Book of Natural Health Remedies* and enjoy your healthy body—the way nature intended.

Doctors? What Doctors?

Every piece of information in this book—a study on red rice yeast and cholesterol, research about the health benefits of meditation or how melatonin works to help you sleep—has been researched, vetted, cited and/or endorsed by a doctor, and then fact-checked by the *Natural Health* writers and editors. The doctors are M.D.s, Ph.Ds., naturopaths, acupuncturists, homeopaths, chiropractors—an entire array. That's why the book is called *The Doctor's Book of Natural Health Remedies*.

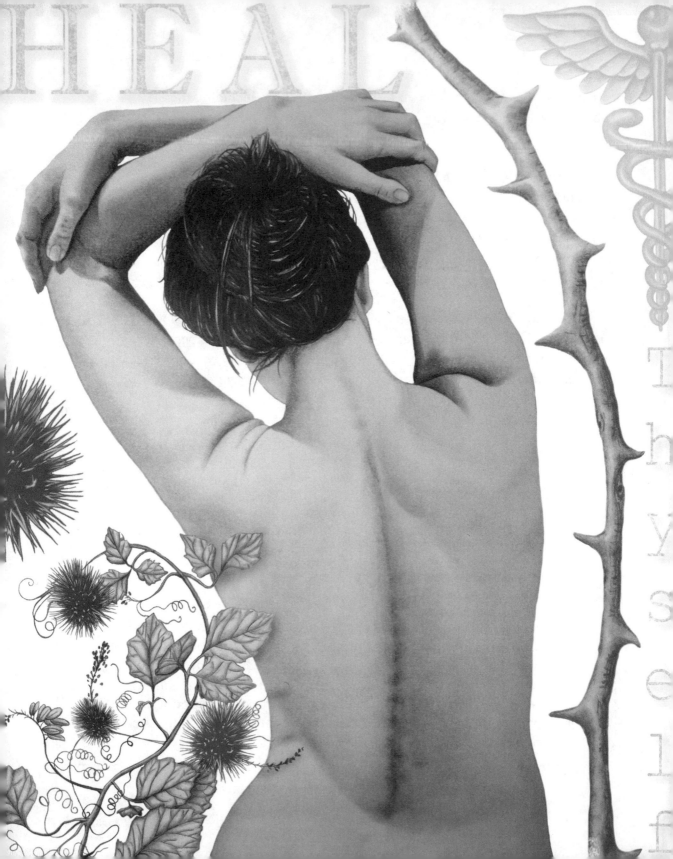

HEAL

Thy self

PART

I

Conditions

America, you're getting sicker.

An obesity epidemic is killing us, and more than one in three of us is overweight or obese. Some 78 million adults have high blood pressure, which could lead to a stroke or heart attack. In 2013, we saw a shocking rise in cancer—more than 1.6 million new cases, according to the American Cancer Society. Even the flu is out of control: Overcrowded hospitals, filled with coughs and sneezes, are forcing some emergency rooms to temporarily shut down. Diabetes, depression, osteoporosis… We could go on. Among Americans, 86% have seen a doctor in the last year.

Read this chapter and you'll go to the doctor less.

We've studied the latest research devoted to curing, healing or relieving problems big (cancer, diabetes) and small, with the cold and flu in between; and we will walk you through the alarming symptoms and the calming remedies—many newly discovered. The result is a compendium of evidence you can use right now, convincing because:

1. THE RESEARCH PROVES IT WORKS.

In each section, we quote the latest breakthrough studies, many from just last year (before publication). Niacin leads to "significant drops in total cholesterol." Coffee could reduce the risk of breast cancer recurrence. And there's hope for the infertile: Doing acupuncture, along with IVF, could increase your chances of conception by 65%.

2. MORE M.D.s ARE WILLING TO WORK WITH YOU.

Let your doctor know what you've read here. An open-minded physician will consider integrating these treatments with the care schedule. This works particularly well with diseases that have awful side effects (like cancer, post-radiation), or last a lifetime (like back pain).

3. YOU WON'T BE ALONE.

"My daughter just turned 8 months old today and was diagnosed with stage 4 neuroblastoma," a type of cancer most common in infancy, writes one concerned parent, on the Fight Cancer Facebook page. "This little angel has touched so many hearts... Pray for my little girl." We all have a friend or relative posting something similar—about themselves, or a loved one. Pages and pages on the Web are devoted to diseases, and dealing with them. We bring them up here because you'll also find more than a few from people fed up with traditional Western medicine. "These Modern Medical Quackery experts are poisoning my poor wife right now," writes another man on the same Facebook page. "Everybody continues to remain blinded from the true nature of healing, which is holistic, not reductionistic."

Fair assessment or not, we get his point. Americans are getting sicker—but are also ready to heal themselves.

ACNE

What's more horrifying than being called "crater face" when you're a teenager? Being called "crater face" *by* your teenager. It's a particularly modern dilemma. "The majority of people used to outgrow adolescent acne," says Richard G. Fried, M.D., Ph.D., a dermatologist and clinical psychologist. After all, it's usually sparked by an increase in testosterone during puberty. Oil and dead skin block the follicles, the tiny sacs that produce hair. Enter zits. "Now about half of adults have acne in some form, and many who never had significant acne develop it for the first time."

Why are so many of us having Oxy moments? Pollution, new medications and hormone-pumped meats are among the potential culprits, experts say. "However, the one common denominator we see among adult acne patients is stress," says Linda K. Franks, M.D., medical director of Gramercy Park Dermatology in New York City. "People are juggling work and family, and generally have busier lives than ever before."

SYMPTOMS

Women are more often affected than men, due to age-related hormonal changes (exacerbated by stress) and increased oil production in the skin (courtesy of the sebaceous glands, which are tweaked by... stress), not to mention certain birth control options, pregnancy, perimenopause and menopause. And ironically, your skin may be drier and less resilient due to the treatments you relied on during adolescence, such as benzoyl peroxide or Retin-A.

Stressed yet?

You're not alone. Forty-five percent of women between ages 21 and 30 had clinical acne, in a 2011 study by Massachusetts General Hospital, as did a quarter of those between 31 and 40. That's on par with a University of Alabama study from a few years previous. Fortunately, a variety of do-it-yourself natural approaches can gently but effectively target acne.

REMEDIES

Topical Treatments

It's important to treat delicate, acne-prone skin gently. Wash your face twice a day, not more, and no harsh scrubbing; choose oil-free non-comedogenic moisturizers and makeup; and try the following:

STEAM

How it works: Opens pores to release blockages, including oil and dead skin cells, that can lead to pustules.

How to use it: Pour boiling water over a handful of strawberry leaves, eucalyptus, thyme and wintergreen. Place a towel over your head to trap the steam and lean over the bowl for 10 to 15 minutes.

NATURAL CLAY MASK

How it works: Also opens pores.

How to use it: Combine a tablespoon of kaolin clay or Fuller's Earth with rose water to form a paste; spread it over your face, leave on for 10 minutes and rinse with tepid water.

TEA TREE OIL

How it works: Antimicrobial action fights the bugs that can contribute to breakouts.

How to use it: Apply a 15% solution to blemishes (unbroken skin only) twice a day.

CALENDULA

How it works: Acts as an antimicrobial and anti-inflammatory; helps heal damaged skin.

How to use it: Apply an herbal ointment or a tea directly to the blemishes.

ALOE VERA GEL

HOW IT WORKS: Contains antibacterial, anti-inflammatory and astringent (pore-shrinking) properties.

HOW TO USE IT: Apply to skin after washing.

Food for Your Face

For years, the common belief was that diet had no effect on acne. That may be wrong, according to recent research.

CHOW DOWN ON COMPLEX CARBS

HOW THEY WORK: Carbohydrates with a high glycemic index (GI) are digested rapidly, causing blood sugar (glucose) and insulin levels to spike. This may influence the development and severity of acne, an Australian study found. Conversely, a diet high in protein and low-GI carbohydrates (complex carbs) seemed to decrease the frequency and intensity of breakouts.

HOW TO GET THEM: Minimize your intake of sugars (sucrose, fructose, corn syrup); processed and refined foods; white rice and bread; and pasta and baked goods made with white flour. Instead, eat plenty of whole-grain products, including breads, cereals and brown rice; beans, lentils and split peas; and fruits and vegetables.

OPT FOR OMEGA-3s

HOW THEY WORK: A report published in the journal *Lipids in Health and Disease* suggests that by suppressing inflammation throughout the body, omega-3 fatty acids may help control inflammatory acne, a severe form of the condition.

HOW TO GET THEM: Cold-water oily fish, such as salmon and sardines; flaxseeds; and omega-3 supplements.

ADDICTION

Most addictions start innocently enough. We turn to an occasional cigarette, glass of wine, sleeping pill or shopping spree to relieve tension. No one would confuse these leisurely activities for a compulsive behavior or addiction—at least not until the psychological or physical need for them starts to interfere and takes control of our lives. Then, Houston (as in Whitney), we have a problem.

If you read *OK!* magazine you'd think the whole world was in rehab; in truth, about 23.5 million Americans 12 years and older needed treatment for drug or alcohol abuse in 2009, according to the Substance Abuse and Mental Health Services Administration's (SAMHSA) National Survey on Drug Use and Health, and only 2.6 million, or 11.2%, entered a drug or alcohol treatment program. NIH statistics from 2011 state that addiction to tobacco, alcohol and illicit drugs costs more than $600 billion a year in health care, lost work productivity and crime. (Note: They include marijuana.) About $137 billion of that number is health costs.

SYMPTOMS

Addiction can seem like a pretty strong word; many of us prefer the term "dependency." But the two aren't the same, says Scott Sandland, C.Ht., a Southern California–based medical hypnotherapist. Dependencies are purely physical; addictions, he says, also have an emotional or psychological component. If you have acute, debilitating pain, you depend on pharmaceuticals to dull it. This dependency makes your stress and pain manageable. When your pain goes away, you no longer need the drug.

But dependencies can turn into full-blown addictions if you continue taking drugs, drinking to excess, gambling or having risky sex despite the destruction this causes—bodily, monetary and long-lasting psychological damage. (Families of addicts regrettably know what we're talking about; the rest of you could watch *Breaking Bad,* or the film *Shame,* or Google "meth mug shots," and be grateful you don't.) Addiction specialists Todd Ritchey and John Montgomery, Ph.D., observe that "Whenever we compulsively behave in ways that are destructive to ourselves and to others, we do so out of addiction."

REMEDIES

The natural remedies and lifestyle changes listed here focus on a certain type of dependency, and may help get your life back on track whether you're just wanting to cut back or have already gone too far. Of course, if you feel your situation is spiraling far out of control, please seek professional assistance; many of the options described here are primarily intended to enhance conventional treatments, such as 12-step programs (12step.org) or psychotherapy, not replace them.

Alcohol

ADDRESS NUTRITIONAL DEFICIENCIES

Chronic alcohol use appears to prevent the body from properly absorbing nutrients, says Thom Lobe, M.D., director of the Beneveda Medical Center, an energy medicine practice in Beverly Hills, Calif. Being deficient in vitamin B and magnesium can cause "DTs" (delirium tremens)—also known as the shakes, or the horrors—and cardiac arrhythmias (serious heart palpitations), which make detoxification from alcohol more difficult.

TRY: Twin Lab's Super B-Complex (8 ounces for $24, vitaminshoppe .com); Natural Vitality's Natural Calm magnesium supplement (8 ounces for $22; vitaminshoppe.com)

RELIEVE DEPRESSION NATURALLY

Excessive alcohol use often masks depression, which omega-3 fatty acids may help relieve.

TRY: New Chapter's Wholemega fish oil (120 1,000-milligram capsules for $55; vitaminshoppe.com)

LAY OFF THE SUGAR

Keeping blood-sugar levels steady by eating a diet that's high in complex carbohydrates and low in simple carbs (such as white bread and sweets), as well as eating a little protein every few hours, will help curb sugar cravings, a frequent problem for people who are giving up alcohol.

TRY: The amino acid L-glutamine, which helps regulate blood sugar and has effectively been used to treat alcohol addiction (for more information, see "Recreational Drugs" on page 10).

Smoking

BREATHE LIKE A YOGI

Ask most smokers why they light up and they're apt to reply, "Smoking calms me down," says Allison Kitchen, L.Ac., a certified addiction specialist with DCMindBody, in Washington, D.C. This is curious, because nicotine is actually a stimulant. But think about the ritual of lighting one up: You remove yourself from whatever you're doing—many times a day—and for several minutes you take long, slow, deep breaths. The problem? You're having your mini-meditation break with "a lethal stick in your mouth," Kitchen says. There are about 8.6 million people who are suffering from some serious illnesses caused by smoking in the United States, according to 2013 data.

When You're Feeling Out of Control

According to medical hypnotherapist Scott Sandland, C.Ht., normal activities—shopping, having sex, even a little recreational gambling—can turn into self-destructive "needs" that closely mirror addictions to drugs and alcohol. Initially, these pastimes bring us pleasure and enhance our sense of well-being. But the more we turn to these activities to get our happy fix, even when we know they cause pain and suffering, the more we get into trouble. Effective solutions include hypnosis and cognitive behavioral therapy (CBT); both can help identify unconscious thoughts and behaviors and replace the emotions that trigger compulsive behaviors with more positive ones.

The solution? Take five without the cigarette—using yoga breathing techniques. Breathe in deeply through the nose, pause for one second, and then exhale slowly and completely, taking longer on the exhalation, which calms the nervous system. Pause at the end of your out-breath for a count of four. Repeat six to 10 times before breathing normally again.

CHOOSE FOODS CAREFULLY

According to a 2013 review of the best ways to quit smoking, a Duke University study found that certain foods and beverages—milk, fruit, vegetables, water and juice—make cigarettes taste worse, while alcohol and, to a lesser extent, meat and caffeinated drinks, enhance their flavor. Reach for some carrot or celery sticks and a glass of water when you feel the urge to smoke; you'll ruin the taste of the cigarette and keep your hands too busy to reach for one more.

TRY HOMEOPATHY

There's a veritable bevy of homeopathic remedies available to help you quit smoking. The following are recommended by Boulder, Colo., certified homeopath Kathy Thorpe:

• Tabacum helps rid the body of tobacco residue and detoxify the effects of tobacco and nicotine. Take 30c twice a day for the first five days of your smoking detox.

• *Lobelia inflata* creates a strong aversion to tobacco. Take three pellets of 6c lobelia at each craving until the urges subside.

• *Nux vomica* can help relieve the irritability, headache, "toxicity" and constipation that sometimes accompany efforts to quit smoking. Take 30c once or twice a day for five days.

• *Antimonium tartaricum* offers relief from the coughing and excess mucus that can accompany withdrawal. Take 6c three times a day for several weeks until your cough eases.

TRY: Boiron Quit Smoking Care Kit contains *nux vomica* and *lobelia inflata* ($14; amazon.com); Hyland's Homeopathic Tabacum ($8 at retail stores); Boericke & Tafel's *antimonium tartaricum* 30X ($5 at retail stores).

Recreational Drugs

Is it 4:20 all day long? Spending too much time with Molly? Been skiing the slopes—every night? A dependence on drugs is no joke. This is your brain—on natural remedies.

GET ACUPUNCTURE, OFTEN

The National Acupuncture Detoxification Association's well-studied protocol uses specific auricular (ear) points to treat drug withdrawal. According to Steve Given, DAOM, L.Ac., dean of clinical education at the American College of Traditional Chinese Medicine in San Francisco, drugs suppress the body's own ability to produce endorphins, which are pain-reducing neurotransmitters. "Acupuncture has been shown to induce the release of endorphins and other neurotransmitters," he says. It calms the nervous system and reduces withdrawal symptoms, cravings and drug-related dreaming. Its effects are cumulative, so consider daily sessions at first.

TAKE AN AMINO ACID SUPPLEMENT

A neurotransmitter deficiency can trigger specific cravings; amino acid supplements can be effective treatments. "We've been using them to treat addiction since the '80s because they work," says Julia Ross, M.A., executive director of The Recovery Systems Clinic in Mill Valley, Calif. A serotonin deficiency (which can cause cravings for alcohol and marijuana) can be treated with L-tryptophan; L-tyrosine can lessen cravings for stimulants like cocaine; a gamma-aminobutyric acid (GABA) deficiency can cause addiction to benzodiazepines (such as Xanax or Valium) and is treatable with a GABA supplement; and L-glutamine, which helps regulate blood sugar, is effective in cases of alcohol and barbiturate

Addicted to Stress?

Because the adrenaline rush from stress creates an unconscious "reward" in the brain, it can become habit-forming, says addiction specialist John Montgomery, Ph.D. Try restorative yoga classes or take slow meditative walks in nature to trigger the brain's release of serotonin, a calming neurotransmitter.

addiction, Ross says. "Don't take a supplement that mixes amino acids in one formula," she cautions; although if you have multiple addictions, you can take separate supplements to address each one.

TRY: Source Naturals amino acids: L-tryptophan (30 capsules for $12), L-Glutamine (50 capsules for $7); L-tyrosine (50 capsules for $7), GABA (45 capsules for $13; sourcenaturals.com)

SMELL THE ROSES

Many essential oils have sedative properties, while others can lift and energize, says aromatherapist Brigitte Mars, author of *Addiction-Free: Naturally.* Use only pure (not synthetic) oils, choose scents you love and switch oils from time to time. Put a few drops of the oil on a cotton ball and inhale deeply, exhaling for even longer. Mars suggests the following:

ROSE OIL (*Rosa damascena, R. gallica*) inspires confidence and lifts depression. Useful during a crisis, such as alcohol or drug withdrawal.

CLARY SAGE (*Salvia sclarea*) helps relieve panic, paranoia and mental fatigue. Good for overcoming cravings for barbiturates ("downers") and marijuana.

BERGAMOT (*Citrus bergamia*) helps relieve anxiety, depression and compulsive behavior. Use to counter addiction to cocaine or other stimulants.

TRY: Aura Cacia Aromatherapy oils (auracacia.com or in stores like Whole Foods Market)

Pharmaceutical Drugs
GET MORE SLEEP

People often turn to prescription drugs like OxyContin, Vicodin or Xanax because they have a lot of pain or anxiety. But withdrawing from these drugs actually intensifies the feelings that likely led to your addiction in the first place, says Jacob Teitelbaum, M.D., medical director for the national Fibromyalgia and Fatigue Centers. Sleep can help relieve the pain and the anxiety. If you can't sleep, the calming herbs valerian, passionflower, wild lettuce, Jamaican dogwood and hops may help.

TRY: Fatigued to Fantastic! Revitalizing Sleep Formula by Enzymatic Therapy ($15 for 30 vegetable capsules; enzymatictherapy.com).

START EXERCISING

Regular workouts of any kind have been shown to be beneficial in treating addictions, especially when paired with other treatment. A 2011 study in *Trials,* for instance, showed exercise worked as part of a treatment program for stimulant abuse, and eased symptoms such as sleeplessness. Strengthening practices with a mindful component, such as karate, can bolster your body's ability to calm itself without replacing one addiction (pills) with another (exercise). Quieter types of exercise like qigong and yoga also help you engage with your body; and the more you get to know your body, the less you'll want to abuse it.

TRY HYPNOTHERAPY

The subconscious mind is always moving you from pain toward pleasure, says hypnotherapist Debra Berndt. If it senses that kicking a drug habit will cause discomfort, your subconscious will steer you toward that addiction, not away from it. Hypnosis can "rewire" this subconscious pattern by using the powers of suggestion and visualization, Berndt says. Commit to 20 sessions (in 20 days, if possible) for the best results. To find a medical hypnotherapist in your area, go to asch.net.

ADHD

These days it's hard to tell what's "attention deficit hyperactivity disorder" (ADHD) and what's just a busy day in 2014. Say you teach yoga, homeschool your children, sing in a choir and remodel the kitchen, all while finishing a novel, redesigning a garden and buying a vintage car—and you do it all with a boundless enthusiasm, tempered by a gnawing restlessness, always moving, moving, moving?

First of all, well done: The kitchen looks awesome. But a behavioral neurologist would inquire about symptoms: Adults with ADHD have difficulty following directions, remembering information, concentrating, organizing tasks, and/or completing work within time limits. Not managed appropriately, these difficulties can cause associated behavioral, emotional, social, vocational and academic problems. And you may be too busy to even notice.

SYMPTOMS

About 4% to 5% of American adults suffer from ADHD, and they work 22 fewer days than their ADHD-free coworkers annually due to their symptoms, according to a national screening survey conducted by Harvard Medical School. According to the Semel Institute for Neuroscience & Human Behavior at UCLA, ADHD is generally a chronic disorder, with 30%–50% of those individuals diagnosed in childhood continuing to have symptoms into adulthood; and there is evidence that ADHD runs in families. "ADHD isn't something that pops up when you're 45 and going through a divorce," says Daniel G. Amen, M.D., founder of Amen Clinics Inc., two-time board-certified psychiatrist and best-selling author of *Unleash the Power of the Female Brain.* "You see there was evidence of it all along."

Adults with past or current symptoms of ADHD are also at a higher risk for other problems. The *American Journal of Psychiatry* found that 59% of ADHD patients suffered from major depression at some point, compared with 40% of the non-ADHD group; the respective ratio for anxiety disorder was 21% versus 8%. All of which means it's essential to look at ways of working with ADHD to harness its creative benefits—and reduce its embarrassing downsides.

Understanding the complexities of the condition and the effectiveness of traditional as well as alternative treatments begins with the acceptance of the diagnosis of ADHD. Originally known, rather alarmingly, as "minimal brain dysfunction" and then "attention deficit disorder," the condition has had one misleading moniker after another. Those with ADHD don't suffer from a deficit of attention—if anything, they have a surfeit of it. Vulnerable to distraction because they perceive too much at once, they are unable to filter out extraneous stimuli and focus on what is most important.

The cause may be a lack of blood flow and electrical stimulation to the frontal cortex—the area of the brain involved in prioritizing, focusing and choosing words thoughtfully rather than blurting them out. Scans of people with ADHD usually show reduced activity in this decision-making area of the brain, notes Amen.

Some researchers suggest that "executive functioning disorder" is a better description. "ADHD people think in a tangential, nonlinear, circular way," says Hal Elliott, M.D., residency program director and associate professor at East Tennessee State University's Quillen College of Medicine in Johnson City. "One thing reminds them of something else, which reminds them of something else. People with ADHD tend to be writers, musicians, visionaries, inventors and people who rock the boat at work—they come up with better ways to do things. There's nothing wrong with being a nonlinear person except that it can make you miserable in this linear world we live in."

Do You Have ADHD?

The principal characteristics of attention deficit hyperactivity disorder (ADHD) are inattention, hyperactivity and impulsivity, according to the National Institute of Mental Health. Behavior can be predominantly inattentive (you make careless mistakes, are easily distracted, leave tasks uncompleted), predominantly hyperactive-impulsive (you feel restless and fidgety, interrupt, blurt out comments, have difficulty relaxing or waiting) or both. Of course, everyone exhibits such tendencies once in a while, but most people quit when these actions become inappropriate or detrimental.

The following self-test questions, developed by the World Health Organization, can help you identify behavior consistent with adult ADHD. Answer never (0 points); rarely (1 point); sometimes (2 points); often (3 points); or very often (4 points).

A score of 11 points or more indicates the potential benefit of getting an ADHD evaluation by a health care provider.

In the last six months:

1. How often have you been distracted by activity or noise around you?

2. How often have you had difficulty getting things in order when you had to do a task that required organization?

3. How often have you had difficulty waiting your turn in situations when taking turns was required?

4. When you had a task that required a lot of thought, how often have you avoided or delayed getting started?

5. How often have you felt restless or fidgety?

6. How often have you left your seat in meetings or other situations in which you were expected to remain seated?

REMEDIES

"Since we still know so little about ADHD, treatment is very trial-and-error," says Hailing Zhang, M.D., a psychiatrist who treats many adults with ADHD. "But the gold standard is stimulant medication." Controlled studies show that drugs like methylphenidate (Ritalin, Concerta) and mixed amphetamines (Adderall) increase mental concentration by making the neurotransmitters dopamine and norepinephrine more available to the brain. Drugs related to antidepressants (Wellbutrin, Strattera) can be successful in treating ADHD, too.

But some of these drugs may cause side effects like insomnia, stomach pain, loss of appetite, irritability, anxiety or heart problems. They

Drain Your Brain

Feeling stressed and overwhelmed? "People with ADHD need time each day without stimulation so they can decompress," says Hal Elliott, M.D. Restore yourself with activities that relieve the mental and emotional strain, such as:

GETTING OUTSIDE
Spending time outside in green settings can be a valuable part of treatment, says a study published in the *American Journal of Public Health*.

PLAYING
It's sometimes easier for those with ADHD to concentrate when they're engaged in pleasurable activities, and there's real therapeutic benefit to be had from achieving tangible results. Having a hobby—gardening, woodworking, knitting, any kind of hands-on endeavor—is a great outlet for ADHD energy.

RELAXING MASSAGE AND YOGA
These give busy minds a vacation by drawing awareness back into the body. "The ayurvedic technique known as Shirodhara involves pouring warm herbalized oil over the forehead in a specific pattern," says John Douillard, D.C., National Ayurvedic Medical Association board member. "This stills the mind and calms the nervous system." Available through ayurvedic practitioners and in some day spas, Shirodhara is sometimes referred to as "bliss therapy."

can even be deadly: Canadian authorities banned the use of Adderall for several months in 2005 due to possible sudden deaths, heart-related fatalities, and strokes in children and adults. And while the FDA considers Strattera an "effective drug" with "low risk," the agency is warning doctors to monitor children and adolescents taking it for suicidal thoughts.

Natural Possibilities

There are alternatives that show real promise. Naturopath and acupuncturist Trina Seligman, N.D., L.Ac., a guest lecturer at Bastyr University in Seattle, recommends a "foundation" of a broad-spectrum, free-form amino acid supplement taken daily to balance a patient's brain chemistry. To target specific symptoms, Seligman uses specific aminos. To improve concentration and diminish restlessness she often prescribes twice-daily single doses of dopamine precursor DL-phenylalanine or norepinephine precursor L-tyrosine; for depression, she chooses serotonin precursor L-tryptophan; and to reduce anxiety and irritability, GABA or L-theanine.

An ayurvedic herb may also help. Two Australian studies published in *Neuropsychopharmacology and Psychopharmacology* found that 300 milligrams of *Bacopa monniera* (aka brahmi) daily improved information-processing speed while slowing the rate at which newly acquired information is forgotten; the herb also reduced anxiety.

Meanwhile, a study in *Progress in Neuro-Psychopharmacology & Biological Psychiatry* determined that zinc sulfate (150 milligrams per day) can reduce some ADHD symptoms. A classic natural therapy may also be beneficial: A Swiss study showed homeopathic treatment comparing favorably to the use of methylphenidate in children with ADHD. Because the condition is so complex, however, there is no advised standard; an experienced homeopath can determine the best remedy for each individual.

The Holistic Approach

Medication and/or supplementation is only part of proper ADHD management. "Taking a whole-person approach to brain health can make an enormously positive difference," says Amen. To which we say, Amen. The following lifestyle adjustments are recommended:

FEED YOUR FOCUS

Keeping blood sugar stable is vital to leveling out symptoms. "If you have ADHD, it can be hard to function on a good day, but if your blood sugar is low or spiking, it makes it even more difficult," says Wendy Richardson, M.A., M.F.T., author of *When Too Much Isn't Enough: Ending the Destructive Cycle of ADHD and Addictive Behavior.* So cut out the processed snacks, eat real meals throughout the day and limit sugar and caffeine. (Caffeine is a stimulant, but it actually decreases blood flow to the brain.) Every breakfast, lunch and dinner should provide complex carbs, quality protein and healthy fats in the form of fresh, whole foods. Avoid preservatives and other food additives, as they may exacerbate symptoms.

PUMP THE BLOOD

Every ADHD expert emphasizes the importance of regular, vigorous movement. "Exercise is not a choice," says Amen. "It boosts blood flow to the brain and helps the brain make new nerve cells." In addition, sustained cardiovascular activity steadies blood sugar, contributes to overall mood and promotes sound sleep—something patients typically need more of. "People with ADHD don't do boring, so do what you enjoy," says Amen. "If you're not sure what to do, walk briskly—don't stroll." Get a physician's OK, then elevate your heart rate for at least 30 minutes, five days a week.

SEEK SUPPORT

ADHD has nothing to do with laziness or a lack of intelligence, yet people with the condition are often pegged as underachievers. Take advantage of psychotherapy, coaching and support groups to clarify the emotional factors involved and help restore your self-esteem.

HONOR WHO YOU ARE

Often, those with ADHD find that meeting their needs as a whole person—eating wisely, exercising, doing yoga, taking herbs and supplements, and getting support—enables them to manage the challenges of the condition. And often they begin to realize that many ADHD qualities—like flexibility, creativity and empathy—are massive strengths.

"The brain is continually adapting to its environment, growing interconnections between nerves and becoming more efficient in response to the stimulation we receive," says Sergio F. Azzolino, D.C., a clinician in San Francisco and vice president of the American Chiropractic Neurology Board. Here are three techniques that can help you reinforce positive brain function:

1. COACHING

While psychotherapy typically deals with thoughts and emotions related to the past, coaching focuses on building the future by developing strategies to attain life and career goals. "Many individuals with ADHD are creative, intelligent people who are frustrated with their lack of achievement," says Pam Milazzo, founder of the SAIL Institute and former chair of the ADHD Awareness Campaign for the Attention Deficit Disorder Association "When they learn strategies that support working memory and executive functioning, they start to see sustained success." (For more information, visit the ADD Coach Academy at addca.com or ADD Consults at addconsults.com.)

2. TAI CHI

A tai chi practice may reintroduce the brain and nervous system to a fluid, sustained state of con–centration. A University of Miami School of Medicine study found that taking two 30-minute classes a week for five weeks re-duced ADHD symptoms like anxiety, daydreaming and hyperactivity. The benefits continued during a two-week follow-up period without classes.

3. NEUROFEEDBACK

The *Journal of Clinical Psychology* published findings showing that neu-rofeedback had an effect comparable to stimulant medication in helping ADHD adolescents and adults intentionally regulate brain activity. This technique uses monitoring equipment to display a visual represen-tation of your brain state. Working with a specialist —a health care profes-sional with additional training—you learn to differentiate between different brain wave types, and independently regu-late brain wave activity for increased concentra-tion and focus.

AGING

Don't fight it, Dorian Gray. Staying younger isn't about turning back time, but enjoying what's left of life—wisely. Eating well, exercising, stressing less and staying positive, plus the latest creams, supplements and, yes, beer, beer!—we've collected the latest advice from the leading experts, and the results will surprise even old-timers bored of the clichés. Herewith, the 25 best ways to always feel under 40. Your longer life starts now.

1. Move it

New research from The Center for BrainHealth at the University of Texas at Dallas claims that 30 minutes of aerobic exercise, three to four times a week, improves short-term memory by increasing blood flow to the medial temporal lobe—where memories are stored. "Learning becomes more brittle as we age," says Sandra Bond Chapman, Ph.D., founder and chief director of the institute. "But the brain's plasticity allows it to grow, change and heal throughout our lifespan, and aerobic exercise helps this happen." The sooner you start, the better: Harvard University researchers recently found that women older than 70 who'd regularly participated in physical activity during middle age seemed to be in better health than those who hadn't.

2. Eat your antioxidants

These free-radical foragers help delay aging and reduce vulnerability to cancer, heart disease and diabetes, so don't just put them on your face. Keri Glassman, M.S., R.D., a New York-based registered dietitian, calls these edible antioxidants "beauty foods": dark chocolate (it contains cocoa flavanols that increase blood flow to the skin); salmon (its omega-3s prevent collagen breakdown and reduce skin-damaging inflammation); and green tea (it's loaded with polyphenols that boost cell turnover to improve skin tone).

3. Be consistent in the kitchen

Don't pay attention to your diet one minute, and then ditch your good eating habits the next. "This can create a sugar imbalance, which causes confusion, headaches, stress and fatigue—characteristic features of aging brain syndrome (ABS)," says Naheed Ali, M.D., author of *Diabetes and You: A Comprehensive Holistic Approach.* Best to keep to a diet that reduces your reliance on processed foods, stick to the good fats found in chicken, grass-fed beef and fish, limit alcohol and caffeine consumption and get rid of the sugar.

4. Pump some iron

The typical American gains a pound of fat and loses a half pound of muscle yearly from the ages of 30 to 60, says Desmond Ebanks, M.D., former assistant clinical professor of medicine at New York Medical College. "Loss of muscular strength is a major reason that elderly people lose mobility and independence," he says. Ebanks suggests an interval-style resistance program for the most muscle-building benefits; brief but intense bouts of strength training, lasting 12 to 20 minutes, have also been shown to help. For example, in a 12-minute bout of intervals you would do about 30 seconds of pushups, then hop on the treadmill for two minutes, then 30 seconds of ab curls, then to the bike for 2 minutes, then 30 seconds of lunges, then 2 minutes on the rowing machine, and so on.

5. Learn how to feel full

Trimming calories can help reduce cellular inflammation, which drives the aging process by causing disturbances in hormonal signaling between cells—thus decreasing the efficacy of every organ in the body. "Reducing excess calories is only possible if you're not hungry between meals," says Barry Sears, M.D., president of the Inflammation Research Foundation. Reach for at least 3 ounces of low-fat protein at breakfast, lunch and dinner, which increase the release of satiety hormones that stop hunger.

6. Think something nice

Researchers in a 2010 University of California, Los Angeles, study found that having social exchanges characterized by strain or conflict in mid-life was associated with poor planning and decision-making later in life. Since you can't always avoid confrontational people, Srini Pillay, M.D., assistant clinical professor of psychiatry at Harvard Medical School, suggests overriding your own cranky thoughts with good ones. "Part of the reason we get annoyed is that when someone is frustrated, our own brain is wired to detect this and sometimes even mimic it," he says. "To stop that from happening, think of something positive about the person—as long as it's true—and your brain will latch on to that thought instead."

7. Eat bitter

Humans recognize six distinct tastes—sweet, sour, salty, bitter, savory and astringent—and each plays a role in feeding your body and mind. In terms of longevity, however, bitter-tasting foods are the best because they balance sugar cravings, support digestion and metabolize fat, says Stephan Dorlandt, C.N., a clinical nutritionist and herbalist in Los Angeles. Tasty bitters include yellow and green veggies like yellow peppers, broccoli rabe, collard greens, mustard greens, radicchio and chicory. Bonus: Bitter foods also help rebalance your taste buds, causing the flavors of natural sugars, like those in milk or apples, to be more pronounced.

LONGEVITY
70 75 80 85 90 95 100
BOOSTER

TAKE VITAMIN D

There's a reason you keep hearing about the importance of getting enough of this "sunshine vitamin": "Vitamin D strongly protects against many kinds of cancer and helps keep bones strong," says Andrew Weil, M.D., author of *Healthy Aging: A Lifelong Guide to Your Physical and Spiritual Well-Being*.

Evidence shows vitamin D also bolsters the immune system, reduces asthma and helps maintain a healthy body weight. Most experts suggest taking at least 1,000 IU a day—but that's often not enough, according to women's health guru Christiane Northrup, M.D. "If you take 1,000 IU a day, you'll prevent rickets, yes. But you'll be far from the optimal dose, which can be between 2,000 and 5,000 IU a day just for maintenance."

8. Replace your morning buzz

Reach for that sweet morning latte and you'll pay for it later, says Jacob Teitelbaum, M.D., *Natural Health* advisory board member and author of *Beat Sugar Addiction Now.* Excess sugar increases your risk of diabetes, blood vessel disease and autoimmune illnesses—all of which accelerate aging. Instead of coffee, Teitelbaum suggests having a daily energy drink with a good vitamin powder (like Enzymatic Therapy's Energy Revitalization System) and adding the special healthy sugar called D-ribose. In a recent study, D-ribose increased energy an average of 61% after three weeks.

9. Eat like a Greek

In a 2011 Rush University Medical Center study, researchers found that the Mediterranean diet, long known to be heart-healthy and reduce risk of diabetes and certain cancers, is now also associated with a slower rate of cognitive decline in older people. This diet—rich in fruits and vegetables, legumes, olive oil, fish, potatoes and moderate amounts of wine—helped prevent Alzheimer's disease and create a sunny disposition in subjects.

10. Take your magnesium

Seventy-five percent of Americans don't get their Recommended Dietary Allowance (RDA) of this important nutrient, which affects age-related conditions like bone, heart and brain health, says *Natural Health* advisory board member Carolyn Dean, M.D., N.D. "Aging-related issues like constipation, memory decline, mobility and sensitivity to loud noises are also helped by magnesium," she says. One of the most inexpensive and absorbable options is powdered magnesium citrate, which you can take with hot or cold water. A serving a day of magnesium-rich cacao, kelp and kale can also help.

11. Whittle your middle

A 2010 American Cancer Society study found that a large waist size doubled one's risk of dying from any cause, regardless of whether you're normal weight, overweight or obese. "Abdominal fat cells actively secrete compounds that increase inflammation and reduce sensitivity to insulin, thus increasing the storage of fat," says Andrew Weil, M.D., founder and director of the Arizona Center for Integrative Medicine. Highly processed and rapidly digested carbohydrates, such as products made with flour, accelerate this cycle. So eat low-glycemic index foods (think whole, plant-based picks), and exercise regularly to fight fat.

12. Beware of calorie trends

New studies show cutting calories leads to longevity in mammals, but Ebanks says to be careful before subscribing to diet fads. "Calorie restriction presumes all calories are equal, but they're not," he says, noting that if you're exercising and consuming an appropriate amount of protein and healthy fat, there's less need to watch calories because you'll probably become satiated before overeating. If insufficient calories are consumed, however, he says you won't have the energy for necessary, vigorous exercise. "Do you want to live better for as many years as you can, or live longer irrespective of the quality?" he asks. The Calorie Restriction Society is a proponent of the "more years" philosophy, but it requires trimming calories by 30% to 40%—a level Ebanks says is not tolerable or sustainable for most people.

LONGEVITY
70 75 80 85 90 95 100
BOOSTER

DON'T FILL UP ON FOOD

Ronald Stram, M.D., founder of the Center for Integrative Health and Healing in Albany, N.Y., has made quite a study of centenarians— those people who have lived to be 100 and older—who are still in relatively good health. One key to their success? They know when to put down the fork. "The people in Okinawa [Japan] practice something called 'hara hachi bu,' which means that they stop eating before they get full," Stram explains. "Eating this way, they are naturally controlling their calorie intake, which has all sorts of health benefits."

But there's more to it than simple weight control. "Traditional Chinese Medicine recommends that you never eat more than 80% of your capacity so you don't overburden your organs of digestion, assimilation and elimination," says Efrem Korngold, O.M.D., L.Ac., codirector of San Francisco's Chinese Medicine Works. "That way there is more qi vital power—available to sustain and nurture the rest of the body and mind."

13. Take your Ls if you're vegetarian

Supplements that start with L, please, Alex. L-glutamine and L-arginine are amino acids found mostly in protein-rich animal sources (chicken, turkey), seafood (halibut, lobster, salmon) and wild game (pheasant, quail). A lack of L-glutamine and L-arginine in vegetarians can make them age faster. To supplement, take 2 grams of L-glutamine and 1 gram a day of L-arginine at night. Studies show these supplements can tighten skin, increase fat loss and help build muscle as we age.

14. Eat your water

Mmm, broccoli. To slow or reverse age-related cellular dehydration, aim to eat three or more fruits and five or more vegetables per day to obtain optimal cell hydration, says Howard Murad, M.D., board-certified dermatologist and associate clinical professor of dermatology at UCLA. In fact, he suggests replacing at least one glass of water a day with a raw veggie or fruit: "Colorful, water-rich produce is the best form of water for your cells, as fruits and vegetables provide structured water and antioxidants, so hydration stays in your system long enough for your body to put it to good use."

15. Get healthy, not skinny

Alice D. Domar, Ph.D., executive director of the Domar Center for Mind/Body Health in Boston, says being thin doesn't necessarily make you live longer. "Being in the middle zone of the BMI scale, somewhere around 24 to 27, is actually associated with the longest life span," she says. Just be sure to choose your calories wisely. A 2011 University of Maryland study says eating relatively high amounts of vegetables, fruit, whole grains, poultry, fish and low-fat dairy leads to superior nutritional status and quality of life in older adults, but those who indulged in sweets and desserts had a 37% higher risk of death.

16. Think young

There's a correlation between how women look (and feel) after having their hair cut and colored, according to a study by Ellen Langer, Ph.D., a mind-body psychology professor at Harvard. Independent volunteers rated women before and after they left the salon, and those ladies who believed having their hair dyed made them look younger actually did look younger after the salon visit. Those who didn't, didn't. The takeaway? "Feeling young makes you look younger," says Langer. "So act your inner age."

17. Prepare your body to sleep

Logging eight hours of shut-eye can make you look as much as three years younger, says Amy Wechsler, M.D., a New York City-based dermatologist and author of *The Mind-Beauty Connection.* If you have trouble relaxing into a sound slumber, prepare for it with a series of bed-time rituals: Don't drink caffeine four to six hours before bed; eat a full meal three hours before and no later; and log off electronics and dim the lights with an hour to go.

18. Snack your way to good sex

Those *Golden Girls* were on to something: Sex is a powerful anti-aging tool. Some studies say it can prolong your life up to 20 years, and others insist getting some reduces your mortality rate by half. So how can you get in the mood for more action? Eat strategically, says Eric R. Braverman, M.D. Foods with phytoestrogens, such as soy and fish, keep sex hormones at younger levels; lean proteins like turkey and duck contain tyrosine and phenylalanine, which boost desire; healthy fats like low-fat yogurt and eggs are packed with choline, a precursor to the brain chemical that controls arousal and lubrication; and high-fiber

LONGEVITY
70 75 80 85 90 95 100
BOOSTER

WALK AND
TALK

Another health factor common to populations who live the longest is good social support. "When you filter through the evidence to look at what is proven to work for longevity, the people who live the longest have good interpersonal connections. They have a reason to be alive," says Domar. Working out with a friend is one easy way to promote interpersonal connections. "I know a lot of women who walked their way through menopause together," says yoga therapist Carol Krucoff. "They benefited from the hormone-regulating effects of cardiovascular activity and had the very therapeutic benefit of spending time with a friend."

Andrew Weil, M.D.'s Best Anti-Aging Advice

Besides adopting an anti-inflammatory diet, here are six simple steps that Weil believes can help you live a longer, healthier life:

- **Get regular physical activity and be willing to adapt it as your body changes.**

- **Make sure to get good rest and sleep; sleep in total darkness.**

- **Find some form of stress neutralization, whether it's meditation or simple breathing exercises.**

- **Maintain good social and intellectual connections.**

- **Seek out people who have the healthful habits you are striving for.**

- **Have fun and play.**

Stress is a big pressure for women, and not recognizing and taking measures to protect yourself from it can be very destructive. Also, because women are judged more on appearance, they tend to invest more energy in anti-aging strategies, instead of learning to age in a healthy way. It's impossible to slow it, so it's better to focus on the positive aspects, namely increased wisdom and experience, more equanimity, depth of character and the ability to roll with life's ups and downs. Studies are even showing that some parts of memory improve with age. Lots of things get better as you get older; focus on those.

vegetables, fruits and whole grains are high in glutamine and inositol, which are precursors to the brain chemical that helps you relax so you can climax.

19. Switch positions

According to Traditional Chinese Medicine, specific areas of the genitals are linked to your internal organs. "This is one way Chinese medicine believes having regular sex affects overall longevity and health," says Jill Blakeway, L.Ac., an herbalist and codirector of Yin Ova Center in New York City. "To achieve inner balance, you must stimulate all of the genital organs and not just one bit of them, which might overstimulate one particular organ at the expense of others." Vary positions during sex to make sure all your insides get the attention they need.

20. Take more naps

"The brain gets slower as we age, in terms of reaction and processing time, but it rebounds when we sleep," says Chapman. "In the long run, sleep staves off those losses." Indeed, a 2009 University of California, Berkeley, study found that sleep helps the brain consolidate ideas. While naps don't count as part of your requisite seven to eight hours, they can help restore brain function if you didn't get your fill the night before.

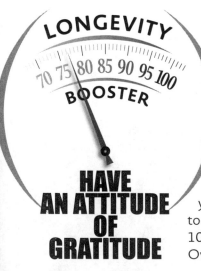

LONGEVITY
70 75 80 85 90 95 100
BOOSTER

HAVE AN ATTITUDE OF GRATITUDE

What's the best predictor of longevity? It's not blood lipids, family history, exercise or diet. According to Mimi Guarneri, M.D., medical director for Scripps Integrative Medicine in La Jolla, Calif., it's personal happiness, joy and appreciation. "If you are the type of person who is focused on doom and gloom—if you're angry, hostile or cynical—you won't live as long," she says. "You need to come to your life every single day and find something to appreciate."

Guarneri recommends creating a practice of gratitude. "If it doesn't come naturally, force yourself," she recommends. "Take a look around you—underneath your negative emotions—and find what you have to give thanks for." One way to do this: Before bed, make a list of at least 10 things that went your way during the day, no matter how small. Over time, you'll see that you do have blessings to count.

21. Believe you're getting better with age

Dilip V. Jeste, M.D., director of the University of California, San Diego's Stein Institute for Research on Aging, says people who think they're aging well aren't necessarily the healthiest physically. "Yet they generally possess a positive, yet realistic, attitude about their lives and an ability to adapt to change," he says. Tend to look at the glass as half empty? Try writing three positive things that happen each day in a journal to redirect your thoughts.

22. Take your herbs

Adaptogenic herbs help the body's ability to adapt to daily stresses, and are often included in Chinese and Western anti-aging medicines. "They help restore and maintain vitality and well-being," says Rosemary Gladstar, founder of the California School of Herbal Studies and author of *Herbs for Longevity and Radiant Well Being.* Start with herbs like rhodiola (which reduces stress and boosts energy), reishi (which protects the liver and heart and reduces cholesterol), and holy basil (which reduces anxiety and mental fog), and talk to a holistically minded doc about the right doses of each for you.

23. Keep working

New data from the United States, England and 11 other European countries suggest that the earlier people retire, the more quickly their memories decline. Researchers found that the longer subjects kept working, the better they did on memory skills tests in their early 60s. Some experts say social and personality skills known to support a healthy aging brain—like getting up in the morning, dealing with others, knowing the importance of being prompt and trustworthy—may play a role here, because these factors are valued in the work environment.

24. Don't be a buzzkill

A 2010 University of Texas study conducted over 28 years found that the way we explain the events in our lives can be a significant predictor of longevity. "Our thoughts, feelings and the way we respond to stress are powerful genetic and immune modulators and affect the way and rate at which we age," says Brenda Stockdale, director of mind-body medicine at RC Cancer Centers of Georgia and author of *You Can Beat the Odds.* So, try to be a little more optimistic and choose to see the good in a situation—or at least talk about what went right along with what went wrong when you're sharing a story.

25. Have a beer. Yes, a beer.

Scientists at the University of California, Davis, found that beer is a substantial source of silicon, which stimulates the production of collagen to keep bones strong and joints healthy by maintaining flexibility in cartilage. The study found that most beer brands contain between 6 milligrams and 57 milligrams of silicon per liter, and those with high levels of malted barley and hops have the most. We say go organic and drink in moderation. If your frat days are over, silicon can also be found in foods like bananas and brown rice.

Get Healthier Every Year!

Forget the "anti-aging" hype that instills fear in women about everything from crow's feet to cancer. Here's how to feel better with every birthday—and embrace aging gracefully in the truest sense.

Making an effort to improve your health *will* improve your health, says Dean Ornish, M.D., pioneering California-based mind-body cardiologist, physician founder and president of the Preventive Medicine Research Institute in California. "We published a study in 2008 that showed that within three months, you can turn on disease-preventing genes and turn off disease-promoting ones," he says. "Within hours, you can have improved blood flow to the brain, you can grow new brain cells and you can feel energized."

That's good for those of us who are feeling time take its toll—and for younger people who want to get a jump-start on lasting health. Here's a guide to aging gracefully in every area of your life, no matter how old you are. Of course, the basics—eating mostly plant-based foods, getting plenty of exercise and incorporating mind-body stress relievers—are crucial. But if you're doing everything right and still looking to feel a little better, read on.

Stay Healthy

In your 20s and 30s

Tune In to Your Cycle

Your menstrual cycle may be flowing like clockwork now, but premenstrual syndrome (PMS) is a common issue for young women—particularly those who are under a lot of stress. To feel your absolute best, take steps to keep this monthly nuisance from derailing your life. "You can often control PMS with lifestyle measures," says Tori Hudson, N.D., author of the *Women's Encyclopedia of Natural Medicine, 2nd Edition*. "Getting regular exercise, and minimizing caffeine, sugar and alcohol will help." If you're having more than just an occasional cramp or breast tenderness—or perhaps your lifestyle is less than optimal—you may need to add a supplement to manage PMS, Hudson says. "Look for a combination formula that contains nutrients proven to offset PMS: vitamin B_6, calcium, St. John's wort, chaste tree berry, chromium and gamma-linoleic acid from either borage or evening primrose oil." Get them all in Vitanica Women's Phase I ($16 for 60 capsules; evitamins.com), designed by Hudson especially for young women with PMS.

In your 40s...

Pump Up the Progesterone

According to hormone guru Christiane Northrup, M.D., author of *Women's Bodies, Women's Wisdom*, the dreaded perimeno-pause starts eight to 12 years before your last period—which means you'll likely spend much of your 40s coping with symptoms like insomnia and irritability. "The bad news for women is that sometime in your 40s, you'll start skipping ovulations," she explains. "That means you'll have less progesterone—the protective, calming hormone—in your system, and you'll begin to see the problematic symptoms of perimenopause." On the upside, it's relatively easy to restore balance with an over-the-counter bioidentical progesterone cream. Look for a product labeled progesterone USP to ensure that it includes a significant amount of the natural hormone, suggests Northrup. Then apply ¼ teaspoon to your skin twice a day when you're not menstruating. Northrup recommends Emerita Paraben-Free Pro-Gest ($29 for two ounces; emerita.com).

Know Your Numbers

If you haven't had a full physical lately, now's the time to get a realistic picture of your health, says Mimi Guarneri, M.D., medical director for Scripps Integrative Medicine in La Jolla, Calif., and author of *The Heart Speaks: A Cardiologist Reveals the Secret Language of Healing.* "In your 40s is when blood pressure, weight and cholesterol start to go up," she says. Numbers to know:

Blood pressure

LDL ("bad") and HDL ("good") cholesterol levels

High-sensitivity C-reactive protein (to check for inflammation in the body)

25-hydroxy vitamin D level

And if you haven't had a mammogram, do it now. When you understand the true state of your health, you can take steps to avoid potential problems.

In your 50s and beyond...

Boost Your Brainpower

In 2009, epidemiologists predicted a coming wave of Alzheimer's disease that will bankrupt the health care system and ruin millions of lives. But don't freak out: You can protect yourself with the right combination of diet, exercise and stress-relief techniques, says Dharma Singh Khalsa, M.D., president of the Alzheimer's Research and Prevention Foundation in Tucson, Ariz. In particular, stave off "senior moments" with a brain-boosting power practice known as "kirtan kriya." Drawn from the kundalini yoga tradition, *kirtan kriya* combines meditation with sound and movement to engage the brain in a uniquely healing way. Studies at the University of Pennsylvania's Center for Spirituality and the Mind have found that practicing just 12 minutes a day is enough to reverse age-related mental decline. "It improves verbal fluency and memory by increasing blood flow to the brain," says Khalsa. Here's how to do it:

- Come to a comfortable sitting position and rest the backs of your hands on your knees.
- Inhale deeply, imagining that you're drawing your breath in through the crown of your head; exhale and send that breath out through the center of your forehead. Continue to visualize this L-shaped breath throughout this exercise.
- Inhale and begin to chant aloud the four-syllable mantra, "Sa-ta-na-ma."
- On the syllable "Sa," touch your index finger to your thumb; on "ta," touch your middle finger to your thumb; on "na," touch your ring finger to your thumb; on "ma," touch your pinky finger to your thumb. Continue these finger movements throughout the exercise (use enough pressure so that your fingertips turn white).
- Chant the mantra aloud for two minutes, then chant in a whisper for two minutes. Next, say the chant silently for four minutes. Then say it in a whisper for two more minutes.
- Finish by chanting aloud for two minutes. The entire meditation takes 12 minutes.

Eat Right

In your
20s and 30s

Set (Pretty) Good Habits

The best move you can make to assure a happy, long life is to adopt good eating habits early—not only for a rockin' body but also for strong bones, a robust immune system and a host of other health benefits. "Your body is forgiving in your 20s and 30s—you can eat junk food, stay up late and party, and get away with it," says Alice Domar, Ph.D., director of the Domar Center for Mind/Body Health in Waltham, Mass. "But the habits you set now will be hard to break later. If you establish a healthy routine in your 20s, you'll be much more likely to be doing the right things in your 50s."

The good-health basics are simple: Stick to whole foods and eat a mostly plant-based diet. Aim to get plenty of fruits and vegetables every day. Forgo processed foods and drive-through windows. But don't get too uptight about it, either, says Domar. "Just aim for an overall healthy diet, and don't get too hung up on the health 'rules,'" she says. "You don't have to be perfect. Just aim for a 'pretty healthy' diet. That is doable at any age."

In your
40s...

Eat Your Phytoestrogens

Of course, continuing to follow the good eating habits you set in your 30s is essential. (And if you're a late bloomer in the healthy-eating department, making changes now will pay off.) One way to mitigate the problems associated with the plummeting hormones of perimenopause is to add phy-toestrogenic foods to your meals. Soy is the classic go-to. "Soy foods mimic the effects of estrogen, and can help treat symptoms like in-somnia, moodiness or hot flashes," says physician and registered dieti-cian Christine Gerbstadt, M.D., R.D.

She recommends two servings a day (½ cup tofu, ½ cup eda-mame and 1 cup soymilk count as one serving each). Berries, beans, nuts and fruits—which include the reproductive organs of plants, es-sentially—are also good sources.

If more help is needed to cope with hormone hell, consider taking a phytoestrogen supplement with the herb black cohosh, suggests North Carolina-based Randine Lewis, Ph.D., MSOM, L.Ac., author of *The Way of the Fertile Soul.* "Black cohosh is especially indi-cated for irritability. It will help you feel uplifted and energized with-out feeling wound-up." If insomnia is an issue, consider a blend that also includes relaxing herbs such as passionflower, valerian root and hops. We like Estroven Nighttime ($11 for 24 caplets; drugstore.com).

Choose Better Snacks

Traditional Chinese Medicine (TCM) has a long history of tonic food thought to improve wellness throughout aging and extend the lifespan. Two to try: pumpkin seeds and goji berries. "Goji berries grow and flourish in Tibet and high up in the Himalayas," says Lewis. "They have the ability to withstand harsh conditions, and they transfer that property to the body. Goji berries help us endure the weather of life." They're most often sold dried and are a tad bitter, so add them to your favorite trail mix recipe if you don't enjoy snacking on them on their own.

Pumpkin seeds nourish the kidney qi—seen in TCM as the primary source of life-force energy. "Kidney qi is our foundation energy, which declines as we age—especially around menopause," Lewis explains. "Pumpkin seeds can restore kidney energy." As a bonus, pumpkin seeds are a premium source of good fats, and have also been found in studies to reduce inflammation and lower cholesterol. Sprinkle some on top of oatmeal or salad.

In your 50s and beyond...

Support Your Structure

With the onset of menopause—which will be happening any day now, if it hasn't started already—bone density takes a big hit. Focus on adding foods rich in calcium and vitamin D, suggests Dawn Jackson Blatner, R.D., author of The Flexitarian Diet. "Low-fat dairy is a good choice because it contains both calcium and vitamin D," she suggests.

Supplements are smart, too—though the best one may surprise you. "Calcium is overrated as a supplement for osteoporosis," says Jacob Teitelbaum, M.D., author of the seminal feel-good manual From Fatigued to Fantastic. Teitelbaum's top pick? Strontium. "There are good double-blind studies that show strontium is effective in increasing bone density and decreasing fractures," he says. If you don't have bone loss yet—or it's very mild—take 340 milligrams a day. If you have full-blown osteoporosis, take 680 milligrams per day. Try EuroPharma Strontium ($20 for sixty 340-milligram capsules; vitaminlife.com).

Move More

In your 20s and 30s

Build Your Bones

In our 20s, we think of ourselves as being all grown up, but in truth our bodies are still developing through our 30s. "In early adulthood, you're still building bone mass," explains Carol Krucoff, ERYT, a yoga therapist and practitioner at Duke Integrative Medicine in North Carolina and coauthor (with husband Mitchell Krucoff, M.D.) of *Healing Moves: How to Cure, Relieve and Prevent Common Ailments with Exercise*. To build strong bones, Krucoff says, you need to do weight-bearing activity and strength training. "The higher impact the activity, the greater the effect on the bones," she explains. "Focus on activities like running, jumping and plyometrics. Racquet sports are particularly good—you're jumping around after the ball, and every time you hit it, you're sending a wave of impact up the arm and through the body." Intimidated by the weight room at the gym? Remind yourself that building muscle will keep your metabolism revved up and help you maintain a healthy weight.

In your 40s...

Strengthen Your Pelvic-floor Muscles

Let's face it: A leaky bladder is a real downer. Dribbling as we sneeze, cough, laugh or jump can happen to the best of us—especially if we've got a kid or two under our belts (so to speak). "The pelvic-floor muscles that govern bladder control naturally weaken as you get older—especially as you start going through perimenopause and there is a fluctuation of estrogen levels," explains Lynn Anderson, Ph.D., N.D., a Los Angeles-based naturopath and creator of *Dr. Lynn's Anti-Aging Workout* DVD series. "You have to make a conscious effort to keep those muscles strong." Do it, she says, and the payoff is huge: Not only do you get to live free from worry about pee-pee problems, but strong pelvic-floor muscles also improve sexual performance and experience.

As you've probably heard before, Kegels are the go-to move to target pelvic-floor muscles. "Imagine that you're urinating and the phone rings and you've got to stop peeing really quickly," Anderson says. "That stopping motion—the tightening of the pelvic muscle—is the Kegel." Do three sets of 10, holding for five seconds each, and end with a set of what Anderson calls "flutters"—quickly squeeze and release 20 times. When you get in the habit of doing Kegels, you can do them anywhere: at your desk, in the car, even at the grocery store.

Up Your Intensity

Weight gain can creep up on you in your 40s, as your metabolism naturally slows and muscle mass begins to drop. Stave it off by adding intensity, says Maryland-based Pamela Peeke, M.D., M.P.H., author of *Fight Fat After Forty*. In your cardiovascular workouts, this means mixing in intervals of increased effort—pick up the pace for a while, even if it takes you out of your comfort zone. In your weightlifting, introduce pyramids—performing three reps of each exercise, increasing the weight each time. "With a bicep curl, do 10 pounds on the first set, 12 pounds on the second set, and the maximum you can lift—maybe 15 pounds, maybe more—on the third set," she advises. "If you can only squeeze out five or six reps on the last set, no matter. What's important is that you're challenging your muscles."

In your
50s and beyond...

Find Your Balance

To maintain a happy, healthy life-style as you age, you have to stay mobile. And that means maintaining both flexibility and balance. When her patients reach age 50, Anderson has three words of advice: yoga, yoga, yoga. "At this age, you have to make a bit more effort to stay in a balanced place," she says. "It will only become more important as you continue to age—a hip fracture is a real game changer, and the number one reason they happen is lack of balance. And flexibility will help you stay walking upright into your 90s."

Along with yoga to improve both balance and flexibility, Krucoff suggests giving yourself a daily foot massage. "I think that by age 50, a lot of women get out of touch with their feet," she says. "Falls might be related to stiff feet and a loss of adequate sensation of their feet on the ground. One of the simplest things you can do is take a tip from ayurveda and massage warm sesame oil into the soles of your feet every day."

ALLERGIES

It's miraculous that spring is considered the randiest, sexiest, "Spring Break!"-iest of seasons, given the red-eyed, hay-fevery, some-times-debilitating allergies that hijack sufferers that time of year. According to American Academy of Allergy, Asthma & Immunology (AAAAI) stats, allergic rhinitis (aka hay fever and seasonal allergies) affects between 10% and 30% of all American adults, and its prevalence is increasing. Thanks to global warming and other factors, the average pollen season is longer (typically running from March through September) and more pollens are being produced, which may be part of the reason we are seeing an increased prevalence of allergic diseases—so says allergist Clifford Bassett, M.D., assistant clinical professor of medicine at New York University School of Medicine and Long Island College Hospital.

Suddenly, your outdoor picnic has turned into an alternate ending for *World War Z*.

SYMPTOMS

Your allergies flare up when your immune system overreacts (mainly to weeds, grasses and trees), the body releasing a substance called histamine to fight off the allergens as if they were a virus. Cue nasal congestion, sinus pressure, sneezing, coughing, a scratchy throat, and red, itchy or watery eyes, as well as fatigue.

What's more, if these allergies are not adequately treated, sufferers often develop related sinus symptoms, ear infections and/or asthma, says Bassett (see "The Asthma-Allergy Connection" on page 40).

REMEDIES

Over-the-counter and prescription meds such as antihistamines, decongestants and corticosteroids (in the form of pills, nasal sprays and eyedrops) can provide temporary relief but can also cause unpleasant side effects, such as drowsiness and dry mouth. Again, spring, romantic—really? While the "big guns" of immunotherapy (aka allergy shots) are often effective, they can be time-consuming and expensive. So before you go sneezing over to the pharmacist or your doctor, try implementing the following lifestyle changes and natural remedies.

Distance Yourself from Pollen

Minimizing the amount of pollen you're being exposed to is your first and simplest line of defense. Here's how:

CHECK THE COUNT

It may be time to finally catch up on that whole season of *Game of Thrones*—guilt-free. When the pollen level is high, it's best to stay indoors, says allergist Andy Nish, M.D., of the Allergy and Asthma Care Center in Gainesville, Ga. Learn the pollen count by checking your local TV weather report or newspaper. Or go to pollen.com and type in your zip code for a four-day forecast. Bonus: You can sign up for allergy alert e-mails or download a smartphone app that will notify you when the pollen count is on the rise.

WATCH THE WEATHER AND THE CLOCK

"Pollen levels are typically higher on sunny, dry and windy days and lower on cooler, moist and windless days," Bassett says. Many grasses and other plants pollinate early in the day, making mornings (particularly between 5 a.m. and 10 a.m.) notoriously bad for allergy sufferers. So wait until the late afternoon or early evening to take the dog for a long walk or weed your flowerbed.

WORK OUT INDOORS

Exercise can often help alleviate nasal congestion so you can breathe better—*unless* you're outside sucking in pollen, says Bassett. Whenever possible, stick to indoor workouts, especially when the pollen count outdoors is moderate to high. And the AAAAI emphasizes that overdoing physical activity could exacerbate symptoms rather than help.

FLUSH OUT THE POLLEN

Recent research shows that using a neti pot to rinse allergens out of your nasal passages can ease congestion and sinus pressure. Elana Gelman, N.D., a naturopathic doctor with the University of Bridgeport Naturopathic Medicine Clinic in Connecticut, recommends filling the device with 8 ounces of warm purified (distilled or deionized) water mixed with ¼ teaspoon salt. Or buy a neti pot that comes with premixed saline. (Never use tap water; doing so was recently associated with a few fatal brain infections in Louisiana.) For best results, use a neti pot in the morning and again just before bed, suggests Gelman.

WASH IT AWAY

In extreme cases, it's best to keep pollen out of your house (and especially your bedroom) altogether by ditching your shoes and changing into clean duds at the door. Put dirty clothes in a laundry bag or hamper with a lid, then wash them in hot water and toss in the dryer (never hang them to dry outdoors!). Rinse your hair nightly so your pillowcase doesn't get covered with the stuff, Bassett suggests.

The Asthma-Allergy Connection

An estimated 20 million Americans suffer from asthma, chronically inflamed airways that swell up and make breathing difficult. And for at least 65% of them, inhaled allergens (such as pollen) can trigger the attacks, says New York City allergist Clifford Bassett, M.D. If you have asthma, getting your seasonal allergies under control should help you. Doing so could even help others avoid developing asthma in the first place.

PROTECT YOUR PEEPERS

Sunglasses (particularly wraparounds) can help keep pollen out of your eyes. Make that snowboarder look work for you!

KEEP WINDOWS AND DOORS CLOSED

Use air-conditioning in your home and car to keep cool, no matter how much you crave fresh air. And don't forget to change or clean your home A/C filters on a regular basis to keep the air pure indoors.

CLEAN LIKE CRAZY

Wash your bed linens in hot water *at least* once a week and vacuum (using one with a HEPA filter is best) carpets and drapes even more often to remove pollen and indoor allergens that could ratchet up your suffering, says Bassett.

VET YOUR PETS

"Outdoor allergens can be carried inside by furry pets," Nish says. Trimming their fur could help reduce the amount that ends up indoors. Or, consider washing off your pet before letting him in and restricting him to one area of the house, Nish suggests. This is assuming your dog isn't a 200-pound St. Bernard named Cujo.

Boost Your Immunity

At the same time that you try to keep pollens at bay, these techniques can help fortify your immune system's response:

ALLERGY-PROOF YOUR DIET

Up to a third of hay fever sufferers experience a worsening of symptoms after eating certain foods, Bassett says. Known as food-pollen or oral-allergy syndrome, this occurs when the body mistakes the proteins in some raw fruits and vegetables, tree nuts, seeds and herbs for the proteins in pollen. Because you never know how *you'll* respond, anyone allergic to tree pollen, such as birch or oak, should be wary of certain fruits (apples, peaches, pears, kiwi, plums, nectarines); vegetables (carrots, celery, fennel, green peppers); nuts (hazelnuts, almonds, walnuts); and herbs and spices (coriander, basil, paprika).

Grass and weed pollen sufferers may want to avoid melons and bananas; cucumbers; certain herbs and spices (echinacea, chamomile, parsley, paprika, oregano, dill, coriander, tarragon, pepper); as well as caraway and sunflower seeds. It may require a bit of trial and error on your part, but once you know your trigger foods, you'll be a step ahead of the game.

To further sidestep symptoms, avoid eating any food that gives you an itchy or tingly mouth or an upset stomach during allergy season. Or, try cooking it—it's typically only when these foods are raw that they cause trouble, according to the AAAAI.

ACUPUNCTURE

Acupuncture can help alleviate hay fever by calming the immune system and decreasing inflammation. A 2012 study published in the *American Journal of Chinese Medicine* found that it reduced symptoms in all the allergy sufferers studied, with no major side effects.

HOMEOPATHY

Choosing the right remedy depends on your specific symptoms, says Christopher Johnson, N.D., founder of Thrive Naturopathic in Alexandria, Va. *Allium cepa* can be effective if you have lots of burning nasal discharge, frequent sneezing when outside, and red, burning and watery eyes. Use euphrasia for bland nasal dripping, burning tears, extremely watery, itchy or swollen eyes, and a daytime cough that improves at night. Sabadilla is for those with intense sneezing, a very runny nose and red eyes.

TRY: *Allium cepa,* euphrasia or sabadilla ($3.80 for 170 pellets; rxhomeo.com) or Sabadil, a mixture of those three remedies ($11 for 60 tablets; amazon.com). Follow package directions to determine dosage. If you're unsure which remedy to try, consult a homeopath or a naturopathic physician, Johnson says.

ACUPRESSURE

Like acupuncture, NAET (Nambudripad Allergy Elimination Technique) aims to rebalance your body's immune system—only without needles. The acupressure treatment takes five to 10 minutes, says Suzann Wang, N.D., a naturopathic doctor at Natural Health California in Palo Alto.

Afterward, you sit holding a glass vial containing the offending allergen for about 20 minutes and then are instructed to avoid breathing it in (by staying indoors or wearing a mask) for 25 hours. About half of Wang's patients report that they no longer suffer allergy symptoms after just one treatment, while it may take several visits for others, she says. NAET is considered a complementary treatment since it combines Western and TCM techniques, and noted integrative physician Jacob Teitelbaum, M.D., swears by it.

ANEMIA

SYMPTOMS

Anemia—and here, we're talking mainly about iron-deficiency anemia—is a sneaky little bugger. Mild symptoms can feel like stress: You're run down even when you get enough rest. You're unable to concentrate or think clearly. Your skin may become pale due to the lack of oxygenated blood that would normally give it a healthy color. So far, so familiar: This may sound like your usual Sunday-morning hangover, cured by a mimosa and the *New York Times Magazine*.

But you may also find yourself craving things like ice, clay or even dirt. (Medical experts have no idea why pica, the desire for nonfood substances, is a symptom of anemia.) And if left undiagnosed, anemia can start to feel like a heart attack: rapid breathing, irregular heartbeat and chest pain from an overworked, oxygen-deprived heart. Wait, what?

It's no wonder, says Lloyd Van Winkle, M.D., a member of the board of directors of the American Academy of Family Physicians. "You're already tired from the lack of oxygen in your blood," he explains, "plus, your body is working overtime with a shortage of blood to try to get oxygen into your cells, which is wearing you out even more." That lack of oxygen stresses every part of your body and can, in fact, lead to heart failure.

Time to take a cue from Tony Stark and channel your inner Iron Man (or Woman).

REMEDIES

Down for the Count

According to the Centers for Disease Control and Prevention, 9% of women ages 20 to 49 have iron-deficiency anemia. If you think you're one of them, ask your health care provider for a complete blood count—to get a reading on your levels of red blood cells, hemoglobin (the protein that contains iron and helps the cells carry oxygen) and hematocrit, which determines the blood's ability to carry oxygen. The lower these numbers get, the more likely you are to experience symptoms of anemia.

"If you're anemic, the first step is to figure out why," says hematologist Bruce Dezube, M.D., associate professor of medicine at Beth Israel Deaconess Medical Center, Harvard Medical School. In most cases, iron-deficiency anemia results from abnormal bleeding due to frequent or heavy menstrual periods, and childbirth can also be a cause. But it can strike men, too. An intestinal disorder such as celiac or Crohn's disease can prevent absorption of nutrients including iron, as can a class of drugs known as "proton pump inhibitors," used to block stomach acid. Internal bleeding from chronic conditions such as stomach ulcers, hemorrhoids and even nosebleeds can lead to iron deficiency. Bottom line: If it bleeds, it leads.

Supplemental Income

If you're diagnosed with iron-deficiency anemia, you'll often be advised to get an over-the-counter iron supplement to bring your levels up to normal. Once downed, you should see improvement within a couple of weeks. For women, "It's especially important to take supplements when you have your period; because you're losing iron, food choices won't always work," says Ashley Koff, R.D., who recommends supplements such as New Chapter Organics' Perfect Prenatal ($49 for 192 tabs; vitacost.com)—even if you're not pregnant or planning a family—or Flora Floradix Iron + Herbs Liquid Extract Formula ($35 for 17 oz.; vitacost.com).

Ten Invincible Sources of Iron

The recommended daily intake of iron for women ages 19 to 50 is 18 milligrams. Pregnant women need significantly more (27 milligrams); men and postmenopausal women need much less (8 milligrams). Although you can find fortified foods that are even higher in iron, here are 10 that are naturally high:

FOOD (amount)	IRON (mg)
Clams, canned, drained (3 oz.)	23.8
Spinach, cooked (1 cup)	6.4
Oysters, cooked (3 oz.)	5.9
Soybeans, mature, cooked (½ cup)	4.4
Pumpkin seed kernels, roasted (1 oz.)	4.2
White beans, canned (½ cup)	3.9
Blackstrap molasses (1 tbsp.)	3.5
Lentils, cooked (½ cup)	3.3
Beef bottom round, lean, cooked (3 oz.)	2.4
Prune juice (¾ cup)	2.3

You will need to keep taking the supplements as long as they are prescribed, often for up to six months, in order to increase your body's store. The most common side effects are stomach discomfort and constipation (hey, that's better than eating dirt), which can usually be relieved with lots of water and exercise. Koff often adds a magnesium supplement like Natural Vitality Natural Calm ($24 for 16 oz.; vitacost.com) if constipation develops.

BE AN IRON CHEF

Although beef, lamb and dark-meat poultry contain the highest concentration of iron, and are more readily absorbed by the body than other sources, iron is found in significant amounts in many other types of foods, too. In fact, legumes and other plant foods like leafy green vegetables often contain more iron than most animal-derived products. Dried fruit, nuts, whole grains, shellfish and enriched rice, pastas and cereals are also excellent sources of the nutrient. (See chart above.)

And cook with a cast-iron skillet. "Many foods, especially those with acidic ingredients such as tomatoes, absorb significant amounts of iron when cooked in cast iron," says Koff. A recent Brazilian study of vegetarians found that cooking tomato sauce in a cast-iron skillet increased the amount of iron in the sauce and improved iron status. In addition, simply serving iron-rich foods with a vitamin C source like tomatoes or citrus fruit aids in iron absorption.

MILK FOR THE BLOCK

Certain substances in foods can negatively affect iron's bioavailability, or the amount that is actually absorbed and used by the body. These "iron blockers" include phosphates in milk and egg whites, calcium in dairy products, phytates in high-fiber foods, and tannins and polyphenols in coffee and tea. Some foods, like spinach and soybeans, are high in iron, but they also contain substances that block iron absorption. "You don't have to avoid these foods, but it's best not to eat them at the same time you're eating foods high in iron if you're focusing on increasing your iron levels," Koff says. "And again, be sure to eat soy and spinach with foods that are rich in vitamin C to help increase iron absorption."

Be conscious of your calcium supplementation, too. The U.K. Thalassemia Society says that calcium taken within two hours of a meal can decrease the body's absorption of iron. (Thalassemia is a condition characterized by irregular hemoglobin production in the body.) Also, if you're using both calcium and iron supplements—unless they're already together in a prenatal vitamin—take them separately, at different times of the day, Koff suggests.

ANXIETY

Living with constant anxiety is like having a Pavlovian in your head—except instead of shocking you every time you smoke a cigarette or take a drink, he shocks you with an irrational thought every time you want a pleasant one. These thoughts usually start with a W: What if he's cheating on me? Zap. Why didn't Donny get into that school? Zap. Was there something I did wrong? Who was that bitch staring at me? What if we all get fired tomorrow? Why, oh why, oh why, me? Zap, zap, zap, zap.

We've all experienced anxiety of some kind. But if you're plagued constantly by anxious thoughts for six months or more, and they've come to dominate your life, you might be suffering from generalized anxiety disorder (GAD), which affects around 7 million Americans, roughly 3.1% of the population.

Many of them bring the pain upon themselves, their nervous systems constantly over-activated, despite the fact that there's nothing motivating it externally. "The anxious feeling you have is actually your body's fear or stress reaction triggered by an inner story or stream of thoughts about something that frightens you," says Jeffrey Brantley, M.D., founder and director of the Mindfulness-Based Stress Reduction Program at Duke Integrative Medicine in Durham, N.C. "In many cases, this is something that has not even happened or may not even be likely to happen. Either way, the frightening thoughts are powerful enough to trigger the stress reaction, and you feel anxious."

But here's one more W: What if you could help yourself get relief? Keep reading.

SYMPTOMS

People who have GAD startle easily and have difficulty concentrating. Other symptoms include difficulty relaxing or sleeping, fatigue, headaches, muscle tension, irritability, sweating, nausea, light-headedness, frequent bathroom trips, feeling out of breath and even hot flashes. Their anxieties often center on family and job responsibilities, and even minor things like car repairs or gardening.

If your mom was a constant worrier, you might be too, since experts believe GAD could have a genetic component; symptoms also can be triggered by trauma or a difficult life event such as a divorce or a death in the family. Perhaps because of interactions between sex hormones and brain chemistry, GAD affects around twice as many women as men. The NIH reports that the average age of onset is 31, but it can start in the teen years, and heighten during times of stress.

REMEDIES

Meditation

Most stress-reduction techniques can help relieve anxiety, says psychologist Edmund J. Bourne, Ph.D., coauthor of *Natural Relief for Anxiety: Complementary Strategies for Easing Fear, Panic, and Worry.* These include abdominal breathing, guided visualizations or even just taking breaks two or three times every day to relax: Do moderate exercise, watch a nostalgic YouTube clip or imagine yourself in a peaceful place.

Mindfulness meditation, which has proven especially helpful in reducing anxiety, is now being taught in many hospitals and health centers across the country. Studies have found that, among other benefits, it can lower breathing rate, reduce levels of the stress hormone cortisol and increase activity in the left frontal area of the brain, which is associated with a positive mental state and lowered anxiety levels. In fact, a Canadian study of cancer patients who participated in a mindfulness-based stress-reduction program found that cortisol levels continued to drop for six months to a year afterward.

The basics of this type (listening to your breath or paying specific attention to various parts of your body) are simple—you'll find a chapter devoted to five different kinds starting on page 325—and one of the easiest is called breathwalking, developed by Jim Nicolai, M.D., medical director at the Andrew Weil, M.D. Integrative Wellness Program at Miraval Arizona Resort and Spa in Tucson (see below). You might even find it addicting, which is a good thing. "The important thing is to make practicing mindfulness a part of your daily life so you'll be prepared when a stressful situation arises," says Brantley.

Go for a Breath Walk

Meditation? Who can just plop down and empty her mind? With breathwalking, you don't have to. It's a way of slowing down, delivering more oxygen to your brain and body and becoming more mindful, diverting your attention to your breath so you can just experience the present moment without judging it. Becoming more mindful is a great way to combat our go-go-go lifestyles—and avoid the resulting stress spiral. Here's how you do it:

Take four short inhales through your nose, and four short exhales through your mouth or nose. Repeat until you've got a rhythm going—four in, four out—then start walking and synch your breath with your strides: Four inhales, four steps, four exhales, four steps.

Once you're got the breathing and walking down, start tapping: Start on an inhale, and touch your index fingers and thumbs (of both hands) with the first inhale, middle finger and thumb with the second inhale, your ring finger on the third and finally your pinkie. On the exhales, repeat this pattern, starting with your index finger again.

If you like, you can add a chant: Jim Nicolai, who teaches this to his patients at Miraval, likes the Sanskrit chant sa-ta-na-ma. Synch each syllable to each of the four inhale breaths, then the four exhale breaths. Always start with the index finger.

Put it all together—it may seem like trying to rub your belly and head at first, but keep at it, and you'll be amazed at how effortlessly you achieve calm. The über delivery of oxygen actually *makes* some people feel high.

Yoga

By combining physical relaxation with controlled breathing, yoga can help you deal with both physical and mental stress, forcing you to *Ommm* out. In a 2010 review of a study published in *The Journal of Alternative and Complementary Medicine,* Boston University School of Medicine found that any type of yoga practice may increase brain levels of the neurotransmitter gamma-aminobutyric acid (GABA), which is associated with relaxation and lowered anxiety. Magnetic resonance imaging showed a 27% increase of GABA in the brains of experienced practitioners following an hour-long yoga session, versus no increase in a group that simply read for an hour.

"People with anxiety often have chronic physiological tension in the body, and the contraction and release of muscles in the active practice of yoga can help," says clinical psychologist, yoga teacher and yoga therapist Bo Forbes, Psy.D., founder of the New England School of Integrative Yoga Therapeutics. "At the same time, yoga requires mindful attention to the present moment, which can break the pattern of worrying about the future."

Cognitive Behavioral Therapy

Repeat after us: "I've got the power." Cognitive behavioral therapy (CBT) refers to any therapies that teach you how to think more realistically so that fearful thoughts don't build into anxiety. While some psychologists view long-term talk therapy as a more effective solution for deep-seated issues, CBT is most commonly recommended for GAD. "For the past 20 years, the standard treatment for all anxiety disorders has been cognitive behavioral therapy," says Bourne. "What we think about an event affects our feelings more than the event itself."

Of course, constant worry can increase your physical symptoms, which may in turn bring about even more worry. But with CBT, you examine the thoughts that underlie those feelings and determine whether or not they really make sense. If they don't, you can replace them with more realistic thoughts. For instance, you might think, "I'm in danger" while walking on a crowded street; the therapist would help you see the situation more clearly, so you instead think something like, "Realistically, the thing I'm most afraid of isn't likely to happen." Therapy sessions are combined with "homework" such as journaling your moods and challenging your negative thoughts during the week. The treatment can last from six weeks to several months, with "booster sessions" recommended afterward.

Conquering your anxiety symptoms can be a huge relief, and ensuring that they don't come back requires practicing the skills learned in CBT on a regular basis, Bourne says. "In some cases, it may be helpful to explore the history of your anxiety issues with traditional psychodynamic therapy," he notes. "Exploring, with a therapist, the history of how some of your problems developed can lead to insights that provide a better perspective on your present life." Look for a therapist who specializes in anxiety disorders, whom you feel you can trust and be completely honest with, and be wary of one who asks leading questions, tries to give you advice or acts like the authority in the relationship. You are the authority; the therapist's job is to help you to explore your feelings and thoughts to the fullest.

Lifestyle Changes

Managing your anxiety can also be achieved by making a few simple tweaks to your everyday activities, including these expert recommendations:

GET MOVING

A study published in the *Archives of Internal Medicine* in 2010 found that, on average, patients who exercised regularly reported a 20% reduction in anxiety symptoms compared to those who did not exercise. "Our findings add to the growing body of evidence that physical activities such as walking or weightlifting may turn out to be the best medicine that physicians can prescribe to help their patients feel less anxious," says lead author Matthew Herring, now a research associate in the department of epidemiology at the University of Alabama at Birmingham.

SUPPLEMENT YOUR SYMPTOMS

Research has linked a variety of nutrients to lower levels of anxiety. In one study, omega-3 supplementation led to a 20% reduction in anxiety symptoms. In another study, supplementing with calcium, magnesium and zinc significantly reduced anxiety and perceived stress. And still another study found that taking 200 milligrams of magnesium plus

50 milligrams of vitamin B_6 for one month relieved anxiety-related premenstrual symptoms.

SLEEP WELL

Getting sufficient nighttime z's allows your nervous system to recover and helps your body to produce the "sleep hormone" melatonin, which helps to mitigate anxiety.

DON'T DRINK OR SMOKE

Caffeine, excess alcohol and cigarettes can all overstimulate your nervous system and affect your sleep, and are all associated with higher levels of stress and anxiety.

MIND YOUR MEDS

Various over-the-counter, recreational and even prescription drugs can cause or worsen anxiety; these include certain cold remedies, diet aids, inhaler medications used for asthma and thyroid drugs. Discuss with your doctor everything you're taking.

Try Herbs

Mild or chronic symptoms, or situational anxiety (related to an exam, for instance) often improve with supplement and herb use, says Boston-based naturopath Cathy Wong, N.D., C.N.S. The options that follow are well worth exploring.

B COMPLEX is a good first step for anxiety relief. "B vitamins are essential for stress management, energy production and neurotransmitter balance," says Wong. Helpful supplements usually include vitamins B_1 (thiamin), B_2 (riboflavin), B_3 (niacin), B_5 (pantothenic acid), B_6 (pyridoxine hydrochloride), B_7 (biotin), B_9 (folic acid) and B_{12} (cyanocobalamin).

DOSAGE: Look for a B-complex containing all eight essential B vitamins or a multivitamin designed for stress support.

TRY: New Chapter Organics Perfect Calm ($46 for 144 tablets; drugstore.com)

GABA, which stands for gamma-aminobutyric acid, has a calming effect on the brain similar to that achieved by medications such as Valium and Xanax. "GABA is a nonessential amino acid and neurotransmitter that blocks stress and anxiety by preventing neurons from over-firing," Wong says. "It's produced naturally in the body but also is available in supplement form." Possible side effects include nausea (especially in doses of 3 grams or more per day), shortness of breath and tingling in the hands and face.

DOSAGE: 500 milligrams to 3 grams daily

ASK THE EXPERTS

How can I ease anxiety?

Soothe your daily stresses in a variety of natural, strategic ways.

An integrative psychiatrist says:

Anxiety is a physiological response to fear; stress hormones cortisol and adrenaline overwork the immune system, causing a racing pulse, hyperventilation, dizziness, brain fog and sometimes lack of consciousness.

TREATMENT: Talk with a therapist to examine the root cause of your fear or stress, which may be current or stem from as far back as early childhood. Seek energy medicine (via body work such as Reiki) and the therapeutic touching of hands about five inches above your chakras to draw nega-tive emotion to the heart chakra, where it dissipates. Do cardio-vascular exercise to boost dopamine and serotonin levels, and avoid stimulants such as caffeine. As soon as an anxiety attack starts, center yourself by placing your hand over your heart for three minutes to stimulate the chakra's warm energy. Get enough sleep, and meditate before bed.

— Judith Orloff, M.D.,
assistant clinical professor of psychiatry at UCLA in Los Angeles, and author of The Ecstacy of Surrender

TRY: Rainbow Light Busy Brain Release ($24 for 60 minitabs; rainbowlight.com)

MAGNESIUM A study published in *Current Medical Research and Opinion* found that magnesium—when combined with *Crataegus oxyacantha* (evergreen hawthorn) and *Eschscholtzia californica* (California poppy) extracts—was more effective than placebo in treating patients with mild to moderate anxiety. It's also effective for easing muscle tension.

A Traditional Chinese Medicine practitioner says:

Anxiety is the blockage of qi, or life energy, in the liver and heart meridians, which can cause insomnia and poor digestion.

TREATMENT: To mobilize qi, get weekly acupuncture along the liver meridian, the energetic pathway that starts on the outside corner of the big toe and runs up the inside of the leg to the rib cage under the breast. Acupressure on meridians will release stagnant qi; try shiatsu-style massage, during which a therapist will press with her fingertips on pressure points. Learn anxiety-easing points from a therapist, so you can perform them on yourself. Snack on longan, a nutty-tasting Chinese fruit similar to lychee, which can be calming.

—Bryn Clark, L.Ac., Dipl. O.M.
(NCCAOM),
of the New Harmony Center for Health & Wellness in Beverly, Mass.

An ayurvedic physician says:

Stress releases the hormone cortisol into the bloodstream. Since cortisol is acidic, it irritates the lymphatic and digestive systems, which then upsets your vata, the dosha—or stress receptors—in the colon that's linked to the nervous system.

TREATMENT: Take adaptogens (calming herbs) like tulsi and ashwagandha in the morning and at night. Try abhyanga, a self-massage that calms the peripheral nervous system, for one or two minutes every day before or in the shower. Use circular strokes to massage herbal sesame oil on your temples, joints and feet, and use longer strokes over your bones. Stimulating the nerve endings in this way increases oxytocin production, which helps fight stress.

—John Douillard, D.C.,
director of the LifeSpa Retreat Center and Clinic in Boulder, Colo.

The essential mineral's most common side effect is loose stools, says Wong. Magnesium may also interfere with the efficacy of certain medications, including ACE inhibitors, diabetes medication and tetracycline. Women taking birth control pills or hormone replacement therapy may need to increase magnesium to see a calming effect.

DOSAGE: 200 to 300 milligrams twice daily

TRY: Twinlab Magnesium Caps ($7 for 200 capsules; vitamin shoppe.com)

PASSIONFLOWER (*Passiflora incarnata*) In an often-cited double-blind study in the *Journal of Clinical Pharmacy and Therapeutics*, giving patients with generalized anxiety disorder 45 drops per day of passionflower tincture was effective in reducing symptoms without impairing job performance (unlike the antianxiety drug Serax, also part of the study); and a recent study found that when passionflower is given to patients before outpatient surgery, no other medication is necessary to reduce their anxiety. Generally considered very safe for relieving stress, anxiety and insomnia, passionflower can cause drowsiness when combined with antidepressants or antianxiety medication, says Wong.

DOSAGE: 40 drops of tincture, up to five times a day, or 400 milligrams divided over the day

TRY: Now Foods Passion Flower Extract ($8 for 90 Vcaps; allstarhealth.com)

RELORA This patented formula combines extracts from magnolia bark (*Magnolia officinalis*) and the amur corktree (*Phellodendron amurense*), both used in Traditional Chinese Medicine. "Magnolia bark contains two compounds, magnolol and honokiol, which are believed to be responsible for the stress-reducing effects," says Wong. Relora seems to work on some of the same receptors as antianxiety drugs without causing sedation. If you're pregnant, nursing or taking prescription drugs, consult your doctor before using Relora.

DOSAGE: 250 milligrams, two to three times a day, taken with food

TRY: Nature's Answer Relora ($11 for 60 capsules; allstarhealth.com)

RESCUE REMEDY British physician Edward Bach designed this formula to be used in times of acute emotional stress. It blends five flower essences: star of Bethlehem (for shock), clematis (for inattentiveness), impatiens (for irritation and impatience), cherry plum (for irrational thoughts) and rock rose (for panic). One of the strengths of Rescue Remedy is that it doesn't interact negatively with conventional medications, says Wong.

DOSAGE: Four drops, four times a day, or two quick sprays, as needed

TRY: Bach Flower Remedies Rescue Remedy Natural Stress Relief ($11 for .7 fluid ounces; rescueremedy.com)

A Prescription Drug Primer

If your symptoms feel overwhelming or are impairing your ability to function, you may need to complement natural treatments with prescription medications. The ones that follow are often effective.

Selective serotonin reuptake inhibitors (SSRIs) are antidepressants that increase brain levels of the calming neurotransmitter serotonin. They include Prozac (fluoxetine), Lexapro (escitalopram) and Zoloft (sertraline). Depression and anxiety often go together, and SSRIs can be effective for both.

Tricyclic antidepressants (TCAs) such as Tofranil (imipramine) are prescribed for panic disorder and GAD, but may cause more side effects than SSRIs.

Benzodiazepines such as Xanax (alprazolam) and Ativan (lorazepam) are tranquilizers that slow the nervous system. Frequently prescribed for serious anxiety, they can be habit-forming and are best used short-term.

Buspirone (Buspar, Vanspar) affects serotonin, dopamine and possibly other neurotransmitters in the brain. It works more slowly against anxiety than benzodiazepines, but is less likely to cause side effects or addiction when taken long-term.

Q How can I reduce my chances of an asthma attack?

*Not being able to catch your breath is like drowning on land.
Here, three experts show you natural remedies
to help you breathe easier.*

An allergy and asthma specialist says:

The main cause of asthma is inflammation of the airways, so anything that reduces inflammation may help. Vitamin D can increase anti-inflammatory molecules in the body; it may also reduce the risk of getting viral infections like colds, which are the most common triggers of asthma. In a recently published study, we found that vitamin D deficiency is associated with hyperreactive airways (when air passages narrow suddenly), lower lung function and poor asthma control.

TREATMENT: Your doctor can measure your vitamin D levels with a blood test to find out if you're deficient (most people are). The Institute of Medicine recommends you get, at minimum, 600 IUs (15 micrograms) of vitamin D every day from foods like oily fish, fortified dairy products, cereals and supplements.

—Manbir S. Sandhu, M.D.,
an allergy, asthma and immunology specialist based in Farmington, Conn.

A naturopath says:

Eating dairy products is often a trigger for respiratory ailments, as it produces a lot of mucus in the body. Gluten is also suspected to be problematic for many people, although the reason isn't yet understood. Asthma sufferers often also have undiagnosed allergies to airborne allergens, such as dust, mold and animal dander.

TREATMENT: Start by cutting dairy products and gluten out of your diet (start with dairy if it's too difficult to do both at once).

Six weeks is the optimal amount of time to omit a food from your diet to test sensitivity to it. Reintroduce the foods and keep detailed notes about how you feel. The herb hawthorn berry, which has anti-inflammatory and anti-allergic properties, blocks the formation of histamine and can open the airways immediately. Have a 1-ounce tincture (you can buy it at most health food stores) on hand at all times; if you start to feel symptoms, take a full dropper of the herb and wait a minute. Try this three to five times, and if it hasn't helped, use your asthma medications. I've had patients who quit eating dairy and used the herbs and were able to stop using their inhalers within three weeks. In more difficult cases, the addition of constitutional homeopathy and adrenal herbs such as licorice root or eleuthero will often turn the case around. Asthma medications containing a steroid component should be discontinued only under medical supervision.

—Deborah Frances, N.D.,
a naturopathic doctor and adjunct professor at the National College of Natural Medicine in Portland, Ore.

An acupuncturist and ayurvedic practitioner says:

Acupuncture can help open the lungs, ease breathing, decrease phlegm and mucus and calm the mind (many asthmatics experience depression and/or anxiety). I also use a variety of other approaches in my practice, including herbal medicine and salt therapy. Salt therapy originated in Russia and Eastern Europe, where they noticed that people who worked in salt mines rarely had respiratory complaints. Salt is antibacterial, and it dissolves or liquefies mucus; if used often enough, salt therapy can help with chronic respiratory problems like asthma. In a salt room, the walls and floors are covered with salt and a special device grinds it into very fine particles that you inhale.

TREATMENT: After a series of acupuncture treatments, patients may be able to decrease their use of inhalers and asthma medications. Let your medical doctor know if you decide to see an acupuncturist, and don't go off your medications cold turkey— you may have to taper off them under a doctor's supervision. If you're unable to find a salt room in your area, you can use a saline solution, either with a neti pot or saline washes, to help cut mucus and fight infections.

—Will Foster,
licensed acupuncturist and certified ayurvedic practitioner at the Traditional Health Clinic in Knoxville, Tenn.

BACK PAIN

It has brought Tiger Woods to his knees (during a tournament in 2013), George Clooney to tears ("I thought I was going to die") and your Uncle Morty under the knife (he'll happily show you the scars). It's back pain, and it doesn't care if you're young, old, rich, poor, fit, fat or starred in *Ocean's Eleven*. With 31 million sufferers, the scourge (often called low back pain) is second only to the common cold among the reasons we seek medical care, and the leading cause of disability in people under age 45.

It follows that treating back pain is big business. According to new NIH numbers, Americans are spending $50 billion a year on physicians, physical therapists, chiropractors and meds. In fact, the U.S. spinal surgery rate is twice that of most developed countries and five times that of the United Kingdom.

SYMPTOMS

Pain. In your lower back. It gets tricky trying to identify the cause. "On an X-ray almost everyone 40 and older will have something that looks abnormal," explains Richard Deyo, M.D., M.P.H., a professor of evidence-based medicine at Oregon Health and Science University in Portland. The same is often true for younger people.

What complicates treatment is the fact that the converse often applies as well: "Only in a minority of people is there a clear-cut underlying cause for the pain," says Daniel Cherkin, Ph.D., senior investigator for Group Health Research Institute in Seattle.

Clooney, for example, was injured on a film set, causing "a two-and-a-half-inch tear in the middle of my back." Your Uncle Morty...?

REMEDIES

"The fact that so many treatments exist is testimony that none is clearly superior," Deyo says. "Lots of claims really aren't supported by scientific evidence, and it is almost always best to use noninvasive treatments first." Back pain sufferers opting to go au naturel often see improvements quickly. "Within 12 weeks, nearly 95% of back pain patients can return to work [without surgery]," Deyo says. A 2009 review of data from a NCCAM National Health Interview Survey found that 17% of Americans who used complementary and alternative medicine (CAM), did so for back pain, which makes back pain the leading reason for seeking CAM. So before you opt for a potentially unnecessary, ineffective and invasive procedure, try these kinder, gentler remedies.

In the beginning

When severe back pain strikes, you may be inclined to stay in bed. But resist that urge and get moving when you can. Deyo advises resting for just a day or two if necessary, along with taking over-the-counter painkillers and applying heat to the affected area. After two days, start taking gentle walks.

If the pain doesn't improve within a few weeks, see your primary care physician for an exam. Depending on what he finds—if he suspects a herniated, or bulging, spinal disk is pressing on a nerve, for example—he may recommend an X-ray, MRI or CT scan. But as we said, such tests are often inconclusive.

If there is no obvious "why" for your pain, your doctor may suggest physical therapy, education about proper movement and an exercise program to avoid reinjury. Once your pain gets a bit better, many alternative or complementary therapies—such as those that follow—can ease muscle tension and inflammation; help prevent long-term problems by improving muscle strength and core stability (weak abdominal muscles may be a big contributor to back problems); and help you cope emotionally.

GO INTO THERAPY

Unlike a large yoga class with one instructor, a yoga therapy session is typically one-on-one, and the postures are specific to your back issues. "Iyengar is the most therapeutically oriented type, but most will work," says Loren Fishman, M.D., medical director of Manhattan Physical Medicine and Rehabilitation in New York City and author of *Cure Back Pain with Yoga.* "Look for an instructor who has at least 10 years of experience as well as education in anatomy and pathology." Fishman says yoga can be particularly helpful if you have arthritis of the spine or piriformis syndrome, in which the psoas, a muscle in the buttock, contracts and compresses the sciatic nerve.

FEEL THE RUB

A recent study funded by the National Center for Complementary and Alternative Medicine (NCCAM) showed that people with back pain who underwent massage therapy were about 70% more likely to experience meaningful improvements in their functioning than people who received traditional medical care. "Surprisingly, both relaxation [Swedish] and structural [soft-tissue] massages were equally beneficial," says Cherkin, who led the study. How to choose a massage therapist? Select one who is certified in your state and has passed the MBLEx licensing exam. If you live in one of the six states that does not currently license massage therapists, look for someone who has passed the National Certification Exam. (See "Massage" on page 254.) Note: Fishman cautions that if you have a neurological problem—such as a stroke, tumor or brain cancer—massage may make it worse.

GET CRACKING

Besides manipulating your spine like a skeletal snake charmer, chiropractors employ other noninvasive therapies that include transcutaneous electrical nerve stimulation (TENS). This causes your muscles to contract, "promoting more profound relaxation in them," says New York City-based Karen Erickson, D.C., director of Erickson Healing Arts. Other options include ultrasound, which uses sound waves to relax muscles, and cold (low-level) laser treatment, which helps damaged muscle cells repair themselves.

When to Bring Out the "Big Guns"

Red flags that should prompt you to seek further medical attention include:

Pain that isn't getting better after six weeks

Pain that travels down your leg

Difficulty controlling your bladder

A history of cancer

Being 55 years or older with a new onset of back pain

Studies have shown that chiropractic spinal manipulation can offer mild-to-moderate relief from low back pain and is as effective as conventional medical treatments. The American College of Physicians and the American Pain Society recommend the technique as well, especially when self-care fails.

HEAD BACK TO NATURE

A naturopathic doctor (N.D.) tends to look for the reason for back pain. "A person might have fallen out of a tree on her back as a kid and it didn't hurt much at the time, but years later she is wondering why her back hurts," says Scottsdale, Ariz.-based Michael Cronin, N.D., of the American Association of Naturopathic Physicians. Naturopaths look at the whole person and offer suggestions for supplements, diet and ergonomic fixes. They often use acupuncture, acupressure, homeopathy and herbs. (See "Naturopathy" on page 376.)

WHAT UP HOMEO?

Homeopathic remedies usually come in the form of small pellets that are placed under the tongue to dissolve. "They are made of highly diluted natural substances that trigger a healing reaction in the body, which may lead to a reduction in pain and inflammation," says Richard

Back Pain Explained

Why so sore? The most common causes are: strained muscles and ligaments from an accident or injury, improper or heavy lifting, or a sudden movement; and structural problems such as a bulging or ruptured disk (sciatica is caused by pressure of such a disk on the large nerve that runs down each buttock and leg); arthritis; osteoporosis; or a pinched nerve. Many of these are a result of age-related changes.

These factors increase your propensity to suffer from back pain:

Being middle-aged or older
Smoking
Obesity
Physically strenuous, stressful or sedentary work
Anxiety or depression

Ezgur, D.C., a chiropractic physician, acupuncturist and homeopath at the Progressive Chiropractic Wellness Center in Chicago. A homeopath can determine the best remedy for your particular condition.

GET POKED

The National Institutes of Health recommend acupuncture as a treatment option for back pain, and given the impressive stats, it's easy to see why. A 2009 *Archives of Internal Medicine* (now the *JAMA Internal Medicine*) study led by Cherkin found that acupuncture treatments, including simulated treatments, worked better to ease back pain than conventional therapy. Clearly, experts feel, there's something beneficial about acupuncture that has nothing to do with needling; of course, research is ongoing.

Supplement your spine

Some natural remedies can help ease your back pain from the inside out. Erickson recommends the following:

BROMELAIN An enzyme that comes from pineapples and reduces inflammation. (Check with your doctor first; it can increase the risk of bleeding.) Take 250 milligrams twice daily.
   TRY: Thorne Research M.F. Bromelain ($28 for 60 capsules; amazon.com)

TURMERIC (*Curcuma longa*) standardized extract. An herbal anti-inflammatory. (Check with your doctor first; it can also increase bleeding.) Take 300 milligrams three times daily.
   TRY: Gaia Herbs Turmeric Supreme ($20 for 60 capsules; pharmaca.com)

GINGER (*Zingiber officinale*) Also an anti-inflammatory. Take 1,000 milligrams daily.
   TRY: New Chapter Organics Daily Ginger ($14 for 90 capsules; iherb.com)

TRAUMEEL The brand name of a topical cream with several natural ingredients, including Arnica montana, a homeopathic remedy.
   TRY: Traumeel Ointment ($17 for 1.76 ounces; drugstore.com)

BLOATING

LAST NIGHT, you looked like Rihanna at the club. This morning, you feel more like a Klump. Chipmunk cheeks and puffy eyes. Rings stuck on fingers. Buttons popping off jeans. And the scale must be wrong, as usual: Somehow, you've gained three pounds overnight. Time for a crash diet? No: Your body is just holding on to water.

SYMPTOMS

Unlike gas, which builds up in your stomach and intestines and causes abdominal bloating, water can swell every part of your body (including your feet, as any woman in heels could tell you). If you feel inflated like an air bag, that's probably gas; if you feel like a waterlogged sponge, that's fluid retention. And although it's often considered normal and is usually temporary, water retention can be annoying and uncomfortable while it lasts.

Body fluid, which accounts for approximately 60% of most women's weight, contains water (obviously), electrolytes (minerals such as sodium and potassium), salts and other substances whose levels are regulated by your hormones and kidneys. "Your body has to maintain a balance between sodium and water," says Joseph G. Verbalis, M.D., chief of the endocrinology and metabolism division at Georgetown University in Washington, D.C., and an expert in body fluid disorders. When the ideal ratio changes, your kidneys hold on to water so they can dilute the sodium. The result is bloating.

Because of hormonal shifts, fluid retention commonly occurs during the premenstrual phase of a woman's cycle as well as during pregnancy. Puffiness that's unrelated to PMS or pregnancy is often due to overeating, which can alter insulin production in such a way that the kidneys retain sodium and fluid, says C. Wayne Callaway, M.D., an endo-crinologist and clinical nutritionist in Washington, D.C.

REMEDIES

By now you've put down that Cool Ranch Doritos Taco. The following lifestyle changes and natural remedies can help flush fluids from a bloated but otherwise healthy body.

Food Solutions

DRINK MORE—YES, MORE—WATER

"It may seem counterintuitive, but this helps relieve bloating. When you don't drink enough water, your body releases a hormone that reduces the amount of urine you produce," says Molly Kimball, R.D., nutrition program director at the Ochsner Clinic's Elmwood Fitness Center in New Orleans. Aim for 64 ounces a day.

SHAKE THE SALT HABIT

While some people are more sensitive to salt (sodium) than others and thus retain fluids more easily, many people experience tempo-rary fluid retention after eating a particularly large load of salt. If this happens, cut back for a while and increase your water intake. Sodium is everywhere, so read labels and try to keep your intake to 2,300 milligrams a day, or 1,500 milligrams max if you are 40 or older, African-American or have high blood pressure. The average American takes in nearly 3,400 milligrams every day. (A Big Mac alone has 1,070 milligrams, but more surprising offenders include deli meats, at 362 milligrams per two slices; a can of chicken noodle soup, with 744 milligrams; and one tablespoon of soy sauce, at 1,024 milligrams.)

EAT PEE-PRODUCING FOODS

Many vegetables, including cucumbers, asparagus, celery, eggplant and fennel, as well as herbs such as parsley, coriander and cardamom, act as natural diuretics, says Leslie Bonci, M.P.H., R.D., director of sports nu-trition at the University of Pittsburgh Medical Center's Center for Sports

Medicine. These foods have high water contents and/or contain minerals such as potassium and magnesium, as well as phytochemicals that promote proper water balance.

DRINK YOUR DIURETICS

Cranberry juice and several teas, including black, green, chamomile and alfalfa, are safe and well known for their diuretic properties. "Dandelion leaf is one of the best herbs for this purpose," says herbalist Christopher Hobbs, Ph.D., founder of the Institute for Natural Products Research in the San Francisco area. He recommends using it in tea or extract form. "Celery seed tea (but not tinctures) can also be safely used."

Commercial diuretic teas, sometimes called dieters' teas, should be used with caution. "If you overdo them, you can lose normal fluid from your bloodstream as well as essential minerals," says Brent A. Bauer, M.D., director of the Complementary and Integrative Medicine Program at the Mayo Clinic in Rochester, Minn. "You could become dehydrated and harm your kidneys or develop an electrolyte imbalance that could trigger fatigue, muscle cramps and even potentially fatal heart rhythm disturbances."

CUT CARBS

Eat fewer high-carbohydrate foods like pasta, bread and pastries, and more lean proteins and vegetables. "Extra carbs are broken down and stored in the body as glycogen, which has a high water content and so contributes to excess water weight," Kimball explains. Protein, by contrast, has a lower water content, and body fluids are used (and passed) in the process of breaking it down.

LIMIT ALCOHOL

Alcohol blocks the release of an anti-diuretic hormone, so heavy drinking can lead to dehydration. This might sound like a good thing when you're bloated, but it backfires by causing your body to hang on to fluid.

MAINTAIN A CONSISTENT EATING PATTERN

Starving yourself because you're feeling heavy from water weight, then overeating when you feel better, can have the opposite effect. "I see serious fluid problems in women who fast as a means to lose weight," says Callaway. "When they eat again, they experience a rebound in fluid retention."

FINE-TUNE YOUR FIBER

Researchers at the University of Minnesota in St. Paul found that people who ate large amounts of inulin (aka chicory root, found in many cereals and cookies) experienced more gas and bloating than those who ate less. Stick to less-processed vegetables, fruit and whole grains.

EAT WARM FOODS

Traditional Chinese Medicine (TCM) recommends avoiding dairy, greasy, sweet, raw and cold foods if you're prone to bloating. "Focus on cooked, warm foods," says Zoe Cohen, L.Ac., an acupuncturist in Oakland, Calif., who treats many women with PMS- and pregnancy-related water retention. "In TCM, cold foods are harder to digest, which creates dampness in the body; water retention is a form of dampness." Adzuki (aka aduki or azuki) and mung beans as well as barley are especially helpful foods, she adds.

Lifestyle Remedies
BREAK A SWEAT

Cardiovascular exercise promotes water loss by boosting circulation, which moves fluid from your extremities back toward your heart and kidneys, where it's turned into urine. It will also make you sweat,

When to Call Your Doc

Several medical conditions, including heart, kidney or liver disease, hypothyroidism and diabetes, can cause significant ongoing fluid retention, aka chronic edema. And certain medications, including non-steroidal anti-inflammatory drugs (NSAIDS), some hypertension meds (such as calcium channel-blockers), steroids, joint supplements (like glucosamine) and some diabetes and anti-seizure meds can also cause persistent, severe bloating. If you press your thumb against your shin and it leaves an indentation that lasts more than a minute, this can be a red flag; contact your doctor.

which helps you excrete both water and sodium. No need to go all Usain Bolt; a fast walk is enough to do the trick.

TAKE THE PLUNGE

Pregnant women know that there's nothing like being submerged in a pool to help relieve fluid retention. The way it works is that the pressure of the water pushes the body fluids back into the blood vessels and on to the kidneys. Even better: Do water aerobics and get two-for-one benefits.

APPLY SOME PRESSURE

"Massage, especially lymphatic-type massage, can help alleviate bloating by moving fluid out of the tissues," says Elson M. Haas, M.D., *Natural Health* advisory board member and director of the Preventive Medical Center of Marin in San Rafael, Calif.

JUST CHILL

While that massage will feel fantastic, it also works to reduce stress. Think about it—when our ancestors were on the run from sabertooth tigers, their guts tightened up, just like yours does in traffic, and digestion was not top priority. Meditation, massage, anything that calms you down will help move things along, a 2009 Canadian review found.

TAKE A LOAD OFF

Elevating swollen feet or ankles above the level of your heart promotes the return of excess fluid to the kidneys. And don't sit with your legs crossed, as this inhibits the removal of fluids from your lower body. Wearing tight jeans can have the same effect. Who said there's no cure for cankles?

Complementary Approaches
STICK A NEEDLE IN IT

No, getting acupuncture won't drain the water from your bloated body, à la Veruca Salt, but TCM can help otherwise. "Acupuncture can stimulate your body's fluid-regulating mechanisms," Cohen says. A number of herbal formulas will also help, she adds; as with acupuncture, the treatment depends on which imbalance is to blame in your case.

TRY HOMEOPATHY

"If you have premenstrual water retention, it's best to choose a homeopathic remedy that takes into account other PMS symptoms that are occurring," says naturopathic physician Tori Hudson, N.D., medical director of A Woman's Time health clinic in Portland, Ore. "Good remedies include Lycopodium, *nux vomica,* pulsatilla, sepia, *Natrum muriaticum,* lachesis, caulophylumm and cimicifuga; Cyclease from Boiron is a good combination product."

CONSIDER SUPPLEMENTS

The balance between certain minerals, like sodium and potassium, or calcium and magnesium, can play a critical role in preventing bloating. If you think you aren't getting enough of these minerals from food, ask your doctor about taking a multivitamin-and-mineral and/or calcium supplement. Research has shown that magnesium (found in nuts, beans, seeds, grains and some vegetables) can reduce premenstrual bloating, and vitamin B_6 is also a natural diuretic, Kimball says. Brown rice and red meat are good food sources of B_6.

If these solutions don't help you feel less, uh, swell, your doctor might prescribe a short course of low-dose diuretics. "[Unless there's a serious underlying medical need] we don't like to put people on long-term diuretics because of the side effects," says Verbalis. These side effects include potassium loss; increased blood pressure and strain on the heart; and "rebound" fluid retention.

How can I get rid of body odor naturally?

Something smells fishy, and it's not this advice. Find out what may secretly be causing your stink.

A dermatologist says:

When the bacteria that grow naturally on your skin mix with water or sweat, the result is body odor. To smell fresh, you need to keep your skin dry and decrease bacteria on the parts of your body that trap moisture, such as the underarms.

TREATMENT: Shower with a body wash that includes a natural astringent, such as tea tree oil, which shrinks pores and limits how much you sweat. Follow with a powder pat-down to absorb moisture. Finish with a natural deodorant that contains potassium or ammonium alum to reduce bacteria.

—Valori Treloar, M.D.,
dermatologist at Integrative Dermatology in Newton, Mass.

A dietitian says:

Foods such as broccoli, cabbage and cauliflower contain the mineral sulfur, which causes an odorous gas that's eliminated through your skin. Other types of body odor are usually a sign that it's time for a nutritional detox.

TREATMENT: Cut hard-to-digest gluten, dairy and red meat from your diet, as these foods increase body odor. In addition, eat at least 25 grams of flaxseeds, chia, hempseed or whole grains each day to boost your fiber intake and encourage bowel movements; and drink eight or more glasses of water to help expel toxins.

—Erica Kasuli, R.D.,
New York City-based dietitian

A naturopathic doctor says:

Yeast infections can give you a fishy scent, as can a genetic disorder called fish odor syndrome, which occurs when your body can't properly metabolize an organic compound known as trimethylamine.

TREATMENT: Zap a yeast infection with 500-milligram capsules of oregano oil, taken twice daily for two weeks. If you're diagnosed with fish odor syndrome, stay away from foods high in trimethylamine, including milk, eggs, liver and peanuts.

—Holly Lucille, N.D., R.N.,
West Hollywood, Calif.-based naturopathic doctor

CANCER

BREAST, UTERINE AND PROSTATE

When Catherine Frompovich was diagnosed with two cancerous tumors in her right breast in 2011, she rejected the breast surgeon's plan of action: surgery and chemo.

"I decided I wanted to go the holistic route from the very beginning," says Frompovich, who was a natural nutritionist and consumer health researcher for 35 years (now retired). She applied her knowledge of food, supplements and other holistic modalities as treatment to fight her breast cancer—despite the surgeon urging her that if she didn't do the conventional treatments recommended, she wouldn't make it.

Today, after embracing a vegan diet, meditation and prayer, Frompovich has confirmation of one tumor gone, as verified by sonograms, and the other greatly reduced. "I'm working with a holistic physician who is allowing me to have input on my protocol—and it feels great to be working as a team," she says.

That proactive attitude is exactly what you need to deal with treatment or to help prevent breast cancer, says Lise Alschuler, N.D., past president of the American Association of Naturopathic Physicians and coauthor of *The Definitive Guide to Cancer* and *Five to Thrive: Your Cutting-Edge Cancer Prevention Plan.* Many women aren't aware of the profound effect that lifestyle changes can have on breast health, she says.

But if you're a cancer sufferer—or know someone who is—you may be concerned that natural remedies are not enough.

REMEDIES

Angelina Jolie's recent preventative double mastectomy (and plans to have her ovaries removed) mirrors many women's determination to do whatever it takes to live. (See our thoughts on Jolie on page 77.)

To that end, we recommend working with your oncologist to integrate natural treatments into more Western therapies. The very first seekers of alternative treatments were cancer patients, and the best cases often use true integrative treatments. As a result, most oncologists are quite familiar with and willing to consider them. You just have to know what you're looking for. To help you be more proactive, we've answered some of the most common questions women have today.

Should I get a genetic test for breast cancer?

If two or more of your close relatives (mother, sister, daughter, aunt, grandmother) have had breast cancer, your risk may be increased. A blood test that analyzes your DNA can determine whether you have a mutation of the breast cancer susceptibility genes, BRCA1 and BRCA2. These mutations are present in less than 1% of the general population, but women who have them—mostly those who have the disease in their family—have a 60% to 80% lifetime risk for developing breast cancer compared to the 12% lifetime risk for women who don't. (Jolie, for example, explained she carried BRCA1, her doctors estimating she had an 87% chance of contracting breast cancer and a 50% risk of ovarian cancer.)

BEFORE YOU TAKE THE TEST: Speak to a genetic counselor (the service is covered by most insurance plans) who can explain the results and walk you through scenarios to consider should your results be positive. The counselor can also help you deal with the emotions afterwards.

IF YOU TEST POSITIVE: A positive test doesn't necessarily mean you will develop breast cancer, just as a negative test doesn't mean you won't ever develop another form of the disease. Still, a positive result should mean more frequent mammograms, breast magnetic resonance imaging (MRI) and clinical breast exams. Some women undergo chemoprevention (using drugs to reduce cancer risk) or even a risk-reducing mastectomy.

In addition, women who test positive for BRCA mutations are also at increased risk for ovarian cancer, and it is often recommended that they have their ovaries and fallopian tubes removed (ideally between ages 35 and 40, and upon completion of childbearing).

Research also shows that removing ovaries by age 40 decreases the risk for breast cancer by as much as 60%. As a result, many women who test positive for the gene have their ovaries and fallopian tubes removed. About half choose intensive breast surveillance; and half choose risk-reducing mastectomies, according to some estimates.

WHERE TO GO: For information on genetic testing or for help finding a health care professional trained in genetics, contact the National Cancer Institute's Cancer Information Service at 800-4-CANCER. To find a naturopathic doctor who specializes in oncology, check with the Oncology Association of Naturopathic Physicians at oncanp.org.

Should I ask for an MRI exam, a BRCA1 or other tests?

An MRI can reveal a tumor that's too small to be detected by a physical exam or is missed by a mammogram. "An MRI is valuable as a secondary diagnostic tool," says Alschuler. "I know several patients who had a suspicious finding on a mammogram and followed up with ultrasound or an MRI and discovered cancer."

That's what happened to Cathy Gergen, 48, a human resources manager for a construction company in Arizona. After she discovered a lump in her right breast, she immediately scheduled a mammogram and ultrasound. When the tests produced conflicting results (the mammogram showed no thickening or lump; the ultrasound did), Gergen's surgeon ordered an MRI, which revealed a tumor. "If I hadn't felt the lump myself, I would have gone for a regular mammogram and thought everything was OK," she says. After reviewing her options with both a traditional surgeon and Alschuler, Gergen had a double mastectomy. She did not receive chemotherapy or radiation and the cancer drug Tamoxifen (the estimated benefit from these treatments was minimal given certain characteristics of her cancer), but she did add 30 minutes of walking to her routine; cut back on processed and fatty foods; and started taking supplements prescribed by Alschuler.

Can vitamin D reduce the risk of breast cancer?

Some research suggests that women with low levels of vitamin D (which the body makes from sunlight) at the time of breast cancer diagnosis had almost twice the risk of their cancer spreading and were nearly three times more likely to die within 10 years. Vitamin D is converted into a hormone that helps to prevent normal cells from becoming cancerous and, in some cases, induces established cancer cells to stop growing and die. Researchers are working to determine whether boosting vitamin D status after a breast cancer diagnosis can lower the odds of cancer spreading. If you're curious about your levels, ask for a 25-hydroxyvitamin D blood test, says JoEllen Welsh, Ph.D., an environmental health sciences professor at the State University of New York at Albany.

DOSAGE: If your 25-hydroxyvitamin D blood test is low, consuming between 1,000 IU and 2,000 IU per day may be needed to get the optimal vitamin D level for cancer prevention as suggested by the research, says Welsh. (Most experts say the government's current guideline of 600 IU per day is too low.) Ask your doctor to administer a vitamin D test to find out what you need.

GET SOME SUN: During the spring and summer, just 10 to 15 minutes of sun per day, three times a week (without sunscreen), is enough to produce the requirement of vitamin D. To protect against skin cancer, avoid the peak sun hours (11 a.m. to 2 p.m.). Depending on where you live, winter sun may be insufficient for vitamin D production, so dietary sources or supplements are especially important for women who live in northern areas.

Do supplements help?

Several supplements have been demonstrated to reduce the risk of developing breast cancer, and some other supplements may help make cancer treatments easier and more effective.

MELATONIN: This hormone, secreted primarily at night, is used to help induce sleep. But it also slows cellular growth, improves immunity and may be effective against tumors, says Alschuler. Talk to a naturopathic physician; a dosage of 3 milligrams to 20 milligrams may be necessary.

GREEN TEA EXTRACT: Epidemiological evidence suggests that green tea can be a potent weapon against breast cancer, particularly in early-stage cancer, says Alschuler. "If you consume more than five (4-ounce) cups of green tea a day, the risk of recurrence may drop 30% to 40%," she says. Green tea is thought to work against cancer four ways: It inhibits tumor growth-signaling pathways; it stimulates cancer-cell death; it inhibits enzymes that cancer cells use to spread; and it alters the metabolism of estrogens. Buy organic green tea, or take two to four 250-milligram to 300-milligram capsules of standardized green tea extract with meals. Make sure they are standardized to 80% polyphenols, of which 50% is EGCG, says Alschuler.

LAVENDER AND CHAMOMILE TEA: For patients with anxiety or sleeplessness, Alschuler suggests melatonin, lavender and/or chamomile tea. Lavender, containing an essential oil extract called silexan, is very effective at reducing anxiety. Just one 80-milligram capsule will significantly reduce anxiety in the majority of people who take it. "Many of chamomile's medicinal properties are in the volatile oils that come out in the steam, so it's important to steep the tea covered," Alschuler explains. Use two bags per cup (look for an organic brand), or buy organic dried flowers and use one tablespoon per cup of boiling water. Let steep 10 to 15 minutes and add honey to taste.

COFFEE: New research from Lund University in Sweden has found that drinking coffee could decrease the risk of breast cancer recurring in patients taking Tamoxifen. Study subjects taking the cancer drug who also drank two or more cups of coffee daily reported less than half the rate of cancer recurrence compared with their non-coffee-drinking Tamoxifen-taking counterparts. The researchers think that something in coffee activates Tamoxifen, making it even more effective.

Should I take extra doses of antioxidants?

Not if you're undergoing radiation therapy. Although antioxidants occur naturally in a healthy diet, some experts believe that taking mega-doses during cancer treatment could interfere with the way radiation

What Would Angelina Do?

Angelina Jolie shocked the world in May 2013, when she announced, via a *New York Times* Op-Ed piece, that she had gotten a preventative double mastectomy. The news went viral instantly: She? Got a what? Oh no. "I hope that other women can benefit from my experience," Jolie wrote movingly, thanking her partner, Brad Pitt. To which many women responded: "Angelina got a mastectomy... Should I, too?"

The short answer is: Depends on your past, and even then, perhaps not. Because Jolie's mother died of breast cancer—and a genetic test for the BRCA1 mutation indicated that Jolie's odds of also getting breast cancer were 87%—she opted for the preventative measure, and will also have her ovaries removed. (Her doctors also estimate a 50% chance she will get ovarian cancer, a much more deadly disease.)

Most women do not fall into this high-risk category. Yes, 50 million women die each year from breast cancer. But 99% of women do not have the BRCA1 mutation and 90% of breast cancer deaths don't have anything to do with it. Most breast cancers have nothing to do with heredity. And some experts even say that the breast cancer one gets as a result of the mutation is not deadly.

The discussion isn't over, and a 1% chance of carrying the gene is worth a long discussion with your doctor, for certain. And maybe even a test. New health care reform will require private insurance companies to cover such testing, if the patient has a family history that indicates a high risk. As Jolie wrote: "I hope it helps you to know you have options."

works. (Antioxidants work to scavenge free radicals; radiation generates free radicals, which kill rapidly dividing cancer cells.) If you're undergoing chemotherapy, avoid antioxidant supplements unless you've consulted with your doctor or your naturopathic oncologist, but do continue eating antioxidant-rich fruits and vegetables (cherries, blueberries, blackberries, red and yellow peppers); they don't contain antioxidants in megadoses and won't interfere with treatment

Will any foods reduce my risk of breast cancer?

Eating a healthy, varied diet based on whole foods remains the best way to prevent cancer and keep it from recurring, says Beth Reardon, R.D., director of integrative nutrition at Duke Integrative Medicine in Durham, N.C. It's also important to include as many colors as possible—colorful plant foods contain a variety of cancer-fighting pigmented compounds called polyphenols. It's also smart to keep your fat intake down (aim for less than 35 grams per day, of which no more than 2 grams should be saturated fat), adds Alschuler, since there's a direct link between breast cancer and extra weight. More specifically, minimize your saturated fat intake from red meat and high-fat dairy, and trans fats from processed baked goods, Reardon says. She also recommends flaxseeds (the ground seeds, not the oil, are rich in lignans, a form of phytoestrogen that the body metabolizes into weak forms of estrogen, which in turn displace the aggressive natural estrogens that stimulate breast cancers); mushrooms (they contain a form of linoleic acid, which appears to inhibit the activity of aromatase, an enzyme the body uses to make estrogen); and some unprocessed non-GMO soy (which can inhibit blood vessel growth in hormone-dependent breast cancer tumors).

How can I ease the stress I feel after my diagnosis?

Learning that you have breast cancer or the gene mutation may leave you feeling frustrated, angry and depressed. And your emotional well-being is a crucial part of your treatment. Negative feelings like stress, pessimism, anxiety and anger can lower your immunity and actually stimulate the growth of cancer cells. Plus, stress creates hor-

Preventing Prostate Cancer

In the United States, prostate cancer is the most commonly discovered cancer in men over 50; it's responsible for 35,000 deaths each year, and an additional 165,000 men are diagnosed each year. African-American men are 40% more likely to develop the disease. About 20% of enlarged prostates are a result of cancer, but an overwhelming majority of cancers do not present as enlarged prostate. Prostate cancer spreads rapidly, but early detection has been very successful in cure rate.

The cause of prostate cancer is not known, but experts believe that hormonal and genetic factors play a huge part, as does age. A few studies have shown that men who have had a vasectomy are at higher risk for both prostate and testicular cancer. There also is evidence that rates are higher among men who have been exposed to toxic chemicals.

Prevention:

PUT. DOWN. THE. CANDY BARS. Keeping the genitourinary tract healthy is key, and good nutrition through an anti-inflammatory diet is crucial. Foods rich in antioxidants such as vitamins C and E help keep the prostate gland and urethra free of microorganisms that might become cancerous cells. Essential fatty acids such as fish oils and olive oil keep the prostate healthy and help reduce blood clotting (clotting can raise the risk of tumors spreading). Also see "The Anti-Cancer Diet" on page 81. Several good studies have shown that decreasing sugar consumption may decrease the risk of prostate and all other cancers. Detox diets also can be protective.

HERBAL REMEDIES are available that keep the immune system strong by stimulating the production and activity of white blood cells, and some even enter cancerous cells and make them more vulnerable to destruction by the immune system. (Saw palmetto, ginkgo and ginseng are particularly helpful.) Exercise is important for general immune strengthening—swimming is an excellent choice—as are sufficient sleep, stress reduction and good sexual hygiene, including use of condoms to protect against HPV. Homeopathy has shown success in treating many prostate conditions.

monal imbalances, says Alschuler, so it's important to support yourself emotionally. The perfect antidote to these feelings is joy and laughter, and prioritizing these emotions—even during the challenges of treatment—is important. Using effective mind-body techniques, such as qigong, Reiki and meditation, can help trigger the release of endorphins, the brain's natural pain relievers, to boost energy, ease any physical pain and help you sleep soundly. Here are two you can do at home, at work or even during your treatments.

DEEP BREATHING

"A proper deep breath is your body's own built-in relaxation mecha nism," explains Carol Krucoff, E-RYT, a yoga teacher at Duke Integrative Medicine and author of *Healing Yoga for Neck and Shoulder Pain.* "When you bring air down deeply into the lungs, it triggers a cascade of calming physiologic changes: The heart rate slows, blood pressure decreases, muscles relax, anxiety eases and the mind quiets down."

TO DO IT: Lie down and place your palms on your lower belly. Relax your abdomen. Take an easy breath in and notice how your belly rounds and your hands gently rise. As you breathe out, notice how your belly relaxes back and your hands fall. Don't strain or force; your body knows how to do this. Count the length of your inhalation and exhalation (for example, 1-2-3-4 inhale and 1-2-3-4 exhale). See if you can make your inhale and exhale the same length. For extra relaxation effect, make your exhale longer—for example, inhale to a count of 4, exhale to a count of 6.

BODY-SCAN MEDITATION

When we're under stress, we're often worrying about the future or ruminating about the past. A body-scan meditation helps bring you into the present moment, which helps calm and center your body and mind, says Krucoff.

TO DO IT: Lie down or sit comfortably, with your body supported. Bring your attention to your breath, and notice the sensations of the breath as it comes into and leaves your body. When you're ready, send your awareness throughout your entire interior landscape, just noticing what's present. Have an attitude of curiosity, self-compassion and nonjudgment. Try not to let your mind spin off into stories about the meanings of any sensation—just notice the sensations that are present and welcome whatever you find.

Does exercise really help?

Despite the complexity of "the big C," some of the natural solutions are smack-your-forehead obvious—Health 101. For example, an analysis of study data published in the *Journal of Clinical Oncology* showed a significant improvement in survival rates among women with stage 1 breast cancer who both exercised for at least 30 minutes per day and maintained a diet that included five servings of fruit and vegetables. Additionally, the American College of Sports Medicine, in 2010, concluded that exercise is safe during and after breast cancer treatments (as long as needed precautions are taken, and the intensity is kept low) and improves physical functioning, quality of life and reduces cancer-related fatigue.

New research from 2012, published in the *Journal of the National Cancer Institute*, shows that exercise can also prevent the disease. Researchers found that just 30 minutes of daily cardiovascular exercise (think moderately brisk walking) can reduce the risk of breast cancer between 40% and 60%.

"Exercise reduces a woman's risk of dying from breast cancer by about 50%, and it reduces her risk of getting the disease in the first place by up to 60%," says Alschuler. "That would be considered a miracle drug if it were in a bottle."

THE ANTI-CANCER DIET
9 Foods that Can Help Prevent Cancer

You have cancer. We all do. But don't panic. We're not talking about the disease. Rather, we're talking about the random cancer cells that regularly pop up in your body just about everywhere—a by-product of eating, breathing and, well, just living. If we're healthy, they get nipped in the bud by our immune system. This process, called apoptosis (also known as programmed cell death) is our body's innate cancer-prevention process. The trouble starts when too many cancer cells get together and figure out how to outfox our body's natural defenses.

"Cancer is like a weed," says Donald Abrams, M.D., director of the Integrative Oncology Research Program, Osher Center, at the University of California, San Francisco. "You need to tend your garden carefully to make the soil as inhospitable as possible so cancer can't take root in the first place."

Step 1 in developing a strong anti-cancer diet is eliminating its "fertilizers," Abrams says. "Dairy, sugar, refined flours and red meat are the top foods for feeding the weed," he explains. These foods also add inches to our waistline, fattening us up and raising our national risk of developing cancer.

Losing excess weight might be the best thing you can do to lower your risk, says Colleen Doyle, M.S., R.D., director of nutrition and physical activity for the American Cancer Society. "People who are overweight have higher levels of circulating estrogen and insulin—both of which are associated with tumor growth," she says.

Moreover, Abrams says, extra fat promotes systemic inflammation in the body. "Excess fat secretes cytokines, which prompt an inflammatory response," he says. "More and more, we are coming to believe that chronic inflammation leads to cancer because it ties up the immune system, undermining apoptosis." Trimming calories is a good idea, but it helps to eliminate the following fertilizers from your diet:

ALCOHOL

"We know that breast cancer in particular responds to alcohol in a negative way—possibly because excess alcohol can raise estrogen levels," says Carolyn Lammersfeld, M.S., R.D., L.D.N., C.N.S.C., vice president of Integrative Medicine at Cancer Treatment Centers of America. "Alcohol also contains a variety of chemicals that may have a carcinogenic effect." Limit yourself to one glass a day.

RED MEAT

A famous study published in the *Archives of Internal Medicine* (now *JAMA Internal Medicine*) found that women who ate 1½ servings or more per day of beef, lamb or pork had nearly double the risk of hormone-receptor positive breast cancer when compared with those who ate red meat just three times a week. A survey released in 2012 confirms the findings. Researchers followed 100,000 subjects for 28 years, and the meat-eaters were definitely dying faster. If the meat is processed, the risk is even higher: A 2012 study found that people who ate one serving of processed meat a day increased their risk of death from cancer and heart disease by 20%. The message? Eat meat sparingly, if at all, and stick to chicken, fish and turkey.

SUGAR

Skip added sugars in all forms, including sweetened and processed foods and drinks. "The link between cancer and sugar isn't clear, but there's an indirect link in that foods high in sugar tend to be high in calories and may lead to excessive weight gain," says Doyle. People who get a lot of sugar in their diets also tend to miss out on nutrient-rich whole foods that are linked to cancer protection.

DAIRY

It's easy to see how cakes, candies and cookies fall under the "sugars" heading, but Abrams adds dairy to the list. "Dairy contains simple sugars that the human body was never intended to digest past the age of weaning. Because we don't digest dairy well, it ends up contributing to inflammation in the body," he says. Milk, in particular, has been linked to cancers of the breasts, prostate and bladder, as well as lymphoma.

The nine most protective foods

You've heard it before: For good health, eat a plant-based diet that's focused on whole grains and organic fresh fruits and vegetables. These are, per nature's design, the most nutrient rich fuel for your immune system. "Any plant that has been grown outdoors organically is one that has had to fight for its life and develop chemical protections against birds and insects and sunshine," explains Abrams. "It turns out that those same protections—phytonutrients—are beneficial for us, too."

When it comes to cancer protection, some fruits and vegetables are better than others. "I encourage people to focus on the three A's: anti-carcinogens, anti-inflammatories and antioxidants," says Carolyn Katzin, M.S., C.N.S., M.N.T., a nutritionist who specializes in oncology and weight management. A good (if well-worn) rule of thumb is to choose the most colorful foods, and aim to get a rainbow's worth of them each day—carrots, grapes, blueberries, spinach, watermelon. "The pigment is where the antioxidants are," says Dave Grotto, R.D., author of *101 Foods That Could Save Your Life*. So, stock up on brightly colored produce as well as these cancer-fighting powerfoods:

1. BARLEY

"The fiber content of many whole grains can block the actions of some carcinogens and promote cell differentiation, making it easier for the body to know which cells to target for apoptosis," says Grotto. Whole oats, corn and brown rice are all good sources, but barley is best.

2. BLACK BEANS

All beans are another good source of fiber, but black beans stand out because of the high antioxidant content in their skin. "Black beans may also block the circulation of estrodiol, a form of estrogen that's a problem for those at risk for estrogen-driven breast cancer," says Grotto. The resistant starch found in the beans is thought to mimic estrogen enough to attach to estrogen-receptor sites, allowing excessive and harmful forms of estrogen to more easily pass through the body.

3. BLACK RASPBERRIES

All berries are good for cancer prevention, but black raspberries are the best. They contain a lot of A's: antioxidants, anti-inflammatory and anti-carcinogenic compounds, plus a fourth A that gives them an edge. "Black raspberries contain a unique form of anthocyanin that has been strongly linked with reduced rates of cancers of the upper respiratory system and digestive tract," Katzin says.

4. BROCCOLI

"Broccoli has more than 300 studies to back its efficacy," says Grotto. The vegetable is among nature's richest sources of sulforophane, a compound that's thought to strongly inhibit cancers. Research suggests that sulforophanes stimulate the body's own cancer-fighting enzymes, slowing the rate of breast and prostate cancer cell growth.

5. GREEN TEA

Switch to green tea for your morning cup, and you'll get a nice dose of support for apoptosis. The key compound, epigallocatechin-3-gallate, seems to work as a signaling agent for inducing programmed cell death. "Drinking green tea helps cells to die at the end of their normal life cycle, which is important because cancer is caused by cells that have continued to grow and mutate beyond their normal lifespan," says Kristin Stiles Green, N.D., former director of naturopathic medicine for Cancer Treatment Centers of America at Midwestern Regional Medical Center in Zion, Ill., now practicing in California. Aim for two to four cups of home-brewed organic green tea per day. Or try the supplement, mentioned previously in this section.

Your Diet During Treatment

Surprisingly, some foods that can help prevent cancer are off the menu once you are diagnosed and treatment begins. Here, what to eat to work with—and not against—your therapy.

TAKE IT EASY ON THE ANTIOXIDANTS The advice seems counterintuitive, but it turns out antioxidants can work against the chemotherapy process. "Antioxidants protect the cell membranes from damage, but in treatment they're purposefully trying to damage the cancer cells," says Colleen Doyle of the American Cancer Society. "If you're undergoing treatment, eating fruits and vegetables is fine, but avoid taking large doses of antioxidant supplements that may interfere with some types of treatment."

PUMP UP THE PROTEIN When undergoing treatment, you need 80 to 100 grams of protein every day. "Protein is necessary for producing hormones and enzymes in the blood cells, stoking the immune system and building muscle mass," says Carolyn Lammersfeld of Cancer Treatment Centers of America.

MONITOR YOUR SUPPLEMENTS Share your vitamin and herb regimen with your medical team, says nutritionist Carolyn Katzin. "Taking the wrong supplements at the wrong time can end up making some drugs more toxic or potentially render them ineffective," says naturopathic doctor Kristin Stiles Green.

6. MUSHROOMS

According to integrative medicine guru Andrew Weil, M.D., mushrooms are on primary cancer treatment protocols in Japan and Brazil. The verdict is still out on whether mushrooms work as a treatment, Abrams says, "but we know mushrooms are anti-inflammatory, and we think they may have an anti-tumor effect." Incorporate them into your diet wherever you can, and consider taking a supplement every day that includes cordyceps, maitake and reishi.

7. SOY

Some studies suggest that consuming soy foods may reduce the risk of breast and prostate cancers, says Doyle. "Soy foods contain several phytochemicals, some of which have weak estrogen activity and may compete with the body's natural source of estrogen, reducing the overall amount of circulating estrogen," she says. Skip supplements and stick to edamame, tofu and tempeh.

8. TURMERIC

If there is a miracle food for cancer, it is turmeric. Studies are showing positive effects in the realms of prevention and treatment (particularly in hard-to-treat pancreatic cancer)—as well as adjunctive therapy for patients going through chemo and/or radiation. For best results, combine turmeric with black pepper. "Black pepper makes turmeric much more bioavailable," notes Abrams. "But because it can increase absorption of other compounds, too—including prescription drugs—you should use it in moderation."

9. WATERCRESS

"It supports liver function, which is crucial for cancer prevention and overall wellness," says Katzin. "As little as three sprigs a day can lead to better outcomes for those at risk for lung cancer."

How can I treat carpal tunnel syndrome?

*Whether caused by too much tennis or too many mice,
carpal tunnel is a pain in the wrist.*

A physiatrist says:

Carpal tunnel syndrome occurs when the arm's median nerve is pinched in the narrow passageway located on the inside of your wrist (the carpal tunnel).

TREATMENT: "I do a clinical diagnosis and confirm my assessment with an electrodiagonistic test. To relieve and control symptoms temporarily, I administer a cortisone injection to the wrist. For severe cases, I may perform surgery to release the ligament on the roof of the carpal tunnel, which expands the passageway and gives more space to the median nerve."

Try ibuprofen or naproxen, nonsteroidal anti-inflammatory drugs that can provide temporary pain relief and reduce inflammation. To prevent a relapse, try wrist stretches (pressing the back of your hand down for 15 seconds and then pushing your fingers back for 15 seconds).

—Meijuan Zhao, M.D.,
instructor of physical medicine and rehabilitation at Harvard Medical School and physiatrist at Massachusetts General Hospital

A yoga therapist says:

Stress on the wrist begins in the upper body, where slouching or a sunken chest may compress and disrupt nerves that link to the arm and wrist.

TREATMENT: "I check your posture and postural habits, making sure your head is aligned with your spinal column and that you aren't leaning too far forward when you sit. I also correct breathing by teaching you how to lengthen the breath and breathe into the belly, which helps mobilize the chest and ribs and reduces stress."

Try a modified version of Downward Facing Dog, placing your hands on a desk with your hips folded slightly. Or, try a simple doorway back bend: Walk into a doorway, and let each hand catch on the door frame. With your feet just forward of the door and hands on the door frame edge behind you, look up and arch your back gently, opening your chest. Hold this pose for at least five minutes.

—Timothy McCall, M.D.,
author of Yoga as Medicine: The Yogic Prescription for Health and Healing

COLDS and FLU

The Natural Remedies for 2014

Every year, Americans suffer 1 billion colds, and as many as one in five people catches the seasonal flu, usually in late fall and winter, according to the National Institutes of Health. It's a germophobe's worst nightmare and Purell's wet dream. And yet brand-new research shows there's A New Hope: certain natural remedies may be the best way to beat the buggers, or at least offer temporary relief. And chances are, you haven't tried them before. Here are the New Remedies for Cold + Flu.

ANDROGRAPHIS

The leaf and underground stem of this South Asian plant is frequently used for preventing and treating the common cold and flu—and a review of seven studies found the herb to be effective for colds in particular. In one trial, cold sufferers who took andrographis reported significant relief from runny nose, sore throat and sleeplessness compared with their placebo-popping peers. "Andrographis appears to be effective in reducing the severity and duration of symptoms if started within the first 26 to 48 hours of the onset of symptoms," says Cathy Wong, N.D., C.N.S., a Boston-based naturopath and author of *The Inside-Out Diet.*

TRY: Nature's Way Andrographis Standardized ($7 for 60 capsules; vitacost.com); New Chapter Organics Perfect Immune ($21 for 36 tablets; vitacost.com)

ELDERBERRY

Preclinical trials suggest that elderberry extract may reduce mucus production and have anti-inflammatory and antiviral effects, says Wong. One study found that elderberry reduced the duration of flu-like symptoms, including fever, by more than 50%. "Elderberry may fight flu-like symptoms, and it's easy for the whole family to take," says Wong, who keeps the syrup stocked in her fridge all year long.

TRY: Gaia Herbs Black Elderberry Syrup ($20 for 3 ounces; gaiaherbs .com); New Chapter Organics Perfect Immune ($21 for 36 tablets; vita-cost.com)

GINSENG

Research suggests that ginseng revs up the immune system—and a University of Alberta study found that subjects taking daily doses of North American ginseng (*Panax quinquefolium*) got fewer colds, as well as colds of a shorter duration and with less severe symptoms, than a placebo group. "North American ginseng may help to fight acute respiratory illness, including colds and flu," says Wong, who does also note that ginseng extracts may have adverse effects such as altering blood pressure, causing insomnia, reducing blood sugar and interacting with anticoagulant or antiplatelet medication. "Make sure to consult your physician before taking this supplement," Wong warns.

TRY: Cold-FX 200 milligrams ($60 for 150 capsules; feelbest.com)

MUSHROOMS

In Traditional Chinese Medicine, mushrooms such as shiitake, maitake, reishi, cordyceps and coriolus are used to boost immunity and fend off colds and flu. "Mushrooms have been found to have antiviral, anti-inflammatory and immune-stimulating properties due to compounds called polysaccharides," says Wong. Indeed, one study found that treating cells with maitake mushroom extract (*Grifola frondosa*) helped to

COLD vs. FLU: What's the Diff?

Symptoms of a cold are very similar to the flu; one big difference is that a cold usually comes on gradually, while the flu hits like a ton of bricks. Also, the characteristics of flu include fever, headache and extreme fatigue, whereas cold symptoms often start with a sore throat and include stuffy nose, sneezing and congestion.

promote the production of proteins that activate the body's immune system in response to infection, potentially helping to slow the growth of the flu virus. "An animal study found that cordyceps polysaccharides may help to fight against flu by moderating the function of macrophages—white blood cells that are key players in the body's immune response to infectious microorganisms," Wong adds.

TRY: Onnit Labs Shroom Tech Immune ($20 for 30 capsules; onnit.com); Gaia Herbs Maitake Defense ($30 for 60 capsules; gaiaherbs.com); Rainbow Light Certified Organics Mushroom Therapy ($30 for 60 Vcaps; rainbowlight.com)

PROBIOTICS

Typically associated with digestive health, probiotics have been proven to boost immunity and may help with cold and flu prevention. "In my opinion, this is the most important supplement of all, as the gut plays such a critical role in our immunity," says Glenn Finley, N.D., a naturopathic family physician and cofounder of New Leaf Holistic Health in Kingston, N.Y., who suggests taking at least 10 billion colony-forming units (CFU) daily for prevention and 10 billion to 20 billion (or more) for treatment of acute flu symptoms, including stomach upset. "We literally have trillions of beneficial bacteria in our bodies, and I recommend rotating through different formulas once a good foundation is established."

TRY: Genestra Brands HMF Intensive ($34 for 30 Vcaps; pureformulas.com); Innate Response Formulas Flora 50-14 Clinical Strength ($36 for 30 caps; amazon.com); MegaFood MegaFlora Plus ($32 for 30 caps; drugstore.com); Klaire Labs Pro-5 ($29 for 60 Vcaps; pureformulas.com). Wong also recommends probiotic-rich foods such as kefir, yogurt and fermented vegetables like sauerkraut and kimchi.

A Homeopathic Flu Shot?

Believe it! Muco Coccinum by Unda is essentially the homeopathic equivalent of a flu shot, but in tablet form, shown to be 88% effective for prevention and 82% effective during an acute episode ($20 for 10 tabs; rockwellnutrition.com). And, of course, people worldwide swear by Boiron's oscillococcinum ($15 for 12 doses; drugstore.com).

EAT FOR IMMUNITY

To ward off bugs and keep your immune system strong, it's important to get enough sleep and exercise; wash your hands regularly; manage stress; and eat the right foods. Here are the top cold- and flu-fighting nutrients recommended by Boston-based naturopath and nutritionist Cathy Wong, N.D., C.N.S.

CAROTENOIDS: These pigments found naturally in foods such as carrots, kale, apricots, mango and papaya are converted in the body to vitamin A, which helps to regulate the immune system, says Wong.

OMEGA-3 FATTY ACIDS: Found in salmon, sardines and other oily fish, as well as flaxseed, hemp seeds and walnuts, these fats can help to decrease inflammation and are important for proper immune function.

VITAMIN C: Get your fill of this antioxidant by eating plenty of citrus, strawberries, kiwi, tomatoes, peppers and broccoli.

VITAMIN E: Another antioxidant that plays an important role in maintaining a healthy immune system, especially among older people, vitamin E can be found in wheat germ oil, almonds, sunflower seeds and hazelnuts.

ZINC: This essential mineral is involved in the production of immune cells, Wong notes. Find it in oysters, baked beans, cashews and chickpeas.

The old standbys

Just how good are those "go-to" remedies vitamin C, zinc, oscillococcinum and echinacea? Here's the latest research:

VITAMIN C: A meta-analysis of vitamin C's effect on colds reported in 2008 by the American Botanical Council shows that vitamin C prophylaxis (meaning taken to prevent symptoms) can reduce duration and

Wet Socks Work Wonders

This naturopathic trick sounds suspicious, but works great for immune, lymph and circulatory stimulation, says Glenn Finley, N.D. Simply wet cotton socks in cool water, wring them out well and put them on your feet. "Cover those with wool socks and go to bed, and your socks will be dry in the morning," Finley notes.

severity of colds, but high doses do not have a significant effect if taken during a cold, and could have adverse effects on one's stomach. One study showed 300 milligrams a day may reduce hospital stays and prevent a cold from becoming pneumonia.

ZINC: A 2011 systematic review by the NIH's National Center for Complementary and Alternative Medicine (NCCAM) found that zinc does help reduce the length and severity of the common cold in healthy people when taken within 24 hours after symptoms start, and has been shown to reduce the number of colds in children when taken for at least five months. But some forms of zinc have side effects: Oral zinc may cause nausea and other gastrointestinal issues, may increase the risk of urinary tract problems and can interact with drugs including antibiotics. The nasal form of zinc may cause anosmia, the loss of a sense of smell.

OSCILLOCOCCINUM: The benefits of homeopathy—based on the theory that "like cures like"—cannot be explained by current scientific methods; so while many thousands around the world swear that oscillo prevents and relieves the flu, this has not been scientifically proven. And beware if you're vegan or vegetarian: It's made from tiny bits of duck liver and heart. Yum?

ECHINACEA: A 2012 randomized controlled study by British researchers found that a special Swiss echinacea formula (Echinaforce) was both safe and effective in helping prevent cold symptoms, findings that are consistent with other clinical trials. NIH reviews have been inconclusive, in part because echinacea products vary widely in terms of plant and species studied and study methods. There has been some evidence that it may cause an allergic rash.

DEPRESSION

Blame the economy, the fast-moving modern world, a brain chemical imbalance or the inescapable, existential, crushing reality of what Prince once called "this thing called life"—regardless of the cause, you are not alone in your depression. And we don't mean to depress you (more), but the news can get scarier—significantly scarier—if you look to Big Pharma for relief: The most commonly prescribed antidepressants, known as "selective serotonin reuptake inhibitors" (SSRIs) such as Prozac, Zoloft and Paxil, stop your body's reabsorption of the "feel-good" neurotransmitter serotonin, causing its levels to increase, which boosts mood. But these meds post a long list of potential side effects, many of them identical to depression symptoms, such as nausea, insomnia, weight gain, fatigue, constipation and anxiety. They often take several weeks to kick in, too, and involve dietary restrictions. Add to those the possibility of sexual side effects, and—depressing.

What's more, SSRIs may be no more effective than a placebo at treating depression. A landmark National Institute of Mental Health study followed 4,000 depression sufferers and found that 75% of them still experienced at least five symptoms after taking antidepressants for three months. And that research is updated constantly; a 2013 review investigated the effectiveness of different combinations of medications based on mood swings and other symptoms, and reported that newer medications had significant efficacy when combined with cognitive therapy, especially for older adults and those with severe depression. But for those with general depression, it's still a complicated issue. Placebo vs. medication studies found that the placebos had anywhere from 30% to 50% efficacy, while those taking the actual antidepressants showed improvement an average of 50% of the time (a range from 31.6% to 70.4%), from 43% to 46.9% of the time, depending largely on the medication.

Are you really depressed?

If antidepressant drugs don't work that well, why are Americans taking 50% more of them than we were 20 years ago? "Many physicians think of antidepressants as a panacea and prescribe them without addressing the underlying causes of the depression or giving people the tools they need to help themselves," says psychiatrist James S. Gordon, M.D., founder and director of The Center for Mind-Body Medicine in Washington, D.C.

They have a surfeit of patients: According to the most recent numbers from the Centers for Disease Control and Prevention (CDC) about one in 10 Americans will face clinical depression at some point in their lives, and 4.1% will experience major depression. Recently, researchers reported in the *Journal of Clinical Psychiatry* that family doctors are prescribing antidepressants to a quarter of patients who exhibit a symptom or two but have not been diagnosed with depression. Another study found that at the same time, fewer people are visiting psychotherapists because insurance offers better coverage for pharmaceuticals.

SYMPTOMS

You're more apt to be depressed if you're between 45 and 64, unemployed or unable to work, have less than a high school education or are divorced. Women have a 70% higher risk than men. Fewer than half of sufferers seek treatment, but if not addressed, depression can seriously impact your productivity, your relationships and your overall health. A recent study found that depression increases the risk of heart disease more than smoking or having a family history of cardiac problems. Worse, depression can become a way of life—a debilitating, accepted and lifelong paralysis.

Your doctor may be quick to write you a prescription without exploring other conditions that have the same symptoms as depression. "You might feel depressed because you love sushi and actually have mercury poisoning. Or you could be a fish hater so you have an omega-3 deficiency," says Mark Hyman, M.D., founder of The UltraWellness Center in Lenox, Mass. "Or maybe you're taking an acid blocker for reflux and as a result your vitamin B_{12} is depleted, which also leads to depression."

According to the Centers for Disease Control and Prevention, you may have major, or clinical, depression if you have at least five of the symptoms below that cluster together, last for at least two weeks and impair your functioning:

- Changes in sleep, appetite or activity patterns

- Fatigue or lack of energy

- Loss of interest in activities that were once pleasurable

- Difficulty concentrating, remembering or making decisions

- Feelings of sadness, hopelessness, helplessness, guilt, worthlessness, irritability or agitation

- Thoughts of death or suicide

Other conditions include low thyroid function, food sensitivities like celiac disease, sugar addiction, systemic yeast infection, adrenal exhaustion, hormone imbalances and nutrient deficiencies. Hyman recommends visiting a naturopathic physician (N.D.) or an integrative M.D. for testing to determine if any of these issues are the real reason you're feeling down.

REMEDIES

Try lifestyle changes and natural remedies before going on meds. For a quicker recovery, combine these holistic approaches, advises Gordon, who has helped depressed patients with mind-body medicine techniques for 40 years. Where should you start? "Ask yourself, 'What am I doing that actually makes me feel better?'" Gordon suggests. To begin, check out the possibilities here and focus on doing what you know helps; then explore additional possibilities.

MOVE YOUR BODY

Exercise is as effective as any antidepressant in reversing depression symptoms and has no negative side effects, numerous studies have found, including research reported by the Mayo Clinic stating that exercise probably reduces depression and anxiety by raising body temperature (which has a calming effect) and releasing feel-good brain chemicals. "If you don't exercise, you won't make 'happy mood' chemicals like serotonin and endorphins or reduce your stress levels," says Hyman, who advises exercising for at least 30 minutes, three to five days a week.

FEED YOUR HEAD

Your brain is mostly made up of fat, primarily docosahexaenoic acid (DHA), so nourishing it with omega-3 fatty acids is essential. If you're not getting enough omega-3s (most of us are deficient), blues-busting brain chemicals won't be properly utilized. Omega-3s also reduce inflammation throughout your body, yet another contributor to mood disorders. Gordon recommends taking 3,000 to 6,000 milligrams of omega-3s daily, at least half of which are EPA and DHA.

TRY: Barleans Omega Swirl Omega-3 Fish Oil Supplement in Mango Peach flavor ($20 for 12 ounces; barleans.com)

GO WITH YOUR GUT

Most of your body's bliss-boosting serotonin is produced in your gut, not your brain. That means the levels of "good" and "bad" bacteria in your intestines may affect your state of mind. Hyman has seen this "second-brain" effect in patients who feel depressed because years of taking antibiotics have altered their digestive flora and affected their "gut brain," which in turn affects their "head brain." You can eat fermented foods like tempeh, sauerkraut or kimchi, or take probiotics.

TRY: American Health Probiotic CD ($30 for 60 tablets; luckyvitamin.com)

Try Side-Effect-Free Supplements

SAM-E: One study showed that when antidepressant users who still exhibited symptoms also took SAM-e, they showed more improvement than those who only tried SSRIs.
  Dosage: 800 milligrams twice daily; but for SAM-e to work, you also need 200 to 600 milligrams of magnesium a day. This mineral also helps relieve anxiety, insomnia and irritability.
  Try: Source Naturals SAM-e Double Strength ($22 for 30 tablets; vitacost.com)

ST. JOHN'S WORT: This herb is well-known for treating mild to moderate depression as effectively as SSRIs. **Note:** Do not take it if you are also taking prescription drugs for various medical conditions, as St. John's wort interacts with many of them and makes them less effective.
  Dosage: 300 milligrams three times a day.
  Try: New Chapter's Mood Take Care ($14 for 30 softgels; amazon.com)

ASHWAGANDHA: This Indian adaptogenic herb helps you stand up to stress, stabilizes your moods and eases anxiety, despair and helplessness.
  Dosage: 20 to 50 milligrams daily.
  Try: Organic India Joy! ($19 for 90 capsules; organicindiausa.com)

AVOID VITAMIN D-FICIENCY

If you live where the sun don't shine or never hit the beach without first slathering on the SPF, low vitamin D levels may be the culprit behind your depression or, in winter, seasonal affective disorder (SAD). The sunshine-triggered vitamin helps regulate an enzyme essential in the production of the neurotransmitters norepinephrine and dopamine. If sun exposure is not an option, research indicates that you should supplement with at least 2,000 to 5,000 IU of vitamin D_3 daily.

TRY: Nordic Naturals Vitamin D_3 ($16 for 120 softgels; nordicnaturals.com)

BE SURE TO GET YOUR B's

Without enough B vitamins, your brain can't properly regulate mood-affecting neurotransmitters. Hyman suggests taking 800 micrograms daily of a food-based folate supplement (not folic acid, the synthetic form); 500 to 1,000 micrograms of B_{12}; and 25 to 50 milligrams of B_6.

TRY: Innate Response Formulas Folate, B_6 & B_{12} ($25 for 90 tablets; pureformulas.com)

FOLLOW AN ANTI-INFLAMMATORY DIET

When followed consistently, this heart-healthy diet has also been shown to lower depression risk by 30%. Staples include cold-water fatty fish like salmon, mackerel and sardines; dark leafy greens, such as spinach, kale and collards; beans, nuts and seeds; and olive oil.

CUT OUT JUNK FOOD

Sugar briefly energizes you until you crash, physically and emotionally, and it also causes inflammation in the brain, Hyman says; the artificial sweetener aspartame has been shown to deplete serotonin; and trans fats cause inflammation and raise depression risk by 48%, a 2011 Spanish study found. You might also try an elimination diet to see if certain foods are not ideal for your body. Hyman has seen longtime depression sufferers drop dairy and gluten—two causes of brain inflammation—and their depression lifts enough that they can go off their meds after having relied on them for years.

DON'T DROWN YOUR SORROWS

While drinking provides a temporary lift, alcohol is a known depressant that alters brain chemistry and mood. "If you're drinking to avoid feeling sad or dealing with your problems, you need to steer clear of alcohol completely," says Meredith Sagan, M.D., founder of Holistic Psychiatry in Santa Monica, Calif. Do not deny yourself wine at a party, but she advises stopping after one glass.

BEWARE OF BPA

Avoid eating foods from cans or drinking water from plastic bottles when possible because of potential bisphenol-A (BPA) exposure. This toxin alters the nervous system, and studies show it may be linked to depression, cognitive decline and schizophrenia.

MEDITATE BEFORE YOU MEDICATE

"We're constantly triggered emotionally by people or situations that send an overwhelming flood of fight-or-flight stress hormones into

If You Need Antidepressants

If you're having suicidal thoughts, the need for an antidepressant outweighs the risk of side effects. Or if you've experienced major life trauma like a divorce, abuse or a death in your family and find it impossible to function, drugs can offer a quick solution, says holistic psychiatrist Meredith Sagan, M.D. The key, though, is to work with your doc to learn alternative techniques that will help you eventually get off the medication. Sagan teaches her patients techniques like meditation to help them cope with and work through the root cause of their depression, something medications cannot do, she says.

According to Holly Lucille, N.D., R.N., a naturopathic physician in West Hollywood, Calif., you also need to detox your liver while you're on an antidepressant. She recommends taking 200 milligrams of milk thistle, standardized to contain 80% of Silymarin, daily. **TRY:** Enzymatic Therapy Super Milk Thistle ($21 for 60 capsules; enzymatictherapy.com).

our bodies," Sagan says. "Meditation can help us become less reactive and more observant of our emotions and stressors so we're not as prone to depression and anxiety as a result." Studies have found that regular meditation can be just as effective as SSRIs in preventing a relapse of depression. (See "Meditation," page 325.)

DEAL WITH YOUR ISSUES

For some people, antidepressants may diminish the ability to feel emotions and don't address what may have triggered the depression in the first place. It's often clear when a life event like losing your job is the cause, but Sagan says that a trauma from childhood can affect how you cope with stressful situations later in life and could predispose you to depression. She advises working through past traumatic events via talk therapy and similar approaches. Many studies have shown that cognitive behavioral therapy—learning to "reframe" negative thought patterns and reactions—is more effective than drugs in easing depression symptoms and reducing relapse.

DIABETES

THERE'S A DIABETES OUTBREAK HAPPENING, right now, as you read this—and you may have the disease without even knowing it. The stats are an American Horror Story: Nearly 26 million of you have been diagnosed with the lifelong condition, more than 8% of our population, as of 2013. Cases soar yearly, striking more kids every day. It's the seventh leading cause of death in the U.S., and any year now, it may be the sixth. Or the fifth. There is no cure.

The uptick can partially be blamed on our genetics, or possibly some unknown virus: Five to 10% of those affected have type 1 diabetes, an autoimmune disorder that usually strikes in childhood or early adulthood; in these cases, the pancreas produces no insulin, a hormone needed to break down glucose (sugar) in the blood. Type 1 cannot be prevented and may be caused by a virus.

Type 2 is more common—and may be our fault. Those with type 2 diabetes either do not produce enough insulin or their body cannot effectively use what it does produce. Throw in a bad diet, full of carbs and sugar, and the symptoms worsen. More than 11% of Americans older than age 20 have been diagnosed with type 2; and after age 60, the figure jumps to 27%, according to the American Diabetes Association (ADA).

Alarmingly, many people with type 2 diabetes don't even know they have it—7 million are undiagnosed—and going without treatment poses risks for serious health complications, including heart and kidney disease, circulatory problems, nerve damage and blindness. And take a Big Gulp—or don't: According to ADA statistics, an additional 79 million Americans are pre-diabetic, meaning their blood sugar levels are elevated but not enough for a diagnosis—yet.

These statistics go hand-in-hand with the rising numbers of overweight and obese Americans, although you don't have to be overweight to develop the disease. This affects the young, especially: The medical profession has abandoned the term "adult-onset diabetes" when referring to type 2, because rates are rising worryingly among teenagers and even elementary school children. It's one reason why governments are introducing new legislation against sugars, like former Mayor Michael Bloomberg's failed attack on supersized sodas in New York City. Diabetes isn't just a large problem—it's a *large* problem.

And solving it will require a big change to the way we live, starting with a more natural way of life.

SYMPTOMS

Frequent urination, exhaustion, extreme thirst, weight loss—or, in some cases, for type 2, there are no noticeable symptoms, partly because it comes on gradually. Things get messier when both types are left untreated: Extra glucose can damage your organs, nerves, basically anything internal, leading to heart disease and stroke, retina damage and blindness, kidney disease, foot ulcers and sexual dysfunction, and amputation, with an increased risk of miscarriage for pregnant women.

REMEDIES
The anti-diabetes lifestyle

The sweet news is that natural solutions can help you both avoid type 2 diabetes and manage either type of the illness if you develop it. What you eat (and don't) and how much (or little) you exercise can have a profound effect on your blood sugar levels and your need for medication. They can also reduce your risk for developing type 2 diabetes.

Here are the most effective strategies, from the world's leading integrative experts:

LOOK BEYOND CONTROLLING CARBS

The American Diabetes Association has released dietary guidelines, which are largely based on restricting calories and controlling blood glucose levels by altering the quantity and type of carbohydrates eaten. But new research shows eating a low-fat vegan diet has proven more effective at lowering blood sugar and body weight.

"The old idea was that carbohydrates were the problem," says Neal D. Barnard, M.D., author of *Dr. Neal Barnard's Program for Reversing Diabetes,* which is based on a study he published in *Diabetes Care.* It was found to be three times more effective than the ADA's guidelines. "The new view is that microscopic droplets of fat build up in the cells and interfere with their ability to respond to insulin. It's like chewing gum in a lock." Taking animal fats out of your diet and keeping vegetable oils low enable cells to get rid of that fat and allow the uptake of insulin.

The ADA's and Barnard's regimens include a variety of different colored, whole vegetables and fruits, rather than refined grains and legumes. These all provide fiber, which helps lower blood sugar. A vegetarian regimen that includes dairy products and eggs can also help with weight control and reduce your risk for type 2 diabetes.

BOIL, DON'T BROIL

If you're too chicken to go vegan or vegetarian, at least cook differently: Some methods of cooking protein are healthier than others for diabetics, according to Steven V. Joyal, M.D., vice president for scientific affairs and medical development at the Life Extension Foundation. He advocates against preparing high-protein and high-fat foods, such as meat, at temperatures higher than 250° F and using the dry methods of frying, broiling, grilling and roasting.

"Any time you brown a food, the sugars in it bind to proteins and a chemical phenomenon called 'glycation' occurs," Joyal explains. This impacts glucose control and is a key factor in the complications associated with diabetes. Instead, cook with liquids and by what Joyal calls "low and slow" methods: boiling, steaming, braising, stewing and poaching.

GET PHYSICAL

It's long been acknowledged that exercise helps regulate blood sugar. However, if you are overweight or suffering the complications of diabetes, a regimen of regular cardio and strength training may be daunting. Try tai chi, the Chinese tradition of meditative physical exercise: A study published in the *British Journal of Sports Medicine* in April

How to Never Get Diabetes

Seven strategies can help reduce your risk for developing type 2:

1. **Lose weight:** We cannot be clearer on this: One of the main risk factors is being overweight or obese, especially if you carry fat around your waist.

2. **Break a sweat:** The Diabetes Prevention Program has shown that 30 minutes of exercise—the kind that raises your heart rate and causes you to perspire a little—five times a week helps prevent or delay type 2 diabetes.

3. **Drink (coffee) to your health:** French researchers discovered that women who drank three or more cups of coffee a day (caffeinated or decaf) had a 27% reduced risk for type 2 diabetes.

4. **Learn to love cinnamon:** A half-teaspoon of this spice daily has been shown in studies to increase glucose metabolism.

5. **Get your vitamin z's:** People who experience insomnia for a year or those who routinely sleep five or fewer hours a night are at increased risk for developing type 2 diabetes, according to research done at Penn State College of Medicine.

6. **Ditch the white rice:** Harvard School of Public Health researchers found that eating five or more servings a week of white rice can increase your risk for type 2 diabetes by 17%, while eating two or more servings of brown rice weekly reduces risk by 11%. Replacing white rice with any other type of whole grain will also work.

7. **Watch your mouth:** Periodontal (gum) disease can cause inflammation in the body, which in turn reduces insulin sensitivity and makes managing glucose levels more difficult. Studies have shown that toothpastes and mouthwashes with bee propolis may reduce plaque formation, bacteria and gum inflammation.

TRY: Nature's Goodness Mouthwash ($9; globalherbalsupplies.com) and Tom's of Maine Fluoride-Free Propolis and Myrrh Toothpaste ($5; tomsofmaine.com). Avoid either if you're allergic to bee stings.

2008 found that tai chi exercises improved blood glucose levels and improved the control of type 2 diabetes and immune system response after 12 weeks of practice. (See "Tai Chi" on page 275.)

Diabetes busters:
The top 6 supplements

Whether you're pre-diabetic or already have type 1 or type 2 diabetes, a variety of herbs, vitamins, minerals and other natural remedies may help you get your blood sugar into the healthy range, especially when used in conjunction with prescription medication. But warning: Taking certain supplements "can alter your insulin levels or sensitivity," says Catherine Ulbricht, Pharm.D., cofounder of the Natural Standard Research Collaboration and a senior attending pharmacist at Massachusetts General Hospital.

As a result, she stresses, if you're taking medication for diabetes, "You must cooperate with your health care provider to see if you need any dosing adjustments." For example, you can end up with low blood sugar, which is also unhealthy, Ulbricht cautions. Bottom line: Never cut down on or go off your prescription drugs or add an herb or supplement to your regimen without medical supervision.

ALPHA-LIPOIC ACID

This is a powerful antioxidant produced in the body. "Many studies have shown alpha-lipoic acid can improve blood sugar levels in type 2 diabetics," Ulbricht says. It may also help with many of the side effects: nerve pain, kidney damage and slow wound healing.

DOSAGE: 600 to 1,800 milligrams a day

TRY: GNC Alpha-lipoic Acid 300 ($15 for sixty 300-milligram capsules; gnc.com)

GYMNEMA

This herb has been used in ayurvedic medicine for 2,000 years as a treatment for high blood sugar. Gymnema has been shown in studies to help manage blood sugar levels "when used as an adjunct to drug therapy," says Ulbricht. Also, if your goal is prevention, it has the effect of lessening your taste for sweets and helping promote weight loss.

DOSAGE: 200 milligrams twice a day

TRY: Nature's Way Gymnema ($12 for sixty 250-milligram capsules; drugstore.com)

CHROMIUM

Chromium deficiency can lead to high blood sugar, and many people don't get the recommended 50 micrograms a day from food. Some studies have shown that supplementing with higher doses can support healthy glucose and insulin levels, and a 2008 study found that while most forms of chromium improve insulin sensitivity, niacin-bound chromium (Cr-N) provides significantly more heart health benefits.

DOSAGE: 200 to 1,000 micrograms daily.

TRY: Puritan's Pride GTF Chromium ($6 for three bottles of one hundred 200-microgram tablets at puritan.com)

MAGNESIUM

Diabetics are often deficient in this mineral. Several large studies have shown that taking magnesium significantly improves insulin sensitivity and blood glucose control. The preferred form is magnesium citrate, says a 2013 report from the NIH Office of Dietary Supplements.

DOSAGE: 160 milligrams three times a day

TRY: Nutricology Magnesium Citrate ($8 for ninety 170-milligram capsules; organicpharmacy.org)

VITAMIN D

The "sunshine vitamin" is associated with blood glucose control, and people with diabetes are often deficient in it. Data from the long-term Nurses' Health Study showed that people with a daily intake of more than 1,200 milligrams of calcium and 800 IU of vitamin D reduced their diabetes risk by 33%.

TRY: Wellesse Calcium and Vitamin D3 Liquid ($17 for two 33.8-fluid-ounce bottles with 1,000 milligrams calcium and 1,000 IU vitamin D3; costco.com)

How can I ease my eczema?

Soothe the extreme itching and irritation of this unsightly inflammatory skin condition with oatmeal wash and omega-3s.

A dermatologist says:

Marked by itchy, swollen, abnormally dry skin, eczema is thought to result from malfunctioning of the immune system and an overactive inflammatory response to irritants. In most cases, symptoms flare up for a period of time, then improve or clear up completely. A number of factors (including stress and exposure to irritating substances) can lead to flare-ups. In addition, bacterial infections (such as strep throat and staph skin infections) can stimulate an immune reaction that may cause eczema to flare up. While eczema most often appears on the inside of the knees and elbows and on the neck, hands and feet, it may affect other areas during flare-ups.

TREATMENT: For the most part, making everyday lifestyle changes is the key to controlling eczema. First, stop washing with soap that contains harsh detergents—it strips away natural oils, dries out your skin and triggers inflammation. You should use soap on areas that carry odor (e.g., your underarms and genitals), but a moisturizing body wash made with soothing ingredients like oatmeal is best for the rest of your body. Hot water can also irritate your skin, so shorten your shower to five minutes and bathe in lukewarm water only. If you're dealing with a flare-up that's making you itch constantly and causing your skin to bleed, getting a topical medicine from your doctor is probably necessary.

For more help in preventing flare-ups, manage your stress with relaxation techniques (such as yoga and meditation) and stave off infections by washing your hands frequently, eating healthy and getting plenty of sleep.

—Lily Talakoub, M.D.,
integrative dermatologist at McLean Dermatology and Skincare Center in McLean, Va.

A dietitian says:

Certain foods can aggravate eczema, while others help fight flare-ups. You can also use your diet to suppress the chronic skin inflammation thought to play a key role in the swelling and irritation associated with eczema. (Typically, the immune system releases inflammatory chemicals to fight off bacteria, toxins and other harmful substances. Chronic inflammation, on the other hand, occurs when the immune system sets off an inflammatory response even when there are no foreign substances to attack.)

TREATMENT: In many cases, intolerance to dairy, coffee, soy, eggs, nuts, wheat and/or corn can contribute to eczema. To figure out whether a food intolerance is at the heart of your condition, try eliminating all of these foods from your diet for two weeks. Next, add the foods back in (one at a time, allowing at least three days before you reintroduce a new food) and see how your skin reacts. If you seem sensitive to a particular item, consider cutting that food out of your diet.

Boosting your intake of foods high in omega-3 fatty acids (including flaxseed and oily fish, such as salmon and sardines) can help tame eczema by curbing inflammation. And there's some evidence that low levels of beta-carotene may be linked to eczema, so make sure to load up on foods like yams, carrots, kale and mango.

—Sharon Richter, R.D.,
New York City-based dietitian

A *skin-care specialist says:*

In people with eczema, the skin has a weakened ability to recover from the loss of oil content that often results from overwashing or harsh environmental conditions. So to protect against the itchiness and irritation that occurs when the skin dries out, it's important to keep your skin hydrated at all times. Because synthetic chemicals tend to irritate the skin as well, you should also strive to select skin-care products made with pure ingredients.

TREATMENT: Soaking for 15 minutes in a warm bath enriched with two cups of sea salt can greatly benefit your skin when you're dealing with a flare-up. Sea salt helps remove dead cells from your skin's surface, which allows moisture to reach new cells more easily and rehydrate your skin.

As soon as you step out of the tub, apply an oil or cream to lock in moisture. A great choice is unrefined olive oil, because it's rich in vitamin E (a nutrient that nourishes the skin). Or try a product that's 99% pure aloe vera (a powerful anti-inflammatory), or a cream made with calendula (an herb that speeds up healing and strengthens the skin's connective tissue).

—Laura Hittleman,
director for beauty services at Canyon Ranch Resort & Spa in Tucson, Ariz.

FIBROMYALGIA

Fibromyalgia sufferers are often accused of hypochondria. Even they'd admit their symptoms are a bit over the top: sinus infection, irritable bowel, constant lower-back pain, fitful sleep, momentary memory problems ("fibro fog"), *C. difficile* (a gut infection typically reserved for the elderly)—not to mention pain or soreness, often after a bout of atypical physical exertion. All those things? Sometimes all at once? Is this a real thing?

Some doctors say no. The offices of the Fibromyalgia and Fatigue Center in King of Prussia, Pa., are typically packed with patients, many of whom have seen dozens of general practitioners and specialists, begging for an explanation or just to be believed. (It may not help that the most famous fibromyalgia sufferer is Sinead O'Connor—a talented singer, but one known for erratic behavior.)

The majority of patients have been dealing with their symptoms for at least a couple of years, some as long as 30 or 35 years, says Andre Garabédian, M.D., formerly the center's national assistant medical director, now president of Garabédian Medical Clinic. Most have seen many physicians and have been told there was nothing wrong with them.

The reasons are complex, Garabédian says. First, doctors want to rule out serious diseases, including diabetes, autoimmune disorders like lupus or multiple sclerosis, and rheumatologic conditions, such as Raynauds disease. Also, reliable fibro research, although accelerating, is relatively new, and little of what has been published has filtered down to the medical community, Garabédian says. Based on what most traditional physicians study in medical school, they have no idea what they are dealing with.

Recent studies are starting to prove it's the real deal, including one reported by the National Sleep Foundation that cited medical studies showing that it is estimated to affect between 2% and 6% of people worldwide.

But there's still a stigma, possibly because most of those affected by fibromyalgia are women, according to the American College of Rheumatology. "You have a disease of [mainly] women who have tests that are technically normal," says Jacob Teitelbaum, M.D., medical director of the national Fibromyalgia and Fatigue Centers and author of *From Fatigued to Fantastic!*, who himself overcame fibromyalgia. "Doctors say, 'I don't know what's wrong with you, so you must be crazy.' There's clearly a sexist component to it."

World of misdiagnoses

The lack of a reliable test also holds back fibro diagnoses. Fibromyalgia is diagnosed based on a host of symptoms and a physical examination to determine whether a patient is suffering from tender points, specific places on the body that are sensitive to touch. One of the major problems is that there are no biological markers or tests that

A Weighty Issue

Because chronic pain causes many fibromyalgia patients to curb their activity, gaining weight is a widespread result. In fact, obesity is common and appears to adversely impact fibromyalgia's severity, according to a study recently published in the *Journal of Pain*. In 2012, researchers at the University of Utah in Salt Lake City found that 47% of 215 fibro patients studied were obese and another 30% were overweight. The obese patients reported the greatest pain sensitivity to tender-point exams, decreased physical strength and lower-body flexibility, shorter sleep duration and more restlessness during sleep.

Brain chemistry may also be a contributor, says Andre Garabédian, M.D. Fibromyalgia patients may not produce enough feel-good brain chemicals known as endorphins, which play an important role in feelings of hunger and fullness. "This causes some sufferers to gain weight much faster and makes it even more important for them to pay attention to their diets and caloric intake."

confirm the diagnosis and say, This is definitely fibromyalgia, Garabédian explains.

These obstacles typically result in patients being sent home with a misdiagnosis of depression and/or a referral to a specialist, such as a neurologist, rheumatologist, orthopedist or endocrinologist, Garabédian says. "Over 90% of my patients have been told that while they may have pain, there's nothing wrong with them or they're depressed," he says. Some have already been given multiple antidepressants.

Seeking solutions in the brain

Garabédian tests his patients' levels of serotonin—one of the essential feel-good neurotransmitters, or brain chemicals—as he believes the root of the problem resides not in the muscles, tendons, joints or other soft tissues but in a segment of the brain called the hypothalamus. "The hypothalamus controls serotonin production," he explains. "It's the main regulator of hormones, sleep, mood, pain sensation and stress management."

He believes that as a result of this lack of serotonin, many fibromyalgia patients develop emotional issues, including obsessive-compulsive disorder, panic disorder, depression and chronic anxiety. "This is why traditional doctors give them selective serotonin reuptake inhibitors [SSRIs]," Garabédian says. Contrary to popular belief, however, these antidepressant medications do not make serotonin. They try to concentrate what serotonin you already have, he explains. "But because most fibro sufferers have very low or nondetectable levels, this usually results in poor response to these medications."

Fibromyalgia patients' adrenal glands also produce less cortisol in response to stress than do healthy people, due to overutilization and resulting adrenal exhaustion, Garabédian adds, pointing out that despite this hormone's negative reputation, small amounts are beneficial because it helps people better cope with stress.

REMEDIES

While treatment differs from patient to patient, a typical Fibromyalgia and Fatigue Center plan involves more than just one strategy.

For example, Garabédian uses nutraceuticals, foods or components of foods or plants that help prevent and treat disease. However, he says, sometimes you need to add prescription drugs or other products to enhance the immune system and increase energy levels. Garabédian says that 85% to 92% of his patients see significant improvement, although it takes an average of six months or longer.

Conventional drugs

A relatively new drug called Lyrica, a medication that has been used to treat the pain from shingles and diabetic nerve pain and spinal cord injuries has shown promise. Garabédian says the good news is not so much that Lyrica is an effective treatment for fibro (although 35% to 40% of patients who take it have an improved pain tolerance, he says) but rather because its presence in the market is helping to provide legitimacy and resources to a syndrome and a community of patients who need them.

SHINE ON

Teitelbaum calls his treatment protocol SHINE, which stands for sleep, hormones, infections, nutritional supplements and exercise. Getting eight to nine hours a night of restorative sleep is recommended. To address the "H," he typically prescribes natural thyroid and adrenal supplements.

Skills, Not Pills

New federally funded research is investigating the effectiveness of teaching fibromyalgia patients strategies to improve their emotional states and ability to manage stress. These include learning how to be cognizant of and then "reframe" negative, self-defeating thoughts. "With fibromyalgia, the brain pathways involved with experiencing pain are overly sensitive," says study leader Mark Lumley, Ph.D., a psychology professor at Wayne State University in Detroit. "The brain is registering pain louder and stronger than it should. Many physicians suggest antidepressants or sleep medication, but we are studying the benefits of skills rather than pills through cognitive behavioral approaches."

TRY: End Fatigue Adrenal Stress-End ($17 for 50 capsules; endfatigue.com) and End Fatigue DHEA 5 milligrams ($5 for 60 capsules; endfatigue.com), as well as ovarian and testicular hormones. (Optimizing thyroid hormone is especially important during pregnancy.)

The "I" might be of particular concern because irritable bowel, sinusitis and *C. difficile* all seem to fall under the category of infection. While the immune system dysfunction associated with fibromyalgia is partly to blame, Teitelbaum says an overgrowth of a strain of yeast called candida is also a significant problem.

To eliminate candida and restore the healthy balance in the gut, Teitelbaum recommends a high-quality probiotic.

TRY: Enzymatic Therapy's Probiotic Pearls ($17 for 30 capsules; emersonecologics.com), or the herbal antifungal mix Anti-Yeast from Nutri Elements ($54 for 120 capsules; endfatigue.com). After a month on a probiotic, add the generic version of the prescription antifungal medication Diflucan (neither this nor the Anti-Yeast should be used during pregnancy). Cutting out most sugar except for dark chocolate is also helpful because sugar feeds yeast; he suggests substituting with Stevia, a natural sweetener.

As for nutritional supplements, both he and Garabédian recommend magnesium and fish oil, which not only decrease fibromyalgia symptoms but also are very important during pregnancy. Both doctors also recommend that patients exercise as much as they comfortably can. "People with fibro often become inactive because of the pain, which

CFS? What's the Diff?

Seabiscuit and *Unbroken* author Laura Hillenbrand has written best sellers about racehorses and track stars—ironic, because she remains mostly confined to her home, with chronic fatigue syndrome (CFS). It's a close cousin of fibromyalgia but they are separate disorders. CFS is characterized by debilitating fatigue and recurrent flulike symptoms, such as muscle and joint aches, sore throat, swollen glands and difficulty thinking. Fibromyalgia is characterized by widespread muscle pain. Yet many experts consider them the same disease. Confused? Your doctor may be also, so new are these disorders.

adds to their deconditioning, pain and stiffness," Teitelbaum says. "It's a vicious cycle."

EXERCISE

Several recent studies have shown that gentle exercise is very effective for reducing fibromyalgia pain. Preliminary findings in the *International Journal of Yoga Therapy* found that participants who did yoga and meditated for an eight-week period saw significant improvement in their overall health and in symptoms of stiffness, anxiety and depression, as well as in the reported number of days they "felt good" and the number of days they "missed work" because of fibromyalgia. A 2012 paper published in *Arthritis Research & Therapy* showed that qigong had similar effects for 100 participants.

ACUPUNCTURE

Acupuncture is another legitimate approach. According to a Mayo Clinic study, patients who got acupuncture for fibromyalgia reported significant improvement in symptoms, especially fatigue and anxiety. The placebo-controlled study gave patients six treatments over a two- to three-week period (half got "true" acupuncture, half got fake treatments), then were questioned about their symptoms immediately after treatment, one month later, then again seven months later. After one month, the patients who got the "true" acupuncture reported significantly less fatigue and anxiety. And a 2011 study showed that acupuncture done on the 18 "tender spots" of fibromyalgia (used for diagnosis) reduced pain over a two-month course of treatment.

The Road Ahead

Pregnancy can be another confounding factor: The hormone fluctuations during pregnancy can cause fibro patients to drastically improve or worsen.

During pregnancy the placenta makes high levels of corticotropin-releasing hormone, which supports the adrenal glands and increases blood volume. That's why people [often] feel pretty good then, Garabédian says. But after pregnancy the hormone levels drop and you start to crash, he says. "The good news is that with proper support, you're not going to crash."

GERD

Heartburn. We've all had it, and if we're lucky, it's mild and occasional, the obvious result of that spicy meatball sandwich on Super Bowl Sunday, or too much pad Thai with the girls. But for more than 8% of Americans, heartburn is a searingly painful and sometimes daily occurrence, and the numbers are growing rapidly: Some studies estimate heartburn and its underlying causes are up by 50% from a decade ago. And now doctors are categorizing frequent heartburn that doesn't respond to nonprescription medications as a symptom of something more serious, called GERD, or gastroesophageal reflux disease. And GERD is on the rise.

SYMPTOMS

Heartburn that occurs at least twice a week is the primary symptom of GERD. It happens when the lower esophageal sphincter (LES), a ring-shaped valve between the esophagus and stomach, becomes lax, allowing highly acidic stomach contents to back up into the esophagus. The esophagus doesn't have the same acid-resistant lining as the stomach. Burn, meet "heart."

Surprisingly, you can have GERD without experiencing heartburn. Some people simply aren't sensitive to the presence of acid in the esophagus. As a result they can unknowingly develop damage there, which in turn can cause esophageal cancer. Other symptoms that can indicate GERD are bad breath, a chronic dry cough, hoarse or raspy voice, lump-in-the-throat sensation and asthma.

Heartburn and GERD cases have risen sharply in recent years; a Norwegian study reported in 2011 places the rise at nearly 50% in the last decade alone. While better diagnostics may be partially responsible, our, how shall we put this gently, "21st-century way of eating" undoubtedly has a lot to do with why so many of us are suffering.

"The higher incidence of obesity in our society is one of the major causes," says Victor S. Sierpina, M.D., a professor of family and integrative medicine at the University of Texas Medical Branch in Galveston and author of *The Healthy Gut Workbook*. As we put on weight, he explains, we develop increased pressure in the abdomen, making reflux more likely. Research shows that obese people are more than twice as likely to have a defective LES and suffer from more frequent and more severe GERD than the general population.

Cuisines like Indian, Thai and Mexican have become dietary favorites, and spicy as well as high-fat foods often trigger heartburn. Over-scheduled, we grab "meals" on the run, often relying on fatty fast food. We're an aging population as well, and heartburn increases with age. But even young people are affected, due at least in part to the rise in eating disorders. "People who induce vomiting, or have in the past, can have an increased risk of heartburn," says Jacqueline L. Wolf, M.D., an associate professor of medicine at Harvard Medical School.

REMEDIES

Americans spend more than $13 billion a year on prescription drugs for this condition, and more than $3 billion on over-the-counter heartburn remedies. (Hence all those ads for tu-tu-tu-Tums.) It's not just a spicy meatball, it's an expensive one. While it's tempting to resort to acid-blocking medications, they're not for long-term use and they can pose serious risks (see "The Downsides of Drugs" on page 117). Before asking your doctor for a prescription or picking something off the drugstore shelf, try these lifestyle changes and natural remedies that can help you avoid GERD in the first place.

Deceptive Symptoms

Heartburn symptoms may actually be due to esophagitis, an inflammation of the esophagus that can be caused by factors besides acid reflux, including allergies, infections or such osteoporosis medications as Fosamax or Actonel. These conditions generally won't respond to antacid remedies; you'll need to see your health care provider for an accurate diagnosis and treatment.

FIGURE OUT WHAT LIGHTS YOUR FIRE

A number of foods commonly trigger GERD. Some work by increasing stomach acid secretion, others by releasing chemicals that relax the LES. Identifying your triggers is crucial. "If you go out for a few drinks and Mexican food every Friday night and you then get heartburn—hello!" says Sierpina. When the triggers aren't so clear, try the following:

GO ON AN ELIMINATION DIET

Start by cutting out fatty and spicy foods, coffee, carbonated drinks, alcohol, chocolate, peppermint, citrus fruits, onions, garlic, tomatoes and tomato-based products. Reintroduce them one by one until you find the culprit.

LOG WHAT YOU PUT IN YOUR MOUTH

If none of the items listed above is the source of your symptoms, keep a diary of everything you ingest to identify what you should avoid. You might find it's not even food but your migraine, osteoporosis or heart medication.

ESPRESSO YOURSELF

Coffee is a frequent culprit, but if you can't stand to give it up, there's good news: Scientists in Europe recently discovered that a chemical generated by dark-roasted coffee beans reduces acid production in the stomach. So counterintuitively, drinking espresso and French and Italian roasts will be easier on you. You can also get your caffeine fix from low-acid coffees.

TRY: Gentle Java ($10 for 12 ounces; gentlejava.com) or Puroast Fair Trade Organic Low Acid Coffee ($12 for 12 ounces; puroast.com).

NIX THE CONSTANT NOSHING

How and when you eat is as important as what you eat. "We're eating food on top of food," says Carolyn Dean, M.D., N.D., *Natural Health* advisory board member and creator of the Future Health Now! Online Wellness Program. She recommends waiting four hours between meals to allow food to properly digest.

AVOID EATING AT NIGHT

Lying down with a full stomach facilitates reflux. Try to wait three or four hours after eating before going to bed.

EAT SLOWLY

Digestion, Sierpina explains, begins in the mouth. Saliva has a neutralizing effect on acid, and chewing food helps ready it for the stomach. When we bolt down our meals, large chunks of food reach the stomach in an unprepared state that's more likely to cause reflux. British Prime Minister William Gladstone famously advocated 32 chews per bite. That might seem excessive, but do make an effort to sit down, eat mindfully and chew thoroughly.

The Downsides of Drugs

If GERD persists after trying lifestyle changes and other remedies, you may need to use drugs such as Tagamet and Zantac that inhibit stomach acid. If these don't solve the problem, more-potent medications such as Prilosec and Prevacid, which completely block acid production, may be useful. While these can provide short-term relief and reduce the need for surgery in ulcer and reflux patients, the U.S. Food and Drug Administration has not approved their use for longer than eight weeks. Why? Because we vitally need our stomach acid.

"As acid is released, it triggers the release of digestive enzymes from the pancreas and bile from the liver," explains Carolyn Dean, M.D., N.D. "If you stop that mechanism with medications, it's to the detriment of your digestion." We also need stomach acid to kill bacteria that can cause food poisoning and to facilitate the absorption of certain medications, vitamin B_{12}, iron, calcium and other essential nutrients. Long-term use of acid-suppressing drugs also puts us at risk for yeast infections, colorectal cancer, anemia, food allergies and various nutritional deficiencies and may even increase heartburn symptoms and GERD. Some studies have found that women who take certain heartburn medications long-term experience bone loss in their spine and an increase in their risk for wrist fractures. It's unclear yet if this is due to calcium absorption problems or a direct effect of the medications on bones. Ladies, be vigilant about taking calcium and vitamin D supplements while on these drugs.

And a recent study published in *Cancer, Epidemiology, Biomarkers and Prevention*, the journal of the American Association for Cancer Research, indicated that prescription meds might even increase the risk of throat cancers in non-smokers.

HEART DISEASE

Ruthless. Predatory. Maniacal. If your body has a super-villian, this is it: Heart disease is the No. 1 killer of both women and men in the United States; 597,689 die every year from heart disease; 813,800 from generalized cardiovascular disease, including stroke. According to a recent *Circulation* study, less than 8% of Americans are considered to be at *low* risk for heart disease, and more than 80 million of us—one in three—have already developed heart disease in one form or another, chiefly high blood pressure and clogged arteries. Obesity, cigarette smoking, sedentary lifestyle, that seventh Cronut you just ate—all are considered risk factors. And if you have a family history? That's the Joker in your deck.

So how to fight back? Live a super-powered life.

"For 80% of us, it's how you live your life that determines whether or not your genes express themselves," says Mimi Guarneri, M.D., director of the Scripps Center for Integrative Medicine. "I've seen identical twins manifest totally different health profiles." The other 20% may need medication, she says, but can still use lifestyle measures to reduce the amount they need.

SYMPTOMS

If you can *feel* your heart beating in a funny way, or have shortness of breath, weakness or sweating, those may be signs of coronary artery disease or arrhythmia, an abnormal hearth rhythm. A heart attack is more familiar (unfortunately): pressure or pain in the chest, a choking feeling, anxiety, difficulty breathing and pain radiating into the back.

REMEDIES

Doctors often suggest that if you do have a family history, you should start taking meds as a preventive measure, as young as your mid-40s, especially if your cholesterol and/or blood pressure numbers are creeping up. Statins, prescription meds that lower cholesterol, are the most prescribed medication in the country.

See the "High Cholesterol" section on page 133 for our take on those "wonder drugs." But long story short, for many people with heart disease risk factors, cholesterol-lowering medications aren't necessarily a cure-all, and may, in fact, be detrimental to overall health, says integrative physician Mark Hyman, M.D., author of the functional-medicine bible *The Ultramind Solution.*

"Doctors are overprescribing medications with the idea that lowering the numbers will lower risk, but that's not the case," Hyman explains. "It has resulted in a generation of Americans who think they can take the pills and do whatever they want and everything will be fine—but if you look at the data carefully, the drugs we're using really aren't that helpful. You can't prevent or treat heart disease without addressing the real causes: poor diet, stress, environmental toxins and a sedentary lifestyle."

The basics are pretty simple: Stop smoking, eat a diet low in saturated and trans fats and simple sugars; don't overdo alcohol; exercise. Beyond that, consider these recommendations from heart-health professionals:

Know Your Numbers

Keeping an eye on your cholesterol can help you troubleshoot cardiovascular problems by showing you what might be out of balance, says women's heart-health expert Tracy Stevens, M.D. Here's Stevens' breakdown of what is generally considered healthy:

Total cholesterol: <190

HDL ("good") cholesterol: >40 for men; >55 for women

LDL (bad) cholesterol: <100 (70 if you have a history of arterial plaque or are diabetic)

Triglycerides: <150

See also "High cholesterol" section on page 133

TREAT TRIGLYCERIDES

These harmful blood fats might be the most dangerous form of cholesterol because they are inflammatory, explains Tracy Stevens, M.D., a cardiologist at St. Luke's Mid America Heart and Vascular Institute in Kansas City, Mo. (See "Know Your Numbers," at right.) She recommends keeping them under control with powerful natural anti-inflammatories: 2,000 IU of vitamin D3, at least 81 milligrams of aspirin and 2,000 milligrams of omega-3 fatty acids daily.

DETOX

Environmental toxins have a profound impact on heart health, Hyman says: "I've seen diabetes cured and heart disease reversed when a patient does a detox." You can do a structured program, or simply eat an organic, plant-based diet, dump your chemical-based household cleaners and otherwise clean up your immediate environment (for more on detoxing, go to naturalhealthmag.com/detox). Even better, take a daily sauna if you can. "Saunas are a great way to sweat out toxins, especially pesticides," Hyman says.

STRESS LESS

"When you get stressed out, a cascade of hormones are released," Guarneri says. The most well known are adrenaline, which can cause skipped heartbeats and raise blood pressure; cortisol, which leads to putting on unhealthy belly fat and suppresses immunity; and aldosterone, which causes the body to hold on to water, raising blood pressure.

Stop the madness by adopting a regular stress-reduction routine. "Try yoga, tai chi, walking or practicing affirmation or prayer," Guarneri suggests. A 2012 study published in the journal *Circulation* found that mantra-based meditation practice was associated with a 43% decrease in heart attacks and strokes among African-Americans.

WHITTLE YOUR MIDDLE

You've heard it before, Slim: More important than how much extra weight you're carrying is where that weight is located. "We have become a nation of egg-shaped people," says Stevens. "Our real health crisis is a crisis of the waistline." Weight gain around the abdomen is associated with metabolic syndrome, a disease process characterized by elevated blood pressure, reduced insulin sensitivity, lower HDL (the "good") cholesterol and higher triglycerides. The treatment is pretty simple, says Stevens: "Focus on your waistline. If you're a woman, keep it under 35 inches; if you're a man, under 40. It's the single most powerful step you can take in reducing your risk for heart disease."

SHAKE THE SALT HABIT

By the end of our lives, 90% of Americans will have developed high blood pressure, or hypertension. Excess sodium (salt) may be the culprit, or at least a contributing factor, and 77% of American salt intake comes from restaurant and processed foods.

"Aim to get less than 2,300 milligrams of sodium per day; 1,500 milligrams if you already have high blood pressure, are older than 40 or are African-American," says nutritionist Jeannie Gazzaniga-Moloo, Ph.D., R.D., a spokeswoman for the American Dietetic Association. Look for canned goods with no more than 150 milligrams and entrées with fewer than 400 milligrams per serving. Better yet, she says, shop for foods that don't have labels at all: Fresh fruits, vegetables and lean meats are naturally low in that evil NaCl.

MOVE YOUR BODY

Aerobic activity is good for your heart? Oh, that's why they call it "cardiovascular exercise." "Aim to get at least three and a half hours a week of aerobic exercise, and add weight training two or three times a week to help keep your metabolism high," suggests says Tori Hudson, N.D., medical director of the Women's Institute of Health and Integrative Medicine and adjunct clinical professor of naturopathic medicine at Bastyr University in Washington.

TURN THAT FROWN UPSIDE DOWN

A 2010 study is the first to show what's long been suspected: A positive attitude has tangible heart benefits. Among the 1,700-plus men and women who participated in a 10-year Columbia University study, those who demonstrated positive emotions had a 22% lower risk of heart disease. Unhappy patients' risks, on the other hand, were 22% higher.

"Happiness should be behind every healthy change you make," says internist Dean Ornish, M.D., founder and president of the nonprofit Preventative Medicine Research Institute in Sausalito, Calif., and author of the game-changing *Dr. Dean Ornish's Program for Reversing Heart Disease.* "In our studies, we found that joy of living is a much more sustainable motivator [to make lifestyle changes] than fear of dying," he explains. "When people make the comprehensive lifestyle changes I recommend, genes that prevent heart disease are 'turned on,' and those that promote it are 'turned off.' Our genes are a predisposition, but they are not our fate."

HEART DISEASE and EMOTIONS

You already know that heart disease remains the leading killer of women and men in the United States—and how does that make you feel? Sad? Angry? Well, for the good of your heart, you might want to just chill out. A growing body of research suggests our mental and cardio-vascular health are intrinsically linked. "We know that anger, depression and even loneliness release stress hormones like adrenaline and cortisol," says Guarneri. "Those stress hormones—both acute and chronic—raise blood pressure and cholesterol, constrict arteries and cause arrhythmia (irregular heartbeat)."

Another stress hormone, cortisol, also contributes to abdominal obesity and type 2 diabetes—both well documented risk factors for heart disease. And, of course, most Americans are all too familiar with the real-ity of emotional eating, not to mention excessive drinking, smoking and physical inactivity, all of which up the risks as well.

Yet these factors are all entirely within your control. "Eighty per-cent of illness is related to lifestyle and environment," says Guarneri. Translation: Genetics are just a small fraction of the equation. If you make healthier choices every day—like the options that follow—you can dramatically alter your outlook and your health. So put your mind to it, and let the healing begin

HEART HAZARD: Anger

The medicine you need may be best served in a glass half full: Healthy women who scored high on a cynical hostility test had higher rates of coronary heart disease (CHD) and mortality than women who tested high for optimism, according to a 2009 study published in the journal *Circulation.* Another study from Johns Hopkins University in Baltimore found something similar: that medical students who became angry quickly when under stress were three times more likely to develop premature heart disease and five times more likely than their calmer col-leagues to have an early heart attack.

Do Hormones Help or Hurt?

If you're a woman approaching menopause, hot flashes are the least of your worries: You can bet your heart health is about to take a turn for the worse. "As estrogen begins to drop, arteries become inelastic, bad cholesterol and inflammatory markers go up, and good cholesterol goes down," says Tori Hudson, N.D., founder of A Woman's Time health clinic in Portland, Ore. "Plus, now we are gaining weight."

So should women consider hormone replacement therapy? The official word is... there is no official word. "As cardiologists, we aren't saying hormones definitely help heart health, but we're also not telling women to avoid them, either," says Tracy Stevens, M.D., a spokeswoman for WomenHeart: The Natural Coalition for Women with Heart Disease.

The Women's Health Initiative hormone study of the 1990s left many women (and their doctors) skittish about hormone replacement therapy. But it's important to note that the population studied was older women well past menopause who took hormones in relatively high doses—plus it was ages ago. Newer research indicates that if there's going to be a positive influence of estrogen therapy on heart health, it may be during perimenopause or the first few years of menopause.

"The current guidelines for hormone replacement therapy are to treat menopausal symptoms, and women should talk with their physicians about the benefits versus risks," Stevens says.

Sure, it's best to let it out rather than bottle it up, but even better is developing more resilient and less aggressive responses to stressful situations. So don't get mad—get glad, with this heart-healthy, anger-management advice:

CALM DOWN

According to a long-term study of subjects with coronary heart disease (CHD), transcendental meditation (TM), which involves allowing the mind to relax and, in essence, transcend thought, rather than attempting to focus on something specific, was associated with a 47% reduction in mortality, nonfatal myocardial infarctions (MI, aka heart attacks) and strokes. "Mindfulness-based stress reduction is good, too, but TM has the strongest evidence in the cardiology literature," Guarneri notes. If meditation is too namby-pamby, take a spa day instead. A recent study published in the *Journal of Alternative and Complementary Medicine* found that deep-tissue massage reduced blood pressure levels and heart rate.

WORK IT OUT

Meditative exercises like yoga and tai chi (see our chapters on both in "Alternative Healing" on page 247) achieve similar results to the aforementioned relaxation practices, but most types of physical activity can help your head *and* your heart—and some research suggests outdoor exercise is particularly effective for combating feelings of tension and anger.

EAT ENOUGH

Deprivation can equal extreme aggravation. According to a 2012 study published in *The Journal of Consumer Research,* people who ate apples for dietary reasons were more likely to watch movies with themes of anger and revenge than individuals who ate chocolate. That may sound like a random fact, but "Exerting self-control makes people more likely to behave aggressively toward others, and people on diets are known to be

Say NO to Sweets

Of course a diet high in saturated and trans fats, cholesterol and sodium isn't good for your heart—but research is increasingly pointing to an even bigger dietary danger: sugar. Several recent studies, including one in the April 2010 *Journal of the American Medical Association,* have found that added sweeteners in foods contribute to heart disease by lowering levels of HDL ("good") cholesterol and raising levels of triglycerides (harmful blood fats). "The body cannot metabolize fructose, which is a component of all sweeteners," notes Andrew Weil. "It deranges liver metabolism and promotes obesity, insulin resistance and inflammation." Weil's advice: "Cut back on all sweeteners, including sugar substitutes and even fruit juice, which is no different from Coca-Cola in this regard." If you can't give up sweets completely, stick to the recently revised guidelines from the AHA, which recommends that women have no more than 100 calories of added sugar daily (for men, it's 150 calories)—and remember to look out for it lurking in unexpected places, from "heart healthy" granola to gluten-free goodies to *literally* to-die-for dressings and sauces.

irritable and quick to anger," the authors said. Just pick your indulgence with your ticker in mind. "Have a piece of dark chocolate—it has emotional and heart-health benefits," says Andrew Weil, M.D., founder and director of the Arizona Center for Integrative Medicine at the University of Arizona in Tucson and author of *Spontaneous Happiness.* And don't skip meals, adds Tracy Stevens, M.D., a cardiologist at St. Luke's Mid America Heart Institute in Kansas City, Mo., and spokeswoman for the American Heart Association (AHA). When you get too hungry and your blood sugar drops, that can lead to stress and anger, as well as making poor food choices (which are frequently not good for your heart), Stevens says. One thing you *can* cut out (and please don't get angry about this): alcohol, which can contribute to high blood pressure, as well as aggressive behavior.

HEART HAZARD: Depression

Sad but true: Cardiovascular disease (CVD) makes depressive symptoms worse, and vice versa. Not only have studies found that depression is common following heart attacks and other coronary events, but in one of many examples, researchers from Washington University School of Medicine in St. Louis recently concluded that a history of major depression increases the risk for heart disease more than genetics or environment. So clear is the connection that the latest guidelines from the AHA recommend depression screening as part of an overall evaluation for CVD risk. Fortunately there are plenty of remedies that help ease depression—many of which are also key ways to boost heart health:

SEE A SPECIALIST

Research suggests that working with a mental health professional—be it a psychiatrist, psychologist or social worker—can be as effective as taking medication in easing depression. Meanwhile, a 2011 study published in the *Journal of the American Medical Association Internal Medicine* found that among people who experienced a coronary heart disease event within the previous year, those who received traditional care plus cognitive behavioral therapy (CBT) had 45% fewer recurrent heart attacks when compared with individuals who received traditional care sans CBT.

Smart Supplements

FLUSH OUT TOXINS

Mark Hyman, M.D., recommends taking a daily konjac fiber supplement, which will bind with toxins and usher them out of the body.

TRY: Physician Formulas Glucomannan capsules ($17 for ninety 500-milligram capsules; physicianformulas.com)

JUST SAY NO

An unsung player in heart health is the gas nitric oxide (NO). "Nitric oxide relaxes the blood vessels and improves blood flow to the tissues, and is especially important for people with high blood pressure and/ or a family history of heart disease," says Janet Zand, O.M.D., L.Ac. and chief technical officer for Texas-based Neogenis Labs, which researches nitric oxide. The body makes its own NO, but production tapers off as we get older, especially after age 40. Offset the loss, Zand says, by eating more NO-rich foods, which include celery, lettuce, spinach, arugula, endive, beets, leeks, parsley, fennel and cabbage. If you just can't stomach the green stuff, consider taking a nitric-oxide-boosting supplement.

TRY: Neogenis Neo40 ($60 for 30 fast-melt lozenges; neogenis.com)

CHINESE HERBS

"Many of the traditional Chinese formulas are aimed at relaxing the blood vessels," says David Scrimgeour, L.Ac., C.H., an acupuncturist based in Boulder, Colo. "Some researchers propose that what they're really doing is improving NO levels." One formula he likes for helping to lower mildly elevated blood pressure is Gou Teng San, a blend of 12 Chinese herbs; take three 500-milligram capsules three times daily. Find it through an acupuncturist or try Brion Herbs Gou Teng San Gambir formula ($15 for one hundred 500-gram capsules; maxnature.com).

MIND YOUR MAGNESIUM

If blood pressure is a problem, boost your intake of this mineral, recommends Carolyn Dean, M.D., N.D., author of *The Magnesium Miracle*. "The muscles in the walls of the arteries get tight and start to contract when they don't get enough magnesium," she explains. Magnesium also helps reduce palpitations, Dean says, and according to a 2013 review of cardiovascular studies dating back to 1937, low magnesium levels are the greatest predictor of all types cardiovascular disease. Magnesium is found in many foods, including seaweed, deep green leafy vegetables, almonds and lentils, but it's difficult to get an effective dose through food alone; Dean recommends taking 600 milligrams of magnesium citrate powder daily.

TRY: Peter Gillham's Natural Calm Drink Mix ($22 for 8 ounces; organicpharmacy.com)

GO FISH OIL

"Whatever cardiovascular mechanism you can think of, fish oil [omega-3 fatty acids] has a positive impact," says Hudson. "It lowers blood pressure and triglycerides, improves insulin sensitivity, regulates heart rhythm, and reduces clotting and inflammation." Hudson recommends taking 1,000 to 2,000 milligrams a day for prevention, and 3,000 to 4,000 milligrams if you have high triglycerides. Look for a brand that ensures purity.

TRY: Nordic Naturals Ultimate Omega ($28 for 60 softgels; nordicnaturals.com)

SIP ON SOY

Soy is a powerful medicine for getting blood fats in line, says Guarneri, who recommends two scoops of soy powder each day. "Combine daily soy supplementation with a diet low in saturated fat, and you can expect to lower your overall cholesterol by 15%, your LDL (the "bad' cholesterol) by 15%, and your triglycerides by an incredible 44%."

TRY: Metagenics UltraMeal Plus 360 ($49 for 26 ounces; healthdesigns.com)

SCORE WITH SUPPLEMENTS

Vitamin D deficiencies have been linked to Alzheimer's disease, depression and cognitive decline, as well as to heart disease—but taking supplements (600 to 4,000 IU daily for depression and 1,000 to 5,000 IU for the heart) can help considerably. Studies show that a lack of omega-3 fatty acids has similar implications for the head and the heart. "Omega-3 deficiency leads to weakened brain architecture and function and strongly correlates with depression," says Andrew Weil, M.D. "It also increases inflammation and clotting tendency of the blood, both of which increase the risk of heart disease." Weil recommends taking 2 to 4 grams a day of a product that provides both EPA and DHA, and looking for products that

 RED FLAGS: The Anatomy of a Female Heart Attack

In both men and women, the most common heart attack symptom is pain or discomfort (think pressure, squeezing or fullness) in the center of the chest—but women also experience a wide range of other symptoms, and studies have found that they are more likely than men to delay seeking treatment, leading to far worse outcomes. If you're experiencing any of the following—even in the absence of chest pain or discomfort—contact your health care provider (symptoms in blue tend to occur in the weeks leading up to an attack) or call 911 immediately (symptoms in red tend to be especially pronounced during the acute phase of an attack):

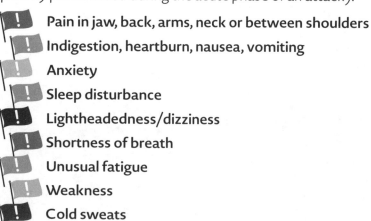

- Pain in jaw, back, arms, neck or between shoulders
- Indigestion, heartburn, nausea, vomiting
- Anxiety
- Sleep disturbance
- Lightheadedness/dizziness
- Shortness of breath
- Unusual fatigue
- Weakness
- Cold sweats

are "molecularly distilled" or otherwise guaranteed to be free of toxins. Many manufacturers—including Nordic Naturals (nordicnaturals.com) and CardioTabs (cardiotabs.com)—offer combined omega-3 and vitamin D_3 supplements.)

FEED YOUR HEAD

Another way to combat both depression and heart disease is with an anti-inflammatory diet, which places a particular emphasis on fresh fruits, vegetables, legumes and healthy fats, plus smaller amounts of whole grains and limited foods from animal sources. "Steer clear of meat and poultry as much as possible, which tend to be high in pro-inflammatory fats, and avoid processed and fast foods and sugary drinks—the fats and quick-digesting carbohydrates in them are strongly pro-inflammatory," says Weil.

BUST A MOVE

Countless studies have found that exercise alleviates symptoms of depression, and the impact of physical activity on heart health is undisputed as well. "As far as natural treatments for depression are concerned, 30 minutes of aerobic exercise five times per week is one of the most effective, and should yield results within a few weeks," notes Weil. That's about how much the AHA recommends for heart health, too. (For more suggestions, see the "Heart-Smart Workout Chart" on page 130.)

HEART HAZARD: Loneliness

The life expectancy for the lonely hearts' club is looking grim. One study of heart attack survivors found that those who scored high on tests of social isolation and stress were four times as likely to die during the three years after their attacks compared with those who had large social networks and less stress. A recent Danish study also reported that people who live alone are twice as likely to suffer from "serious heart disease" as those living with partners. Meanwhile, a survey of more than 200 people in Chicago found that blood pressure was 30 points higher among lonely people than among those who felt more connected to others. But there is hope for the Ross- and Rachel-less out there:

IMPROVE YOUR PARTNERSHIP

According to one University College London study, being unhappy with a significant other is a strong predictor of coronary events, while recent research from the University of Rochester in New York found that happily married people who underwent coronary bypass surgery were more than three times as likely to be alive 15 years later compared with their unmarried counterparts. Most forms of psychotherapy can help. "Relationships break down for all kinds of reasons, including issues of self-esteem, guilt, shame and a lack of communication," says Judith Orloff, M.D., assistant clinical professor of psychology at the University of California, Los Angeles. "Talking things through with a professional—individually or as a couple—can help partners delve into the underlying issues and work towards correcting them."

KEEP IN TOUCH

Modern technology—texting, e-mailing, social networking—is supposed to bring us closer together, but in many ways it has accomplished the opposite. "Hearing somebody's voice and laughing out loud together, not just LOL-ing from one keyboard to another, connects you in a deeper way," says Malissa Wood, M.D., codirector of the Corrigan Women's Heart Health Program at Massachusetts General Hospital in Boston. So pick up the horn or, better yet, schedule some *real* face time with friends and family members.

The Heart-Smart Workout Chart

Regular cardiovascular exercise is a crucial part of keeping your heart healthy—but it's not the *only* kind of workout that keeps your clock ticking. "There is some evidence that strength training, Pilates, tai chi and yoga all have an effect on peripheral circulation, which lowers overall blood pressure after exercise," notes Andrew Wolf, M.Ed., an exercise physiologist with Miraval Arizona Resort and Spa in Tucson, Ariz. "All forms of exercise can lower stress as well—and that will in turn reduce inflammation and improve heart health." Of course, you should make aerobic activity your primary focus (give it at least 50%, but up to 70%, of your exercise time each week, Wolf suggests), but sprinkle in these other activities liberally for a healthier, happier heart.

EXERCISE TYPE	WHY TO ♥ IT	TRAINING TIPS
Cardio/ aerobics	Helps you to maintain a healthy weight, strengthens the heart and lungs, boosts the body's ability to use oxygen, and can help lower your resting heart rate and blood pressure.	Strive for at least 150 minutes of moderate—or 75 minutes of vigorous—activities like walking, jogging, swimming or biking each week. Wolf suggests also varying the intensity and duration from one day to the next. "When you ask the heart to make some adaptations, it becomes a better pump," he explains.
Pilates	Keeps the midsection tight and toned which, when combined with cardio, helps to combat central adiposity (associated with increased risks for heart disease). Also good for improving circulation and lowering stress levels.	Can be done on the same day as cardio or on noncardio days in place of strength training. To get a great at-home workout, check out the new CoreBody Reformer by Nautilus ($279; corebodyreformer.com).
Weight training	Improves heart and lung function, enhances glucose metabolism and lowers coronary disease risk factors. Stronger muscles equal less stress on the heart, too, keeping blood pressure and resting heart rate down.	Aim for a total-body workout two to three times a week, focusing on multimuscle moves and using enough weight so that you can't do more than 12 reps per set. See *Men's Fitness* or *Shape* magazines for workout ideas.
Tai chi	Reduces stress, anxiety, depression and mood disturbance, according to research.	Try to make it a daily practice, if only for a few minutes each morning or evening. Check out *BodyWisdom Media: Tai Chi for Beginners*, featuring sequences lasting from 10 to 30 minutes.
Yoga	Helps to achieve higher heart rate variability and parasympathetic control (both signs of a healthy heart), as well as lower levels of cytokine interleukin-6 (or IL-6, part of the body's inflammatory response that's been linked to heart disease, stroke, type 2 diabetes and other chronic diseases) when done regularly, studies suggest.	Aim for a short or more meditative yoga practice on the same day as cardio and/or in place of your strength-training workout. (Go to naturalhealthmag.com for routines or see the "Yoga" section in this book.)

GET A PET

This is so true, it's nearly a cliché: Studies suggest that companion animals are beneficial for both emotional and physical health. A review of research published in 2013 by the American Heart Association stated that owning a dog was associated with a reduced risk of heart disease (Americans own 70 million of them, and 74 million cats). One study of New York City stockbrokers who were on angiotensin converting enzyme (ACE) inhibitor medication (used to treat hypertension)—and all of whom had lived alone for five years—found that those who were given a cat or dog remained significantly more stable during stressful situations than test subjects in a no-pet group. "If you have high blood pressure, a pet is very good for helping you during times of stress, and pet ownership is especially good for you if you have a limited support system," says study author Karen Allen, Ph.D., professor of medicine at the University of Buffalo in New York.

GIVE A LITTLE BIT

The reasons for social isolation often are self-inflicted. "Some evidence even suggests that susceptibility to heart attack correlates with how often people use the words 'I,' 'me' and 'mine' in casual speech," notes Weil. On the flipside, a review of studies released by the Corporation for National and Community Service found that people who volunteer have greater longevity, higher functional ability, lower rates of depression and less incidence of heart disease. The opportunities to help others are limitless; there's even a national support group for people with heart disease, Mended Hearts (mendedhearts.org), which forges connections between heart patients. "Helping others creates connections that bring you joy," says Guarneri. "When you do something for someone else and you see that you've made a difference, you never forget that. Your heart is truly full."

HIGH CHOLESTEROL

I f you've got high cholesterol, chances are your doctor has prescribed a statin, hailed as the wonder drug of the 21st century— brand names include Lipitor, Crestor and the like (you've seen the ads). The sexy little numbers slow down the production of cholesterol and increase the liver's ability to remove LDL (or "bad") cholesterol, thus reducing the chances of a blocked artery or a heart attack. About 32 million Americans take statins, says Harvard Medical School. What could go wrong?

Famous last words. Statins also come with a slew of heart-stopping side effects, including muscle pain and soreness, digestive problems, skin rashes, liver damage, type-2 diabetes—a 2013 study linked them to cataracts. One of the scariest is a rare but life-threatening muscle damage called rhabdomyolysis (so frightening, it's hard to pronounce: rab-doe-mi-OL-ih-sis), according to the Mayo Clinic. Rhabdomyolysis can cause severe muscle pain, liver damage, kidney failure and death. It can occur when you take statins in combination with certain drugs, or if you take a high dose.

In short, even if you believe the hype, you don't want to be on statins forever. Experts say the best results for lowering your cholesterol are taking them combined with some classic therapies: lifestyle changes such as diet, exercise, weight loss and nutritional supplements. That's where we come in.

SYMPTOMS

Here's a truth that might surprise you: We all need cholesterol. A naturally-occurring molecule, it helps produce hormones and vitamin D, stokes bile production, which breaks down fats and digests foods, and even strengthens our cell membranes. But like any deal with a devil, this comes with a hitch: have too much, and the waxy substance begins to build up along the artery walls, which restricts blood flow to the heart, resulting in blood clots, angina, heart disease or heart attacks. Most doctors recommend keeping cholesterol numbers at or below 200 mg/DL (milligrams per deciliter of blood). But 106.7 million Americans ages 20 and older exceed this optimal level.

REMEDIES

Before you refill your Lipitor prescription, consider opting for a cholesterol-lowering supplement instead. Natural treatments can not only decrease your overall number, but also optimize your lipid profile (that is, increase "good" HDL and lower "bad" LDL and triglyceride levels). Combining the right supplement with exercise and a healthy diet can help you keep cholesterol under control without growing a third nipple. "On top of a strong lifestyle foundation, supplements can often make the difference in pushing cholesterol into a satisfactory level," says Brent A. Bauer, M.D., FACP, director of the Complementary and Integrative Medicine Program at the Mayo Clinic in Rochester, Minn.

Here are *Natural Health*'s picks for the best cholesterol-lowering supplements. Talk to your doctor about which are right for you, and how to take them—especially if you're taking any medications—some of these supplements work as blood thinners, and may interact with prescription drugs.

1. Niacin

Niacin, a B vitamin, gathers extra "bad" LDL cholesterol in your blood and delivers it to your liver for disposal, like nature's Wall-E. "In some studies, very significant drops in total cholesterol have been achieved with niacin," says Bauer. However, niacin can cause side effects, such as liver irritation and flushing, when taken in high doses, Bauer notes. "But used carefully, niacin can be very effective," he says.

DOSAGE: Take up to 2 grams a day of an extended-release formula, but talk to your doctor to determine the optimal dose for you. People with liver disease should avoid this one, and if you are already taking a statin, stop because niacin can interact with the statins.

TRY: Nature's Bounty Flush-Free Niacin ($11 for fifty 500-milligram capsules; drugstore.com)

2. Red yeast rice extract

Red yeast rice, a byproduct of fermented and cooked rice, contains monacolin K, a natural substance known to inhibit the synthesis of cholesterol in the body. "Some authors speculate that red yeast rice might be one way of getting the benefits of statins without the side effects," notes Bauer. "Since multiple studies have shown efficacy, red yeast rice is a good first-choice supplement to discuss with your doctor." A study published in the *Annals of Internal Medicine* in 2009 showed that a red rice yeast supplement worked as well to lower LDL ("bad") cholesterol as prescription statin drugs.

However, red yeast rice is not without controversy: While the FDA compares red yeast rice favorably to the cholesterol-lowering medication lovastatin, it warns that the amount of active ingredient can vary widely from product to product despite labeled dosage, and that certain brands contained trace amounts of the toxin citrinin. In addition, the FDA insists that labels inform consumers about the potential side effects of red yeast rice and how it can adversely interact with other medications and supplements. Buy yours from a reputable source.

DOSAGE: Take 600 milligrams three times daily. People with hepatic or renal disease should check with their health care provider before using red yeast rice.

TRY: Bluebonnet Nutrition CholesteRice Red Yeast Rice Complex ($47 for 90 capsules; luckyvitamin.com)

3. Psyllium

Commonly known as a cure-all for constipation, soluble fiber-packed psyllium reduces cholesterol absorption in the intestine. Studies show that taking 5 to 10 grams of soluble fiber a day can lower LDL by 5% (and—bonus—keep you regular). "It's something that you can incorporate in your daily life that doesn't cost much," says Julie Anne Chinnock, N.D., M.P.H, a researcher and naturopathic physician.

DOSAGE: Take 5 grams of psyllium seed husk (about a teaspoon) twice a day in a full glass of water. Supplemental fiber may affect the absorption of other oral medications, so ingest them at least two hours apart.

TRY: Now Foods Whole Psyllium Husk Powder ($15 for 12 ounces; iherb.com).

Power Pick

Get a heart-protecting, cholesterol-lowering three-for-one with **Nordic Naturals Omega LDL with Red Yeast Rice and CoQ10** ($30 for 60 1,000-milligram softgels; nutritiongeeks com).

4. Soy protein isolate

Though researchers aren't quite sure why it works, studies have shown that soy intake can decrease LDL by 12% and triglycerides by 10%. If you don't like soy-rich foods like miso, soy flour, tempeh and soymilk, try hiding a daily dose of a low-sugar supplemental soy protein in a yummy fruit smoothie. Make sure to get a soy isolate, which has undergone a process to remove most of the fat and carbohydrates but leaves protein intact—it tastes better and is less likely to cause gas.

DOSAGE: 50 grams day (a glass of soy milk has about 10 grams, 1/2 cup of tofu has 20 grams). Add to juice, smoothies, or sprinkle on cereal.

TRY: Bob's Red Mill Isolated Soy Protein Powder ($25 for 14 ounces; bobsredmill.com)

5. Omega-3 fish oil

While fish oil has been touted as a panacea for everything from depression to ulcers, researchers found that it really does regulate cholesterol. "There is strong evidence to show that fish oils can decrease triglycerides and LDL and increase HDL, in part by reducing liver production and release of VLDL [very-low-density lipoprotein, one of the three major types of lipoproteins]," says Chinnock. Since contamination can be a concern with fish oil supplements, she recommends "getting it from a good source that tests for heavy metals and pesticides."

CoQ10 Eases Statin Side Effects

While this antioxidant doesn't reduce cholesterol on its own, it's important to incorporate if you take statin drugs, which tend to deplete CoQ10 levels. "There is good evidence to show that CoQ10 supplementation may decrease muscle pain associated with statin treatment," says Chinnock.

Dosage: In general, take 150 milligrams a day to offset symptoms. Check with your doctor to discuss dosage and interaction possibilities.

Try: Life Extension Super Ubiquinol CoQ10 ($58 for one hundred 50-milligram softgels; vitacost.com)

DOSAGE: For best results, take 2 to 4 grams of fish oil every day. If you're bothered by the fishy aftertaste, try using a flavored oil and keep it refrigerated.

TRY: Carlson's Very Finest Fish Oil Lemon Flavor ($24.90 for a 200-milliliter bottle; carlsonlabs.com)

6. Artichoke extract

Artichoke extract works by increasing bile production in the liver, which in turn increases cholesterol excretion—meaning that any excess is eliminated rather than absorbed. One recent study found that an over-the-counter artichoke leaf extract (ALE) from the globe artichoke plant can lower cholesterol in otherwise healthy individuals with moderately raised levels. "Artichoke extract is an exciting complementary therapy for the prevention and treatment of arteriosclerosis and coronary heart disease," says Chinnock, who points to several studies showing positive effects on total cholesterol and LDL.

DOSAGE: Take 500 milligrams three times daily

TRY: Enzymatic Therapies Artichoke Extract ($26 for 45 capsules; vitaminshoppe.com)

7. Phytosterols and phytostanols

These compounds, which occur naturally in some plant sources, can also be taken as supplements. "They seem to work at lowering cholesterol by competitively inhibiting the absorption of dietary cholesterol," says Chinnock. Even if your diet includes plenty of foods that naturally contain phytosterols and phytostanols—like fruits, vegetables, nuts, seeds, legumes and vegetable oils—Chinnock recommends adding a supplement to your daily regimen if cholesterol is an ongoing problem.

DOSAGE: Recommended doses vary from product to product; ask your health care provider or follow package instructions.

TRY: Source Naturals Cholesterol Rescue ($31 for 50 tablets; sourcenaturals.com)

For more ideas, see our "Heart Disease" chapter on page 118.

HORMONE IMBALANCE

Erica Kelly, a 35-year-old marketing executive, couldn't believe there could be a simple solution to her chronic fatigue and depression. Two years ago, she felt tired and cranky all the time. "Around my period my symptoms were always worse," says Kelly. "I went to one doctor who put me on 10 supplements; another specialist I went to said I needed 10 different ones. I bought books, and I tried journaling to track my moods and symptoms. Nothing worked."

Then she went to see integrative internist Erika Schwartz, M.D., author of *The Hormone Solution* and *The 30-Day Natural Hormone Plan*. Schwartz was able to identify the common denominator underlying Kelly's problems: hormone imbalance. Yes, at age 35.

If you saw that one coming, you're one step ahead of many Western doctors. "We're trained to address symptoms of hormone imbalance rather than putting them into context and treating the causes of the symptoms," says Schwartz.

SYMPTOMS

In healthy women—and forgive us if we sound a little *Our Bodies, Ourselves* 101 for a second—the ovaries and the adrenal glands produce various hormones that equalize the ebb and flow of everything from menstruation to metabolism to sleep, after which they're broken down by the liver and then excreted by the kidneys and digestive tract. But if any part of the chain isn't working properly, your hormones aren't in balance, and the whole body can short out.

"Many female health issues are due to hormone imbalance," says

Susan Lark, M.D., a San Francisco-based clinical nutrition and preventive medicine specialist. And for most women, the problem boils down to one cause: estrogen dominance. "If you're among the millions of women in the 35 to 55 age bracket experiencing headaches, sleep difficulties, fluid retention, anxiety, irritability, mood swings, cramps, weight gain, breast tenderness and heavy bleeding," says Lark, "you're likely to be affected by estrogen dominance."

Estrogen is a wonderful hormone. In the right amount, it makes conception and pregnancy possible; it's also a natural mood lifter and skin toner. But many women have too much of a good thing for too long. In addition to the unpleasant symptoms of PMS and perimenopause, too much estrogen can lead to fibroids, benign uterine disease and some female cancers.

Progesterone is the estrogen police; it helps balance estrogen. In the right ratio, the two hormones help the body burn fat for energy, act as an antidepressant, aid in reducing fluid retention, assist metabolism and promote sleep. Estrogen dominance occurs when a woman's body doesn't have enough progesterone to keep the estrogen in check.

So what causes this excess of estrogen? Beyond our bodies simply making too much, probable causes include environmental toxins, rampant stress, nutritional deficiencies and the estrogens introduced into the food supply.

"Commercially produced meat, eggs and dairy products can be full of hormones, which are often injected or fed to the animals to promote faster growth," says Loretta Lanphier, NP, CN, a naturopathic practitioner and the CEO and president of Oasis Advanced Wellness in The Woodlands, Texas. "The hormones start in the grains we feed animals, then make their way up the food chain and into our bodies." The concern compounds over the years. "By the time I see women in their 30s, their bodies are often a mess, hormone-wise." (And not to scare you husbands, but estrogen levels—particularly of estradiol—rise in men as they age.)

REMEDIES

To stabilize your body's levels of estrogen, you need to reduce its production, block its ability to bind to tissues and assist its breakdown and elimination. By taking a natural approach—a combination of diet and lifestyle changes, bioidentical hormone therapy and supplements—you can see results in as quickly as 30 days. And begin now. "Don't wait until you get steamrolled like your mother did," Schwartz says. "Starting young can set you in a healthy pattern for the rest of your life." To balance your hormones, take these five simple steps:

1. Start with a test

Women should first determine their hormone levels. A blood, urine or saliva test can be ordered from online suppliers; Lanphier likes one available from ZRT Labs at salivatest.com.

Typically, these tests will determine your levels of five different hormones (estrogen, progesterone, testosterone, DHEA and cortisol). "If any one of these is out of balance, the entire body can feel out of balance," says Lanphier. "But the frequent mistake women make when they get their results is to run out and take more of everything they're deficient in. That's not the best way to achieve balance." For many women, if their progesterone-estrogen ratio is out of balance, the addition of bioidentical progesterone can be enough to alleviate symptoms and help achieve balance, she explains. But the best bet is to always consult a knowledgeable practitioner, who can help you interpret your test results and apply them to your overall medical picture.

2. Eat hormone-friendly foods

"It's impossible to exaggerate the importance of good nutrition in controlling hormones," says Lark. "No medication can entirely overcome the effects of a poor diet." What's the connection? A diet high in sugar and starch moves into the bloodstream quickly and causes insulin to spike—and high insulin levels trigger an increase in estrogen levels. Also, most women with PMS experience a drop in serotonin levels, which triggers cravings for carbs because the body uses carbs to make serotonin. A study in the *British Journal of Nutrition* showed that women who suffered from PMS consumed significantly more cakes, desserts and high-sugar foods before their periods; a 2013 study published in the *American Journal of Epidemiology* analyzed data from this study to reach the conclusion that foods rich in non-heme iron (vegetables) and zinc have also been linked with lower risks of PMS.

Schwartz recommends eliminating soda, sugar, caffeine, alcohol and highly processed foods; Lark adds saturated fat, red meat, dairy products and white flour to the no-no list. At the very least, look for organic meat and dairy products that are certified free of hormones, she says.

On the other hand, foods like complex carbohydrates break down slowly and help keep blood sugar levels stable. So, Schwartz says to load up on plant-based proteins, whole grains, healthy fats, colorful fruits and vegetables, green tea and "good" sweeteners (think natural organic honey, brown sugar or stevia). Soy foods, buckwheat and ground flax meal are particularly beneficial, Lark adds. "If your symptoms are mild to moderate, you can be a little less rigid. But if your symptoms are severe, dedicate yourself to the diet until you begin to get relief."

3. Keep stress in check

"When we're under severe stress, we're less likely to ovulate," says Lark. If you don't ovulate, you don't produce progesterone during the second half of your cycle. Without enough progesterone to keep estrogen in check, the negative effects of estrogen can become more pronounced. Stress also raises levels of cortisol, which causes other hormones to get out of balance.

If it's immediate relief you're after, try meditation or yoga—or an attitude shift. "When a stressful situation occurs, remember that you can't control the situation, but you can control your reaction to it," recommends Schwartz. "Try to keep cool, or at least accept that you can't change the situation."

4. Boost progesterone

The most direct way to offset high estrogen levels and regulate other hormones is to take in more bioidentical progesterone. Many doctors offer synthetic hormones in the form of hormone replacement therapy (HRT) or birth control pills, but be wary: The practice has been linked to increased risk of stroke and female cancers. Women can get the same benefits without the side effects by using bioidentical hormones—that is, hormones extracted from wild yams or soy oil that are molecularly identical to those produced by the human body. These are best applied as a cream. Patients rub on a small amount where skin is thin: the neck, upper chest, underarms or wrists.

Low-dose progesterone creams are available online and at health food stores, and most medical practitioners recommend using progesterone cream once a day for the two weeks before your period starts, which often coincides with the worst symptoms. Generally, the bloating, headaches, mood swings and insomnia abate within two menstrual cycles of using the cream.

After three months, women should stop hormone therapy and see how they feel; many patients can cease using the cream if they're maintaining good lifestyle habits. After applying the cream for several months, Belson now finds she can maintain her hormonal equilibrium simply by watching her diet and exercising.

It's safe to treat yourself with progesterone, Lanphier says; if you use too much, the worst side effect is fatigue. However, while younger women will do well with progesterone alone, women in their late 30s or older may need to combine progesterone and estrogen under the supervision of a physician.

5. Supplement your efforts

In addition to lifestyle changes, Lark advises women—particularly those with estrogen dominance—to add the following supplements to their daily diet:

FLAX: Take 2 tablespoons of flaxseed oil or 4 to 6 tablespoons of ground flax meal to help promote more frequent ovulation, and thus more progesterone production. Supplementation will also provide essential fatty acids necessary for reproductive health.

VITAMIN B COMPLEX: Take 25 to 100 milligrams of a good multi-B formula to help support the liver so it can process estrogen more efficiently.

VITAMIN C: A premier antioxidant, vitamin C helps clean up toxins created by the body in nearly every one of its chemical processes, including the manufacture of hormones. Take 600 to 2,000 milligrams.

MAGNESIUM: This mineral is critical to helping the body produce energy and for keeping the cycle of hormone production and excretion in check. Take 500 to 600 milligrams.

CALCIUM: Essential to maintaining healthy bones, calcium also helps reduce moodiness, food cravings and water retention, especially when combined with magnesium. Take 1,000 to 1,200 milligrams. Give these changes a try. If you notice that between days 15 and 28 of your cycle you're less edgy and crave fewer sweets, you're on the road to natural balance.

IBS

Interesting: In this tell-all era of oversharing, live blogging and Instagrammed what-I-had-for-dinner pics, only about 10% of Americans with irritable bowel syndrome (IBS) discuss their symptoms with their doctors, let alone anyone else. It seems some conditions are simply too embarrassing: abdominal pain, cramps, bloating, flatulence, mucus in the stool, food intolerances and constipation or diarrhea (often alternating between the two)—stuff straight out of that scene in *Airplane!* Except not funny. (You try working, eating or having sex with constipation or diarrhea.)

"Some people don't find their IBS symptoms bothersome or unusual, and some may be shy about talking to a doctor about bowel problems," says gastroenterologist G. Richard Locke, M.D., professor of medicine at the Mayo Clinic College of Medicine. Experts including the NIH estimate that about 20% of Americans (that's 60 million people, most of them women) have IBS. We know you're out there. Lucky for you, help is in here.

SYMPTOMS

Once called "spastic colon," and even "nervous stomach" IBS is thought to be the most common functional gastrointestinal (GI) disorder in the world, and experts believe its numbers are growing.

What causes IBS? Do I have it?

IBS is believed to stem from a disturbance in the interaction between the digestive tract, the brain and the autonomic nervous system. As a result, the colon can move too fast, resulting in diarrhea, or too slowly, resulting in constipation; sometimes it's spasmodic. "IBS used to be called spastic colon or spastic colitis, but those terms are not accurate," says Lin Chang, M.D., professor of medicine in the division of digestive diseases at the University of California, Los Angeles, David Geffen School of Medicine.

The diagnostic criteria include having abdominal pain or discomfort for at least 12 weeks out of the previous 12 months, not necessarily consecutively. Generally, pain is relieved by a bowel movement; the frequency of bowel movements alters when pain or discomfort begins; and/or there are changes in the form or appearance of the stool. "For most people, symptoms occur now and then, a couple of days a week or so," says Locke. "To meet the definition of IBS, you have to have the symptoms 25% [or more] of the time."

The good news is that IBS has not been linked to more serious bowel problems; nor does it raise the risk of colon cancer. "IBS is not a life-threatening condition, but it is a nuisance," says Keith Bruninga, M.D., a gastroenterologist at Rush University Medical Center in Chicago. And it can take a financial and emotional toll, with patients reporting missed work, sleep problems, low energy, reduced sexual interest and feelings of nervousness or hopelessness. "You don't know when it's going to come on," notes Chang. "You don't know how long it's going to last, and you don't know what might trigger it. It's constant anticipation."

Who is at risk?

IBS affects two to three times more women than men, and chronic stress—including current stressors as well as a history of physical, sexual or verbal abuse, parental divorce or parental alcoholism—seems to be a contributing factor. "We think there is an early, adverse life event [that boosts IBS risk]," says Chang.

The condition isn't "all in your head," but stress and emotions can affect the colon, since its many nerves connect it to the brain. "People who are prone to anxiety, who hold stress in, tend to be more likely to have problems with IBS," says Peter Galier, M.D., a physician at UCLA Medical Center, Santa Monica. Experts also believe that our super antiseptic lifestyle might be to blame for IBS: Past generations grew up getting dirty, and had a lot more contact with all kinds of bacteria. Grandma's system was just that much better at handling strange invaders.

REMEDIES

It's a bit of a—forgive us, please—crapshoot. No single treatment for IBS works for everyone. "The initial management of IBS is really about managing your lifestyle," says Locke. "People need to pay attention to stress in their lives. Regular exercise is also crucial, as is eating smaller amounts of food frequently rather than large meals," he adds.

After that, treatment is based on whether diarrhea or constipation is predominant. For mild symptoms, Locke says, you can self-treat, using milk of magnesia for constipation and nonprescription Imodium (loperamide) for diarrhea. If symptoms worsen, consider the following options:

ELIMINATE THE TRIGGERS

Steer clear of foods that exacerbate your symptoms. Among the common culprits are greasy foods, milk, grains, alcohol, chocolate and caffeinated beverages. "Up to 50% of patients will relate a worsening of symptoms to specific foods," Chang says.

Baby's Got Too Much Bac!

An alarming-sounding diagnosis might be hiding behind your IBS. Researchers, including Cathy Wong, N.D, are finding more evidence of something called "bacterial overgrowth," and it can cause symptoms that mimic IBS, such as gas, bloating, constipation and/or diarrhea. Researchers at Cedars-Sinai in California studied 202 people who met the criteria for IBS and gave them a test for bacterial overgrowth and found that 157 of the 202 people (78%) had bacterial overgrowth. When the unwanted intestinal bacteria were eradicated, symptoms improved in 48% of the subjects, particularly diarrhea and abdominal pain. Conventional treatment is with antibiotics; natural remedies include a low-carb diet, probiotics and enteric coated peppermint oil, grapefruit seed extract, goldenseal and olive leaf extract.

FOCUS ON FIBER

It might sound counterintuitive, but increasing fiber aids both diarrhea-predominant and constipation-predominant IBS. "Fiber has water-holding capacity, so it bulks up the stool," Bruninga says, explaining how it can ease diarrhea. "And it can also help bring fluid into the bowel," lessening constipation.

Eat plenty of fiber-rich foods, such as fruits, vegetables and whole grains, chia or flaxseeds, or consider adding a fiber supplement.

TRY: Garden of Life's Detoxifiber ($15; gardenoflife.com), an organic food-based blend with a balanced ratio of soluble and insoluble fiber that's free of gluten, psyllium and harsh laxatives. Since taking too much fiber too quickly can cause bloating, gradually work your way up to the dosage recommended on the package.

GO PRO(BIOTICS)

These microorganisms, believed to make the intestinal environment friendlier by populating it with "good" bacteria, are worth a try. Several studies presented at the American College of Gastroenterology's annual scientific meeting in 2008 found probiotics to be effective at normalizing bowel habits after 28 days of use; however, there was not enough information to determine whether any one strain was particularly effective or whether combinations are required.

One study found that IBS sufferers who took *Bifidobacterium infantis* and *Lactobacillus acidophilus* for four weeks had fewer symptoms and a higher quality of life; no side effects were reported.

TRY: American Health Priobiotic CD ($30; americanhealthus.com), a vegetarian supplement with 12 billion bio-active microorganisms, including *Bifidobacterium infantis* and *Lactobacillus acidophilus*

SNAP UP GINGER

This herb is often recommended as a general aid for digestion and a remedy for diarrhea and stomach upset. Take a daily dose of 2 to 4 grams of the fresh root, ¼ to 1 gram of the powdered root or 1½ to 3 milliliters of tincture.

TRY: New Chapter Organics Digestion Ginger Honey Tonic ($15; newchapter.com), a liquid supplement you can mix with sparkling water

INCONTINENCE

No one wants to be the woman in a Depends commercial, the lady who can't enjoy a Kristen Wiig movie or time with her grandkids because she's wet herself. Embarrassing stains, soiled panties, padded diapers—you only expect this when you're a baby, or pregnant with one.

But time has other plans. The decades between pregnancy and old age are when you're likely to leak, bulge, sag or otherwise experience pelvic trouble—and thus the most important time to attend to your bladder and adjacent organs, muscles and ligaments. "Women are shocked when it happens. They hit 50 and say, 'Oh my gosh, I survived pregnancy, but now this,'" says Missy Lavender, founder of the Women's Health Foundation, a Chicago-based nonprofit that educates women about pelvic health.

SYMPTOMS

About 28% of women age 50 and younger experience urinary leakage, rising to 34% for women older than 50, according to a 2013 NIH review of 22 studies. And 20% to 30% of all women suffer from some degree of pelvic organ prolapse—slippage of the uterus, vagina, bladder or rectum—because the surrounding muscles and ligaments no longer provide enough support. (Likelihood increases with age.) Urinary incontinence can be a symptom of prolapse, though you can have leakage without prolapse and vice versa. Other prolapse symptoms include a feeling of pressure or discomfort in the vagina or pelvis, back pain or painful intercourse.

"Women who have had kids get a double whammy," says Diana Quinn, N.D., a naturopathic physician and founder of the Hygeia Center for Healing Arts in Ann Arbor, Mich. "First the mechanical and structural changes that happen during labor and delivery, then the diminishing estrogen levels after menopause cause thinning and irritation of the bladder wall." But even women who have not delivered babies can develop incontinence as well as prolapse, due to gravity, age and hormonal changes. There are surgical options for both problems, including mesh "sling surgery," but complications are common and results do not always last.

Now—finally—for the encouraging news: Natural approaches—Kegels, physical therapy, acupuncture, dietary changes and herbal remedies—work well both to prevent and treat incontinence. And a pelvic-floor workout program (see "Less Leakage, Better Sex" on page 152) also can slow or even improve symptoms of both incontinence and prolapse while making sex more pleasurable, Lavender says.

REMEDIES
Stress incontinence

If you leak when you sneeze, cough, run, jump or lift weights, you have stress incontinence, caused by pressure—"stress"—on the bladder. You're especially prone if you had a long or difficult vaginal delivery, such as one involving forceps or other interventions that can injure pelvic nerves and muscles.

Being overweight doubles the risk of stress incontinence because the extra poundage puts pressure on the bladder, and losing weight appears to help. In a 2010 *Journal of Urology* study of women with daily leakage episodes, those who lost 7.5% of their body weight after one year reported a 65% reduction in episodes of stress incontinence.

If you leak urine only when you exercise, you may want to be fitted for a pessary, a small silicone disc that is inserted like a diaphragm and holds the pelvic organs in place (your gynecologist fits and prescribes one). A pessary also can be helpful for women with severe uterine prolapse, pelvic pain or feelings of heaviness or bulging from the vagina, Lavender says.

If stress incontinence interferes with your daily life and you are not a candidate for, or interested in, surgery, what then? First: Kegels. Then, more Kegels. (And by the way, Kegel rhymes with "bagel," not "legal.") Kegels work both to prevent and treat stress and urge incontinence by strengthening the pelvic floor, a thick, wide band of muscle that stretches across your pelvis and acts as a hammock, supporting the bladder and uterus.

Kegels can help women who develop stress incontinence because their pelvic floor is too lax. "You know how your arms are no longer taut and toned like they were when you were 18? The same thing is happening to the muscles in your pelvis," says Melissa Nassaney, M.S., DPT, a pelvic-floor physical therapist at Women & Infants Hospital in Providence, R.I.

How to Do Kegels Correctly

Most women squeeze the wrong muscles or fail to contract them long enough, physical therapist Melissa Nassaney says. Here's how to make Kegels worthwhile:

→ Start by lying down in a quiet place so you can focus.

→ Try to imagine that the muscles of your vagina are like the doors of an elevator. Gently close the doors and lift the elevator up to the next floor, then bring the elevator back down and open the doors. Do not lift your hips.

→ If you have difficulty finding your pelvic-floor muscles, place a finger or two inside your vagina, squeeze the surrounding muscles and make sure you feel a tightening. You also can locate these muscles by stopping the flow of urine as you pee, but only try that once: Doing it regularly can wreak havoc on your urinary system.

→ Once you get comfortable with contracting and relaxing these muscles, you can try doing Kegels in other positions.

→ Remember not to hold your breath or squeeze other muscles, such as your buttocks or inner thighs.

→ Do 10 to 15 repetitions three times a day. Work up to holding each contraction for 10 seconds.

→ Do Kegels daily for six weeks, and then two or three times a week—forever.

You can, and should, do Kegels on your own. However, if you have persistent, bothersome leakage when you laugh, cough or sneeze, or if you are experiencing urinary urgency, you might want to see a specially trained physical therapist, who may use exercises and/or biofeedback to improve your pelvic floor muscle strength and endurance. These techniques may also help reverse symptoms of pelvic organ prolapse, according to a 2010 article published in the *American Journal of Obstetrics and Gynecology.*

Urge incontinence (overactive bladder)

Are you the type who always sits on the aisle at the movie theater? If you have urge incontinence, also known as an overactive bladder, you get the urge to go, though your bladder is barely filled, and you leak en route to the restroom. (Having frequent urges without the leakage is called urinary frequency and often has the same causes.) Urge incontinence is heavily influenced by dwindling estrogen levels after menopause, and the more babies you've delivered, whether vaginally or via Cesarean section, the higher your risk.

A huge percentage of women have mixed incontinence—both stress and urge—and the only reliable way to distinguish between the two is to undergo urodynamic testing at a urology clinic. (It's also important to rule out other causes, such as urinary tract infections.) Bladder-retraining exercises help for urge incontinence, and there are also several drugs available, but their effectiveness and side effects vary widely, so it pays to explore other options first. Because urge incontinence is often triggered by bladder irritation or inflammation, the following approaches can be helpful:

DIETARY CHANGES

Bladder inflammation is often caused or aggravated by certain beverages and foods, such as coffee and black tea, alcohol, spicy foods and acidic foods like citrus and tomatoes. Eliminating wheat or dairy may help some women. "Identifying food sensitivities can make a big difference," says Quinn. A blood test as well as an elimination diet can indicate how your immune system responds to certain foods and help you decide which foods or beverages to cut out.

AMINO ACIDS

"The two key ones are L-glutamine and N-acetyl glucosamine," Quinn says. She also uses the herbs zea mays (cornsilk), uva ursi and marshmallow root. "They are protective of all the mucous membranes in the body and have a particular affinity for irritation and inflammation of the bladder," she explains. These products and the toning herbs below should be prescribed by a qualified practitioner, such as a naturopathic physician (N.D.) or an osteopathic physician (D.O), who can diagnose your specific problem and determine the right doses and combinations.

TONING HERBS

Herbs such as passionflower and chamaelirium can help tone the pelvic tissue, says Pina LoGiudice, N.D., L.Ac., a naturopathic physician at InnerSource Natural Health in Huntington, N.Y. "Also, an herb called equisetum helps strengthen the whole pelvic floor and helps with nighttime urinary frequency."

Less Leakage, Better Sex

If you are experiencing urinary leakage or are intent on preventing it, try the Total Control Pelvic Wellness Workout ($20; totalcontrolprogram.com). The 60-minute total-body routine includes a six-minute segment that targets your body's three most ignored muscle groups: the levator ani of the pelvic floor, the transverse abdominals (the deepest "core" muscles) and the multifidus, which run along your lower and middle spine. "These are the most important muscles that you never work," says Missy Lavender, founder of the nonprofit Women's Health Foundation, which produced the video.

In one study, 25% of women who completed the program stopped leaking within seven weeks, and many others saw tremendous improvement. On average, the women reported a 40% improvement in their quality of life. This workout also may help minimize vaginal dryness, a cause of painful sex, says Lavender:

"Exercising these muscles builds blood flow in the vagina, which increases lubrication. It absolutely helps with arousal and stronger orgasms."

ACUPUNCTURE

"Traditional Chinese Medicine looks at imbalances in the body, and incontinence is an energy-deficiency problem," says LoGiudice, who is also a licensed acupuncturist. "By stimulating various points you can strengthen a patient's qi, or energy, so the bladder regains its strength and doesn't spasm." LoGiudice recommends weekly treatments for eight to 10 weeks.

PERCUTANEOUS TIBIAL NERVE STIMULATION (PTNS)

Among the most promising treatments for urinary urgency and frequency is this technique in which an acupuncture needle transmits a mild electrical current at the ankle. "We've seen surprisingly good results, mainly among women who couldn't tolerate overactive-bladder medication or didn't respond to it," says Roger Goldberg, M.D., director of urogynecology research at the University of Chicago NorthShore University HealthSystem. "The main downside is that the results aren't permanent," he adds.

If you have any degree of bladder or other pelvic-area problems, says Quinn, "First consult with your holistic health provider, then get a referral to a physical therapist and a urologist with a big-picture attitude."

The Vagina Workout

Want to find out how strong (or weak) your pelvic muscles are, then strengthen them? The Myself Pelvic Muscle Trainer ($99; themyselftrainer.com), a battery-powered gizmo, actually makes a vagina workout kind of fun (no, not in that way—though you don't want to do this in front of the kids). Lying down, you insert a super-tampon-sized plastic sensor, then press a button to inflate a balloon inside it. A handheld device that resembles an oversized iPod guides you through a five-minute workout, instructing you when to squeeze and relax. A series of bands on the screen indicates how strong your pelvic-floor muscles are, and three strength levels keep you motivated to improve.

INDIGESTION

As kids we were taught that bacteria was a bad thing: germy, dirty and dis-*gus*-ting. But bacteria is trendy these days. Sexy even. The reason? Probiotics. In recent years, these "good" bacteria superstars are the hottest commodity on store shelves—U.S. sales were an estimated $1.1 billion in 2010, according to a report in the *Oxford Journals' Clinical Infectious Diseases*, and seemingly they're the key to good digestion, which in turn is key to overall good health. And experts are becoming convinced that indigestion means more than a rumbling stomach. If you're suffering from migraines, allergies or chronic disease, the reason may be rooted in your poor digestion. Could these miracle bugs be the real deal?

Digestion—the process by which your body breaks down food into nutrients, absorbs those nutrients and eliminates the rest—isn't just about simple mechanics. Recent research has homed in on the digestive system's most abundant inhabitants: trillions of beneficial bacteria that colonize the GI tract starting from the moment we're born. These "good bugs" support digestion itself (by manufacturing certain vitamins and aiding peristalsis, which is the wave-like muscular movement of food trough the gastrointestinal tract) and affect health in myriad other ways, starting with our immunity.

"Many people don't realize that the lining of our intestines is one of the biggest parts of our immune system," says Boston-based naturopathic doctor Cathy Wong, N.D. Indeed, with its massive surface area— if stretched out, it's actually the size of a football field—the GI tract is continually under attack by harmful bacteria and viruses present in the food we eat and the air we breathe.

SYMPTOMS

Optimizing both your gut health—its ratio of "good" to "bad" bacteria—*and* the digestive process are two of the best things you can do for your body. When the good bugs are plentiful, they keep the bad ones at bay; healthy flora release acid, making the environment inhospitable to harmful microbes. Plus, researchers are still uncovering more ways in which our inner ecosystem affects our health, with studies linking bacterial imbalance in the gut to everything from allergies to obesity to heart disease to the reason for this chapter: indigestion, aka dyspepsia. That's when you may feel full when you shouldn't, or bloated or burpy.

REMEDIES

To start, eat a plant-based diet with plenty of fiber and healthy fats, fermented foods like yogurt and miso, and minimal sugar and processed foods. And try to relax because the body's stress response inhibits digestion. "Stress can change the bacterial balance in the gut, giving harmful bacteria the upper hand," says Wong. Beyond the basics, you can help your gut get healthy by giving the following supplements a go.

PROBIOTICS

Antibiotic use, excessive sugar and stress can alter the bacterial balance in the gut. As we've said, probiotics can help restore this bacterial balance, strengthening immunity and potentially preventing or treating a wide range of health issues, including yeast infections. "There's good data that probiotics improve symptoms of allergies, irritable bowel syndrome (IBS), eczema and colic," says Patrick Hanaway, M.D., an integrative family physician in Asheville, N.C. A recent Tufts University School of Medicine report confirms that randomized, double-blind studies are finding great results for diarrhea (including antibiotic induced) and food allergies. Preliminary research has also shown that probiotics activate an immune response in mucous membranes, which helps prevent colds and flus, notes Wong. The probiotics with the greatest number of proven benefits are *Lactobacillus rhamnosus* strain GG and *Saccharomyces boulardii*. (For more on probiotics, see "Supplements" on page 415.)

DOSAGE: Look for a mixed-strain product that includes bifidobacteria and lactobacillis and follow package directions.

TRY: Dr. Ohhira's Probiotics Original Formula ($40 for 60 capsules; drohhiraprobiotics.com)

GINGER

According to ayurveda, ginger increases *agni*, or digestive fire, the body's most essential "ingredient" for good health, says Kate Gilday, an herbalist and ayurvedic consultant in Cold Brook, N.Y. Impaired *agni* (caused by overeating, eating the wrong foods for your constitution or eating while stressed or upset) can lead to impaired metabolism and immunity, over time putting you on a slope toward chronic illness.

DOSAGE: Before meals, try either a cup of ginger tea or a thin slice of ginger with a squeeze of lime juice and a pinch of sea salt. Note: Those with heartburn should avoid ginger because the herb aggravates the condition.

TRY: Traditional Medicinals' Organic Ginger Aid ($6 for 16 tea bags; traditionalmedicinals.com)

L-GLUTAMINE

Normally, only nutrients pass through the intestinal lining. But if the lining is compromised (often due to improper diet or flora imbalance), food particles can pass through the lining into the bloodstream (known as intestinal permeability or leaky gut syndrome). When this happens, immune cells may react to these unwanted proteins and chemicals, causing inflammation, food allergies or an immune disorder. L-glutamine, an amino acid found naturally in the GI tract, "promotes the growth of intestinal cells, repairing the lining of the gut," says Wong.

DOSAGE: If you have leaky gut syndrome, supplement with L-glutamine under the guidance of a health care practitioner. The usual dose is 2 grams of the powder mixed in 6 to 8 ounces of any fluid. Drink on an empty stomach once a day.

TRY: Jarrow Formulas L-Glutamine ($14 for 100 tablets; vitamin-shoppe.com)

GROUND FLAXSEED

Ground flaxseed is a prebiotic, a nondigestible nutrient that serves as "food" for good bacteria in the gut, helping them grow and flourish. What's more, it's high in fiber, which means it helps digested food move through your system—and that can help prevent (and even treat) a range of GI issues, including IBS and leaky gut syndrome. (When stool sits in the colon, the bile acids become more concentrated, irritating the lining of the colon and triggering these conditions.) A 2009 NIH report confirms that the soluble fiber in ground flaxseed is well tolerated and has a laxative effect.

DOSAGE: Store ground flaxseed in the refrigerator or freezer (it's prone to rancidity). Mix 2 tablespoons into yogurt or sprinkle on cereal daily.

TRY: Bob's Red Mill Organic Brown Flaxseeds ($5 for 24 ounces; bobsredmill.com)

DANDELION ROOT

A true multitasker, this age-old herbal remedy is a wonderful digestive tonic. Its mild bitter taste increases salivation, which primes the GI tract for digestion. The herb also increases bile flow and hydrochloric acid production (both crucial for digestion), supports the liver's detoxing functions and increases the production of digestive enzymes. Regular use is great for those who have trouble digesting fats (which can lead to liver problems) or who experience constipation, says Gilday.

DOSAGE: Mix ½ teaspoon of dandelion root tincture in warm water and drink about 15 minutes before meals.

TRY: Gaia Herbs Organic Dandelion Root ($12 for 1 ounce; gaiaherbs.com)

DIGESTIVE ENZYMES

Probiotics' costar, digestive enzymes, are gaining popularity as people understand what they do. The body's digestive enzymes help break down food into components that our cells can use, says Wong. Because many people are enzyme-deficient, supplemental enzymes help with nutrient absorption. Taken with meals, these extra enzymes help food digest more fully, easing a wide range of digestive symptoms, including gas and bloating, heartburn and indigestion. They can also be beneficial for those with food sensitivities or intolerances, because they allow for more complete digestion of food, which lessens irritation in the small intestine.

DOSAGE: Look for a broad-spectrum enzyme supplement (with lipases for fat digestion, proteases for protein digestion and amylases for carbohydrate digestion), and take with meals three times a day.

TRY: Enzymatic Therapy CompleteGest ($24 for 90 capsules; vita-cost.com)

PEPPERMINT OIL

The essential oil of the peppermint plant has anti-spasmodic properties, says Wong. This helps relax the digestive system's muscles, which can prevent the onset of bloating and gas. Peppermint oil has been shown to ease IBS, and also helps probiotics colonize.

DOSAGE: Look for enteric-coated peppermint oil (the coating keeps the oil from being released in the stomach, which can cause heartburn). Take one or two .2-milliliter capsules a day, after meals.

TRY: Nature's Way Pepogest ($14 for 60 softgels; vitaminshoppe.com)

TRIPHALA

This classic ayurvedic remedy, a combination of three fruits, helps with the three crucial aspects of the digestive process—digestion, absorption and elimination. It's also a prebiotic, which helps the good flora in the body flourish. Triphala also boosts *agni* and helps the body detoxify by regulating bowel function, protecting the intestines against inflammation due to toxin damage and protecting and supporting the liver. The Deepak Chopra Center in San Diego promotes its use for cleansing and detoxing without the irritating effects of many laxatives; it also strengthens and nourishes bone and the nervous system.

DOSAGE: Triphala comes in powder or capsule form. Take ½ teaspoon of the powder once or twice a day, mixed in water, or 1,000 milligrams in capsule or tablet form. Some people take triphala for short-term indigestion or detoxing, while others take it long-term. (Do not take it if you're pregnant.)

TRY: Planetary Herbals Triphala Gold ($12 for 60 tablets; planetary-herbals.com)

INFERTILITY

There might be nothing tougher on a marriage than infertility—the onslaught of hormone treatments, the sex on demand (sounds fun, but it really isn't) and the expensive, invasive (and, some fear, even cancer-causing) in vitro fertilization (IVF) treatments have many couples looking for a blend of holistic and medical solutions. "Nope," they say, mournfully placing another Clearblue into the trash, "not this month."

It's like this for one in eight couples in the United States today: Blame pesticides in food or hormone-disrupting stress or blocked fallopian tubes—experts point to a host of medical, environmental and social factors, although a 2013 report from the National Center for Health Statistics says rates are stable or possibly declining.

Chief among the fertility-zappers is age. According to the Centers for Disease Control and Prevention, 20% of American women now have their first child after age 35. Unfortunately, about one-third of them will have a hard time, thanks to diminished egg reserves or a heightened risk of other reproductive challenges. But while one-third of infertility problems can be traced to the female partner, the same number can be attributed to the man (see "Sperm Zappers" on page 165). Both partners have issues 10% of the time, and 20% of cases are frustratingly labeled "unexplained."

So let's look instead at the causes.

SYMPTOMS

Most female infertility stems from ovulatory issues, including hormone imbalances or polycystic ovarian syndrome (PCOS), a hormonal disorder characterized by irregular periods, excess hair growth and acne. Others face infections or thyroid disease; mechanical issues like blocked fallopian tubes; or endometriosis, a painful disorder in which the uterine lining grows outside the uterus. Certain culprits, including blocked tubes, require surgery or assisted reproductive techniques like in vitro fertilization (IVF). Some experts believe that IVF cases are on the rise in the U.S. and worldwide because techniques are becoming more high-tech, and the perception (purely anecdotal) is that they are more successful.

But some fertility specialists say a quick-fix mentality on the part of both patients and physicians has contributed to an overreliance on IVF, which costs about $12,000 per cycle and can be exceptionally taxing on a woman's body and emotions.

"Approximately 50% of women who are undergoing IVF don't need it," says Sami S. David, M.D., assistant professor of reproductive medicine at Mount Sinai Medical Center in New York City and author of *Making Babies: A Proven 3-Month Program for Maximum Fertility*. "Lifestyle is a huge factor," adds David, one of a growing number of practitioners who are advocating a blend of holistic care with mainstream reproductive endocrinology.

REMEDIES

While you can't change your age, you can control the foods you eat, the way you handle stress and your environment. We asked the experts—many of whom used a combination of traditional and complementary approaches to surmount their own fertility challenges—for their top recommendations. Choose the methods that suit your physical or emotional needs; if after three months you've seen no improvement, consult a reproductive endocrinologist.

Stress Less

Many experts believe chronic stress has hijacked our primitive fight-or-flight response, causing the pituitary gland to unnecessarily release endorphins that suppress reproductive hormones. A landmark Harvard Medical School study found that women who participated in a 10-week mind-body program, including relaxation and yoga, were nearly three times more likely to conceive than women who didn't take part. The research was lead by Alice Domar, Ph.D., executive director of the Domar Center for Mind/Body Health at Boston IVF and author of *Conquering Infertility*.

STRIKE A POSE

"Yoga reduces the stress hormone cortisol and induces the relaxation response," explains Tami Quinn, a registered yoga teacher and cofounder of the Chicago-based holistic fertility center Pulling Down the Moon. Specific poses, such as Viparita Karani (Legs up the Wall), can also increase blood flow to the ovaries and uterus, potentially thickening the uterine lining; this can aid with embryo implantation. Stick with gentle hatha or restorative yoga and avoid breaking a sweat—this is not the time for Bikram yoga.

PICTURE THIS

Guided imagery is a therapeutic technique that allows you to enter a deeply relaxed state of mind, then focuses your attention on specific images that work to calm you. Mind-body expert Bernie Siegel, M.D., author of *Love, Medicine & Miracles,* suggests tailoring this brain game to your conception goals: "Like rehearsing for a performance, when you visualize your egg being fertilized, your chemistry changes and the body responds as if fertilization is happening."

ON PINS AND NEEDLES

A 2008 *British Medical Journal* study found that women who underwent IVF and acupuncture together were 65% more likely to conceive than women who only underwent IVF. According to acupuncturist-herbalist Jill Blakeway L.Ac., it works by promoting uterine blood flow. It can also quiet post-IVF uterine contractions, encouraging implantation and decrease levels of cortisol (a "stress hormone") and prolactin, both of which are known to disrupt reproductive function.

Send In Patch Adams?

Laughter might be good medicine for infertility. An Israeli study found that women who were visited by "medical clowns" immediately following IVF embryo transfer were more likely to conceive than patients who missed out on the laughs.

Eat to Conceive

Jorge E. Chavarro, M.D., Sc.D., an assistant professor of nutrition and epidemiology at the Harvard School of Public Health and author of *The Fertility Diet*, followed 18,000 participants in the long-running Harvard Nurses' Health Study who were trying to get pregnant. Among his findings:

GET YOUR PROTEIN FROM PLANTS

Foods that elevate insulin levels contribute to fertility-zapping ovulatory disorders. "Not all proteins are digested the same," Chavarro explains. "Animal proteins require more insulin to be secreted." Beef and poultry, specifically, were associated with infertility. The good news: Replacing 25 grams of animal protein with 25 grams of plant protein (beans, peas, nuts) was related to a 50% lower risk of ovulatory infertility.

BAN TRANS FATS

Found primarily in packaged baked and fried foods, trans fats elevate insulin levels. Monounsaturated fats, like those found in avocados, nuts and olive oil, are associated with a decreased risk of infertility.

AVOID SUGAR SPIKES

Quickly digested carbs, such as white bread, potatoes and soda, spike your blood sugar, promoting insulin secretion. Carolyn Dean, M.D., N.D., dislikes "white" carbs for another reason: They encourage yeast overgrowth. "Yeast toxins can cross-react with hormones necessary for pregnancy, blocking their receptor sites," she says. Dean recommends eliminating sugar and white flour, eating fiber-rich, slowly digested complex carbohydrates and incorporating plain yogurt or probiotic supplements to encourage the growth of healthy gastrointestinal bacteria, which favorably compete with yeast toxins for space.

TRY: Culturelle Probiotics ($15 for 30 capsules; vitacost.com) or Lifeway plain organic kefir ($5 for 32 ounces; lifeway.net)

LIMIT LOW-FAT DAIRY

Chavarro's research found that low-fat dairy foods appear to heighten the risk of infertility, while women who consumed one daily serving of whole milk or full-fat ice cream were 27% less likely to experience infertility.

TEA UP

A study published in the *American Journal of Public Health* found that tea drinkers doubled their odds of conceiving, perhaps because of their antioxidant content. Note: Blakeway advises avoiding red raspberry leaf tea because it is linked to miscarriage.

Supplement Smartly

Certain supplements and herbs may help you on your conception quest.

MELLOW MAGNESIUM

The mineral is thought to keep the fallopian tubes relaxed, facilitating the travel of sperm to meet egg. In IVF, it can calm the uterus to encourage implantation; during pregnancy, it may help prevent miscarriage. Dean, who is the medical director of the Nutritional Magnesium Association, suggests 750 milligrams daily. The mineral is also found in seaweed, cacao, leafy greens, nuts and seeds.

TRY: Natural Calm Magnesium Citrate ($23 for 16 ounces; calmnatural.com)

SOMETHING FISHY

Holistic nutritionist Sally Kravich, M.S., CNHP, recommends fish oil (800-plus milligrams EPA and 500-plus milligrams DHA per day) to balance your hormones and encourage healthy fetal brain development.

TRY: Nordic Naturals Ultimate Omega ($60 for 180 softgels; vitaminshoppe.com)

HELPFUL HERBS

Chinese herbs are often used in conjunction with acupuncture to address elevated follicle stimulating hormone (FSH) levels, repeat miscarriage, unexplained infertility and PCOS, says Oakland, Calif.-based acupuncturist and herbalist Zoe Cohen, L.Ac. Single herbs are rarely prescribed; instead, multicomponent formulas are tailored for each patient based on her diagnosis. Herbs traditionally sold raw, dry or as powder are available in pill or tincture form. Cohen explains that herbs can be deceptively powerful and may interact with fertility drugs, so it is crucial to work with a licensed herbalist experienced in treating infertility.

BLEND IN A BOTTLE

Not ready to jump head-first into Chinese herbs? Stanford University School of Medicine researchers found that FertilityBlend, a combination of prenatal vitamins and fertility-enhancing herbs, increases your chances of conceiving. (FertilityBlend for Men boosts sperm count.)

TRY: FertilityBlend for Women ($30 for 90; fertilityblend.com)

Clean Up Your Act

Every day, we're exposed to hundreds of chemicals, from our shampoo to our water bottles to car exhaust. Research has found that many of these products contain endocrine-disrupting compounds called xenoestrogens (bisphenol-A, or BPA, and phthalates are two examples), which mimic estrogen in the body, meddling with the body's sensitive hormonal milieu by blocking real estrogen from doing its work. High blood levels of the chemicals used in nonstick cookware and waterproof clothing have been shown to significantly increase a woman's risk of infertility.

David suggests eating organic foods and keeping your home as green as possible: Avoid microwaving food in plastic containers, steer clear of cosmetics containing phthalates or parabens and include dietary phytoestrogens, such as flax seed or soy, in your diet; they'll bind to the estrogen receptor sites before xenoestrogens get the chance.

AVOID WEIGHT EXTREMES

According to the American Society for Reproductive Medicine, 12% of female infertility cases are a result of a woman weighing too little or too much. That's because estrogen is produced in fat cells. Too little body fat and the body can't produce enough estrogen to fuel ovulation; too much and the body reacts as if it were on birth control. Gaining just six to eight pounds (if underweight) or losing 10 to 14 pounds (if overweight) may be enough to boost your baby-making odds.

EXERCISE IN MODERATION

Similarly, it's important to strike a balance between overdoing it and not doing enough on the exercise front. David says gentle exercises like walking, swimming and yoga promote blood supply to the pelvic region and reduce stress. But he recommends avoiding "workout intensities that elicit an endorphin rush, as this can suppress egg and ovarian hormone production." A landmark study in *Obstetrics & Gynecology* found that IVF patients who reported exercising four hours or more per week for one to nine years were 40% less likely to have a live birth than women who did not exercise. Women are advised not to work out while undergoing IVF treatment because doing so could harm the ovaries, but a study that followed 118 IVF patients from June 2009 to March 2010 found that 12% of them were ignoring the exercise warnings from their doctors.

Sperm Zappers

The average American man has half the sperm count of his grandfather's generation, says Jill Blakeway, L.Ac. We can partly blame our *Mad Men*-era moms: "Research suggests that the damage gets done in utero because the mother has been exposed to so many toxic chemicals." Fortunately, men can benefit from lifestyle modifications in as few as three months, as they continually regenerate new sperm (women are born with all the eggs they will ever have). Encourage your man to adopt changes like the following to turn his men into the Michael Phelps of sperm.

STOP SMOKING Sucking on cigarettes damages sperm DNA, which can increase your miscarriage risk.

CHECK OUT THE MEDICINE CHEST Calcium channel-blockers used to treat high blood pressure can lower sperm count. Other common culprits include diuretics and peptic ulcer, epilepsy and antifungal medications.

REDUCE STRESS A 2010 study published in *Fertility and Sterility* found an inverse relationship between stress and sperm quality.

KEEP 'EM COOL Heat and sperm don't mix. Swap briefs for boxers, keep the laptop off the lap and the cellphone out of the pants.

BE FRUITFUL AND MULTIPLY Antioxidant-rich, produce-heavy diets (as well as antioxidant supplements) have been shown to improve sperm quality.

INSOMNIA

Some people are born to sleep. Neither alarm clocks nor earthquakes nor a good *Jimmy Fallon* will keep them from passing out. Insomniacs think about these people often—because they have a lot of time to think, usually at 2:41 a.m., as they scan Twitter, or watch a bad movie, or toss and turn. Three hours till it's time to get up for work. Now two. Now one. Maybe tomorrow night will be better.

Maybe not.

SYMPTOMS

Insomnia affects more than 60 million Americans each year, and the problem tends to worsen with age. Eight out of ten will suffer what experts call "situational insomnia," meaning restorative sleep becomes temporarily elusive because you're changing jobs, buying a house or coping with a relationship gone sour. But when situational insomnia becomes chronic, it may lead to numerous health problems, including insulin resistance and weight gain.

If you're looking for a super-quick fix, drugs like Ambien definitely work, but some rather freaky side effects, such as sleep driving, ordering and eating food, as well as hallucinations have been reported. If you're looking for effective relief that's still quick but nonpharmaceutical, read on.

REMEDIES

If your doctor has ruled out medical or psychological roots for your wakefulness, these techniques could be your Fast Pass to dreamland.

1. Need the kneads

A professional full-body massage is a no-brainer, especially when it's part of a weekly or monthly routine. "If you're getting regular treatments, you'll be much more relaxed and you'll sleep better," says integrative physician Ann Marie Chiasson, M.D., author of *Energy Healing*. But it can get expensive. Instead: "For insomnia, a light self-massage is also effective," she says. Here are simple techniques to try at home, to bring your systems into balance and help you fall asleep naturally:

FOOT PRESS: Any type of foot massage is extremely relaxing and grounding, and helps prepare you for sleep, especially if you add a light aromatherapy oil to your feet, ayurvedic experts say. While sitting or lying down, place both thumbs on top of one foot near the toes, and the fingers of both hands on the bottom of the foot. Squeeze the foot for two seconds and release for two seconds. Work your way from the toes (in between the toes) to the ankles, then switch feet and repeat. Even better? Recruit an energetic friend.

SHAMPOO STROKE: Lying in bed, gently massage your head and neck as if shampooing your hair. Continue until you begin to feel relaxed.

SCALP ROLL: Touch the top of your head with your fingertips, rolling the scalp skin forward and back over your skull in a light, rhythmic motion. Continue as long as the movement feels comforting.

THUMB PRESS: Cradle the back of your head with your hands so that your thumbs come together at the occipital ridge (the protrusion where the skull meets the neck). Using your thumbs, gently press upward on the skull in a circular motion, gradually working your way over to your ears. Press with your fingers and find the tender places. Press lightly when you feel a tight spot and breathe.

GET HELP: To find a licensed massage therapist near you, see our "Massage" chapter on page 254, or visit the American Massage Therapy Association at amtamassage.org. Make sure the therapist has the proper certifications and licenses—L.M.T., N.C.M.T., C.M.T.—but these vary so widely that they alone don't guarantee a great massage therapist. Best to call, ask them to describe their work and tell them what you are looking for.

2. Practice in pajamas

In a study in the *Indian Journal of Medical Research*, yoga postures and deep breathing helped seniors fall asleep faster, stay asleep longer and feel more rested in the morning. To experience the effects, try a bedtime ritual designed by massage therapist John LeMunyon, L.M.T., founder of Heartwood Yoga and Body Centered Therapies in Birmingham, Ala. "Start a half hour before you go to bed and direct your attention inward," LeMunyon advises. Just before climbing into bed, apply cream or calming oils to your body, brush your hair or perform other self-care, but skip any deep reading or screen surfing.

TRY THIS ASANA: Lie on the floor and prop your calves on the seat of a chair or on the edge of your bed with your knees directly over your pelvic bones and both bent legs forming a 90-degree angle. Place both arms out to the sides and turn your palms upward. Observe your breath as you inhale, and lengthen your exhalations. With each breath, increase your exhalation by one second and repeat until you've reached a comfortable maximum. Stay at that length for 12 breaths or longer, then return to normal breathing, and finally, get into bed.

GET HELP: Go to a local class, start practicing daily yoga online at gaiamyogastudio.com or turn to our "Yoga" chapter on page 344.

3. Press your points

Applying gentle acupressure to targeted points on the body can release stress and promote deep relaxation, says Michael Reed Gach, Ph.D., founder of acupressure.com. According to a Taiwanese study published in the *American Journal of Chinese Medicine,* subjects who received 15 minutes of either acupressure or transcutaneous electrical stimulation three times a week for a month experienced better sleep and superior moods than those in a control group. "Two important and effective acupressure points are between the ankle bone and the heel," Gach says. "Place your thumb on one side of the ankle bone and your fingers on the other side. Squeeze between the anklebone and the heel. Hold for two to three minutes with firm pressure." Repeat with the opposite hand and foot, then stretch both arms overhead and back to induce a deep yawn; for further instructions, visit acupressure.com.

ROLL ON A BALL: If you're carrying knots of tension between your shoulder blades, try this tension tamer from Gach that stimulates 20 acupressure points: Put a couple of tennis balls in a sock and place them on your bed. Lie down so the balls are directly between your shoulder blades, or where the tension is greatest. Hold this position for two or three minutes with your eyes closed, breathing slowly and deeply. Afterward, stretch your arms and legs to induce a deep yawn.

GET HELP: Visit the American Organization for Bodywork Therapies of Asia at aobta.org, or book a weekly shiatsu or Thai massage at a local day spa because these also zero in on pressure points.

4. Dream about herbs

There are several available Chinese remedies for treating insomnia, according to Drew Francis, O.M.D., founder of Golden Cabinet Medical Healing Center in West Los Angeles, Calif. "These herbal formulas have been used successfully for a thousand years throughout China," he says. (His caveat: no alcohol and no caffeine when you take them.) The formulas are available from Traditional Chinese Medicine (TCM) practitioners, in shops within metropolitan Chinatowns or via suppliers such as chineseherbsdirect.com.

GET HELP: To find a credentialed TCM practitioner, visit the National Certification Commission for Acupuncture and Oriental Medicine at nccaom.org. See Traditional Chinese Medicine on page 263 for tips on choosing a TCM practitioner.

If symptoms...	Take...
include waking with menopausal night sweats	Tian Wang Bu Xin Dan, eight to 10 capsules one hour before bed
are marked by low energy, sluggishness or poor appetite	Gui Pi Tang, four capsules twice a day, the last dose one hour before bed
accompany nervousness or anxiety	Suan Zao Ren Tang (or Zizyphus combination), four capsules twice a day, and eight more capsules one hour before bed

5. Tune in, turn in

Listening to music can trigger the relaxation response, a state of deep rest marked by reductions in blood pressure, muscle tension and heart rate, says Chiasson, who teaches at the Center for Integrative Medicine at the University of Arizona. A 2009 study in the *Journal of Advanced Nursing* showed that sleep improved for slumber-challenged participants who listened to 45 minutes of music each night at bedtime. Other studies found that listening to music helped women fall asleep faster, experience fewer nighttime awakenings and feel more satisfied with the overall quality of their snooze.

What kind of music works best? Chiasson finds success with patients who use drumming, chanting and Native American songs for sleep induction. The optimal solutions are tailored to your own personal tastes, however. "Find the calming piece of music that speaks to you and allows you to take deep, relaxing breaths and leave the stress of the day behind," she says. "The aim is to get lost in the music, and I've even used Lady Gaga and Eminem's rap songs to help patients fall fast asleep."

GET HELP: A certified therapist uses music interventions in a clinical setting to accomplish individualized goals. To find one near you, visit the American Music Therapy Association at musictherapy. org; or purchase a guided "Energy Healing Meditation" with Chiasson at soundstrue.com; or set up a sound machine with noises that lull you.

How can I feel less irritable?

Maybe you're not actually annoyed at your husband.
Maybe, instead, it's the food.

A naturopath says:

Food allergies may trigger irritability. When you're allergic to a certain food, the body releases histamine, which can make you feel stuffed up and sluggish, depressed and cranky. Even a sensitivity to certain foods can make your insulin and blood sugar levels rise more quickly, creating a sense of agitation.

TREATMENT: The most effective way to find out if certain foods bother you is to go on an elimination diet for about two to four weeks, avoiding anything suspicious, as well as the typical red flags: wheat, dairy, corn, soy, nightshade vegetables, citrus and meat. Then reintroduce the targeted foods for one or two days, a little bit at every meal, and see if there is an ensuing reaction. Generally, people during the summer tend to feel best when they eat cooling foods (think raw, moist, hydrating picks, like salads and fruits). Big, heavy meals slow digestion, which can also make you feel tired and cranky.

—Paul Anderson, N.D.,
faculty member at Bastyr University's School of Natural Medicine in Kenmore, Wash.

An integrative doctor says:

The raging hormones at play in both premenstrual syndrome (PMS) and premenstrual dysphoric disorder (PMDD) often cause irritability. PMS, which relates to the more physical symptoms associated with the onset of menstruation such as back pain, bloating, cramping and breast tenderness, can make you grumpy thanks to sheer physical discomfort. PMDD makes you more sensitive to everything— lights, noise, emotions— contributing to your short fuse.

TREATMENT: In addition to regular exercise and relaxation practices, certain supplements can make a significant difference in your mood. Vitamin B_6 has long been recognized as an antistress vitamin, and taking 50 milligrams to 100 milligrams a day can get you on a more even keel. The herb St. John's wort (take 300 to 600 milligrams three times daily) or the amino acid 5-hydroxytryptophan (take 200 to 300 milligrams in divided doses of 100 milligrams) are also particularly effective ways of nipping crankiness in the bud.

—Shelley Wroth, M.D.,
integrative medicine physician and assistant professor of obstetrics and gynecology at Duke Integrative Medicine in Durham, N.C.

An ayurvedic doctor says:

In ayurveda, there are three doshas—vata (air), pitta (fire) and kapha (earth)—that govern everyone and everything. During hot summer months (the pitta time of year), these doshas can get thrown out of balance. A person's internal heat, combined with the sultry weather, often produces an inflammatory response in the body that can trigger emotions like anger and irritation.

TREATMENT: First, take a look at your lifestyle. Pittas tend to overextend themselves, a recipe for burnout. Second, go easy on the caffeine and alcohol, which are warming, and choose cooling drinks like coconut water; and mint, chamomile and lemon balm teas. A favorite yogic trick for staying calm and collected in the heat is sitali breathing: Make an "O" shape with your mouth and curl your tongue, inhaling through your mouth and exhaling through your nose with long, slow breaths. Do this for two to five minutes a day.

—Hillary Garivaltis,
dean of the Kripalu School of Ayurveda in Stockbridge, Mass.

How can I improve my memory?

Ever find yourself walking into a room, then forgetting why you're there? Take some omega-3s so you don't forget this.

A neuroscientist says:

The best way to take care of your brain is to apply the same strategies involved in taking care of your heart, such as eating healthfully and exercising regularly. Exercise triggers an increase in the number of new cells in the hippocampus, which is ground zero for making new memories. People who continue to stimulate themselves with new intellectual challenges have been shown to age more successfully.

TREATMENT: Learning to play a musical instrument, for example, helps engage the parts of the brain involved in detecting patterns. Read challenging books or learn a new language. Being in an environment with a lot of stimulation—new sights, smells, and tastes—nourishes the brain as well. The brain thrives on change, so you have to constantly throw new challenges at it.

—Julian R. Keith, Ph.D.,
director of neuroscience for Memory Assessment and Research Services, Wilmington, N.C.

A dietitian says:

To maximize your memory, maintain a balanced diet that includes healthy fats, plenty of fruits and vegetables, and whole grains. Inflammation may promote memory loss.

TREATMENT: Getting omega-3 fatty acids through salmon, walnuts and flaxseed helps brain cells reduce inflammation. Spices like turmeric and ginger also reduce inflammation—try cooking with the fresh or freeze-dried versions. B vitamins help the body use fatty acids, so make sure to eat B-rich foods like beans, and whole-grain bread and pasta. In mice studies, researchers have found that an antioxidant in green tea may protect memory. And in general, deeply colored fruits and vegetables like blueberries, beets, radishes and broccoli provide phytonutrients that may boost brain health.

—Dee Sandquist, M.S., R.D.,
spokeswoman for the American Dietetic Association

A naturopath says:

A top supplement is phosphatidyl-serine [PS], which helps keep cell membranes intact and enables cell communication, preserving memory. When researchers studied older individuals with dementia and Alzheimer's disease, they found diminished levels of the clinically beneficial fatty acid DHA in the patients' brains.

TREATMENT: I suggest 300 milligrams daily of PS, along with a daily omega-3 supplement, either fish oil or vegan. *Ginkgo biloba* is considered one of the best herbs for memory; it increases blood flow to the brain and acts as an antioxidant. Daily doses vary from 120 to 240 milligrams. The ayurvedic herb *Bacopa monniera* has been used for centuries to improve alertness, boost cognitive functioning, and sharpen memory. The standard dose is 200 to 400 milligrams daily. If you don't eat fish, consider supplementing your diet with 500 to 1,000 milligrams daily.

—Keri Marshall, N.D., M.S.,
spokeswoman for the American Association of Naturopathic Physicians

MENOPAUSE/ PERIMENOPAUSE

Want to *not* be the cool kid at your next party? Say the word "menopause." Hot flashes, night sweats, vaginal lubrication, cooling off in front of the fridge, "The Change," "The Big M." Yeesh. Menopause makes *you* feel vulnerable—and reminds everyone else that they can't stay young forever. No one wins.

But guess what: If you're a woman (or love one), menopause could be coming up faster than you think. Now's the time to prepare your body, with the exercise and supplements you need to face it with grace. And maybe in the process, we can destigmatize the whole thing. Because somehow, Helen Mirren and Meryl Streep got through it, and you'd party with them, right?

SYMPTOMS

Menopause isn't officially reached until you haven't had a period for an entire year, and when you get there is largely determined by the one thing in this chapter you can't control: genetics. For most women it tends to hit closer to the mid- to late-40s. (About two million women each year reach menopause—that's 6,000 every day.) But many woman start seeing symptoms of perimenopause—the five- to twelve-year transition that leads up to menopause—as early as their 30s.

Wait, five to twelve *years*? Yes, your hormones can go haywire for that long, thanks to fluctuating estrogen levels. Erratic periods are usually the first sign of perimenopause, says gynecologist Sara Gottfried, M.D., founder of saragottfriedmd.com, a virtual integrative medicine practice based in Berkeley, Calif. They can get closer together or farther apart, heavier or lighter, longer or shorter.

According to a 2010 study published in the *Journal of Mid-Life Health,* 20% of women in perimenopause report severe symptoms; 60%, mild symptoms; and 20%, no symptoms. "Your ovaries are making less progesterone, a hormone that calms the nervous system," says Gottfried, "so you may become more irritable or anxious, and see your PMS go from bad to worse."

And yet, "You can actually sail through this transition," says Christiane Northrup, M.D., author of *The Wisdom of Menopause.* "And if you enter menopause in optimal health, your symptoms will not be as severe or you may not even experience any at all." It all comes down to paying attention to certain health and lifestyle habits that make good sense no matter how young (or old) you are.

REMEDIES

Given the uncertainly of hormone therapy—and the high price of health care—natural remedies are more relevant than ever. So instead of reaching for Advil, Ambien or Paxil to treat hot flashes, cramps, insomnia and other symptoms, try the techniques below. "Treating yourself with lifestyle and home remedies is the easiest, least invasive and some times the most effective treatment," says Rosemary Gladstar, founder of Sage Mountain Herb Center in Barre, Vt., and author of the classic *Herbal Healing for Women.*

Strengthen Your Adrenals

Stress. You don't outgrow it, so there's no stopping the constant flood of the fight-or-flight stress hormone cortisol, which depletes the adrenal glands. This can make fatigue, brain fog and hot flashes particularly bad during perimenopause, says Susan Doughty, A.P.R.N.-C.N.P., an OB-GYN nurse practitioner and cofounder of New England WomenCenter in Portland, Me. "That's because when estrogen levels dip, the adrenals increase cortisol production," she says. Basically, you're getting a double whammy of the stress hormone during the transition to menopause. Also, cortisol levels are normally highest in the morning, then drop throughout the day. "But in perimenopause, cortisol stays elevated, so falling and staying asleep become difficult," Doughty says.

ACTION PLAN: Ease stress, reduce cortisol production and facilitate sleep with relaxation techniques such as meditation, breathing exercises, yoga, tai chi or massage, Doughty advises. We all know that cardio can also alleviate stress, but don't overdo it: "Pushing yourself so hard that you're left feeling depleted can weaken your adrenals even further," Northrup says.

Holly Lucille, N.D., a naturopathic doctor in West Hollywood, Calif., also advises patients to support exhausted adrenals with adaptogenic (aka stress-busting) herbs such as licorice root, ashwagandha and rhodiola. Try Gaia Herbs Adrenal Health ($30 for 60 capsules; gaiaherbs.com).

Cut Out White Foods

Wonder Bread, not wonderful. Northrup notes that foods high in simple carbohydrates, such as white flour, pasta, bread and rice, as well as sweets and processed foods, raise cortisol levels. As noted above, this can exacerbate perimenopause symptoms, including exhaustion, mental fogginess and hot flashes. Eating too many of them also spikes blood sugar, which can lead to cravings and overeating; the resulting weight gain makes certain symptoms worse (see "3 Perimenopause Pointers" on page 181).

ACTION PLAN: Choose carbohydrates in their whole-food form such as vegetables and whole grains over white-flour pasta, crackers and cookies, and include quality proteins and healthy fats at each meal, advises dietitian Ashley Koff, R.D. "Eating flaxseeds, which are high in omega-3 fatty acids, and cruciferous vegetables helps your body metabolize estrogen, which will balance its fluctuating levels," she adds. Other good omega-3 sources include wild salmon, hemp or chia seeds, and walnuts. A 2011 study in the journal *Menopause* reported that omega-3s decreased depression, hot flashes, brain fog, vaginal dryness and night sweats in women approaching menopause.

Think About Your Thyroid

During perimenopause, estrogen that's not counterbalanced by progesterone can slow the production of thyroid hormone, triggering weight gain, fatigue, depression, mental fogginess and other symptoms.

In fact, about 25% of women discover they have low thyroid, or hypothyroidism, during perimenopause.

ACTION PLAN: Have your thyroid hormone levels tested by an endocrinologist or naturopathic physician, Northrup advises. Low levels are easily remedied with thyroid medication.

Embrace "The Change"

"If a woman believes she will have a difficult time [with menopause], it can become a self-fulfilling prophecy," notes Doughty. Indeed, according to a 2011 study published in *Clinical and Experimental Obstetrics & Gynecology,* menopausal women who exhibited negative attitudes about entering menopause experienced more severe symptoms.

ACTION PLAN: Northrup suggests looking at perimenopause as an opportunity to make positive changes by dealing with issues and problems you may have been ignoring for years. "At perimenopause, you come to a crossroads in your life where you have to choose between one path that says 'grow' and the other that says 'stagnate,'" she says. As such, it's often an ideal time to assess things like your career, relationships or general health and well-being and take proactive steps toward self-improvement. She also advises seeking the guidance and support of women you know who are thriving after menopause.

If the prospect of menopause is really taking a psychological toll, try working with a therapist who specializes in cognitive behavioral therapy (CBT), advises Marianne Brandon, Ph.D., a clinical psychologist in the Washington, D.C., area. "CBT retrains your brain to let go of anxiety and self-defeating thoughts and subsequent reactions," she says.

Beware of the Pregnant Pause

Sometimes a missed period or two means pregnancy, not perimenopause. If you don't want to have a baby, continue using birth control until you haven't menstruated for a full year. While fertility is greatly reduced during perimenopause, a "surprise" pregnancy is possible as long as you're still ovulating.

Try Supplements

While healthy lifestyle changes will likely lessen the severity of peri-menopause symptoms, you may still experience them to some degree. If any of the following hit, try the corresponding natural remedies.

HOT FLASHES/NIGHT SWEATS

Solution: Sage (*Salvia officinalis*)

"Sage has been passed down from generation to generation in Western herbal tradition as the surefire cure for hot flashes," explains Sheila Kingsbury, N.D., of Bastyr University in Kenmore, Wash. It's such an effective astringent that it has been approved in Germany as a treatment for excessive sweating for both women and men. "Sage was also used in Native American cultures to clear negative energy so it may help ease some of the irrational fears that can cycle through your head during perimenopause," says herbalist Margi Flint, author of *The Practicing Herbalist*.

DOSAGE: Steep one tablespoon dried sage in one cup of hot water for 15 minutes or longer to make a tea; strain and cool. Drink up to three cups a day. If you don't like the taste, put the tea into a spray bottle (after it has cooled completely) and spritz it on your neck.

Also, the black cohosh in Remifemin has been found to reduce hot flashes, night sweats, mood swings and irritability by 70%.

DOSAGE: Lucille 20 milligrams twice a day for 12 weeks

TRY: Remifemin ($20 for 60 tablets; remifemin.com)

And omega-3 fatty acids have also been found to lower the frequency of hot flashes.

DOSAGE: 1 tablespoon daily

TRY: Spectrum Essentials Organic Flax Oil with Cinnamon, a blood-sugar stabilizer ($10 for 8 ounces; amazon.com)

HEAVY PERIODS

Solution: Yarrow (*Achillea millefolium*)

Yarrow is the go-to herb for menstrual bleeding, says Gladstar. "It slows excessive bleeding, relieves pelvic congestion, reduces cramping and flushes out the liver so estrogen and progesterone are processed more efficiently," she says.

DOSAGE: Two droppers of tincture every 30 minutes until bleeding slows

TRY: HerbPharm Yarrow ($33 for 4 ounces; amazon.com)

INSOMNIA

Solution: Valerian (*Valeriana officinalis*)

Many studies have affirmed the safety and efficacy of valerian for treating garden-variety insomnia—a common problem during perimenopause. "It works in the same way that Valium or Xanax do, but the effect is much milder. There is no hangover afterward nor any risk of addiction," says Kingsbury. There's just one catch: "It's a reliable sedative for most people, but a small percentage will get jazzed up instead," she cautions.

DOSAGE: Two 500-milligram capsules one hour before bedtime as needed

TRY: Nature's Way Valerian ($11 for 90 capsules; vitamanshoppe.com)

CONTRAINDICATION: Do not take valerian if you're taking prescription sleep aids.

FATIGUE

Solution: Ashwagandha (*Withania somnifera*)

In ayurvedic tradition, ashwagandha is the great revitalizer, says ayurvedic practitioner Will Foster of Knoxville, Tenn. "It's an adaptogen that helps balance out scattered energy, which means that when stress or hormonal changes leave you feeling drained, ashwagandha can help fill up your tank." The herb means "smell of horse," a deliberate nod to the strength and vitality of horses, says Foster. "Take ashwagandha when you need to boost your horsepower." It also may boost libido.

DOSAGE: Two 500-milligram capsules two times every day

TRY: Putian's Pride Ashwagandha Standardized Extract ($12 for 60 capsules; puritan.com)

BRAIN FOG

Solution: Water hyssop (*Bacopa monnieri*)

Used in Western European, Chinese and Indian herbal traditions, water hyssop is called *brahmi* in Sanskrit, which means "consciousness." It can help if you feel particularly distracted before or during your period; it's also good for everyday focus. "*Bacopa monnieri* can sharpen concentration, memory and overall intelligence, and it also improves longevity," says Foster. "Its ability to improve mental performance [by enhancing nerve impulses between cells in the brain] has been documented in multiple studies in the United States and abroad."

DOSAGE: One 500-milligram capsule twice daily. Foster suggests starting off slowly—perhaps with a 100-milligram dose twice per day—and increasing the dosage in 100-milligram increments up to the recommended 1,000 milligrams a day. "If the herb makes you feel spacey [or increases existing feelings of spaciness], contact your ayurvedic practitioner for guidance on dosing," he advises.

TRY: Nature's Answer Hyssop Herb ($6 for 90 capsules; iherb.com)

Also, several studies have found that omega-3 fatty acids improve memory and cognitive functioning in older adults.

DOSAGE: 1,000 milligrams of fish oil supplements daily

TRY: New Chapter Wholemega Whole Fish Oil ($9 for 30 softgels; amazon.com)

MOODINESS, IRRITABILITY, BLOATING

Solution: Magnesium and calcium

DOSAGE: Experts recommend a combination of magnesium (150 to 300 milligrams daily) and calcium (500 to 600 milligrams twice per day).

TRY: Natural Vitality Natural Calm Magnesium Plus Calcium, Raspberry-Lemon Flavor ($16 for 30 packets; drugstore.com)

LOW SEX DRIVE

Solution: Peruvian maca root

Studies have found that Peruvian maca root can increase sex drive as well as ease anxiety.

DOSAGE: 500 to 1,000 milligrams daily

TRY: Navitas Naturals Raw Maca Powder ($25 for 16 ounces; navitasnaturals.com)

VAGINAL DRYNESS

Solution: Kudzu

Studies show that *Pueraria mirifica*, or Thai kudzu, exhibits an estrogen-like effect that boosts vaginal elasticity and lubrication, similar to hormone replacement therapy.

DOSAGE: Follow package recommendations.

TRY: Solgar PM PhytoGen Complex ($17 for 60 tablets; amazon.com)

3 Perimenopause Pointers

Here's some additional advice that can make the "Big M" feel smaller

1.
Maintain a Healthy Weight

Women who are overweight are more likely to suffer more hot flashes during perimenopause than women with a body mass index of less than 25, according to a study published in *Obstetrics & Gynecology*. "When women are out of balance in their life, stressed, not sleeping, not exercising and not eating well, they tend to gain weight as a stress response," notes Shelley Wroth, M.D., an integrative medicine physician and assistant professor of obstetrics and gynecology at Duke University in Durham, N.C. "This can lead to a vicious cycle with perimenopausal symptoms, as women produce more estrogen if they have higher levels of body fat. But being physically active, having a relaxation practice and eating an anti-inflammatory diet are all known to improve the perimenopausal transition."

2.
Stick with Exercise

A new Finnish study of women ages 45 to 63, all of whom were experiencing menopause symptoms, found that those who walked and did other forms of aerobic exercise for 50 minutes a day, four days a week for 24 weeks reported reduced mood swings, irritability and night sweats.

3.
Limit the Booze

"Besides contributing to weight gain, alcohol spikes blood sugar, boosts cortisol, increases hot flashes, contributes to depression and ups breast cancer risk," says Christiane Northrup, M.D. "It also causes an almost immediate imbalance of too much estrogen relative to progesterone."

MIGRAINE

More than 36 million Americans suffer from painful, disorienting headaches known as migraines, their days hijacked by a blinding, full-body assault. Worse, they hit when you least expect them. A storm moves in? So does a migraine. Miley too loud? Throbbing agony. A period due? A stressful presentation? Ted from sales wearing Drakkar Noir? Here comes the boom. "I'd never heard of them before," tennis champ Serena Williams once said about menstrual migraines, which cost her a first-round match. "They were really splitting headaches. Mine went from the left to the right side of my head... and I couldn't focus. I was so dizzy and nauseated, and I was really tired."

SYMPTOMS

Left untreated, migraines typically last from four to 72 hours and can be accompanied by neck pain and nausea, followed by exhaustion. And episodes can strike two to eight times per month (or more), according to the National Headache Foundation. While the tendency runs in families, the exact cause of migraines, which affects more women than men, is unknown. One theory says migraines are kick-started by abnormally low levels of serotonin, a brain neurotransmitter that regulates pain perception.

"Think of your migraine as a wave," says Carolyn Bernstein, M.D., assistant professor of neurology at Harvard Medical School in Boston. "When one hits, it sets off a cascade of cellular events throughout the brain, triggering responses that may differ from a regular headache. For some people, it's nausea; for others, it's pain in the face or jaw."

And that wave is more like a tsunami: Headaches are the number two cause of disability in the United States and one of the top causes for the loss of workplace productivity. More than 18% of women and 8% of men between the ages of 18 and 55 will suffer from what is technically defined as a migraine, and it's likely that still more suffer from a milder set of symptoms.

REMEDIES

The key to stopping them may involve a bit of *Minority Report* detective work: trying to prevent a crime before it starts. Here's how to plan your anti-migraine strategy:

TRIGGER HAPPY

Your first step is to be familiar with the list of possible triggers. They include—but aren't limited to—barometric pressure changes, too much or too little sleep, stress, bright sunlight, intense heat or cold, muscular tension, hormonal shifts, loud noises, chemical odors or perfumes, over-exertion and a broad range of foods that includes aged cheese, chocolate, caffeine, canned foods, artificial sweeteners, MSG, red wine, beer and processed foods of all sorts.

KNOW YOUR SYMPTOMS

Next is recognizing your personal symptoms. A lucky few will be able to identify one or two triggers. For most, it's not so clear. Common symptoms include auras—bright, wavy lines of light or blind spots in your vision—vomiting, widespread muscle pain, dizziness, ringing in the ears, even partial paralysis. Others may include numbness or tingling in the extremities, extreme drowsiness or sudden irritability preceding a full-blown attack.

GET READY

The third part of the migraine solution is arming for battle with an arsenal of natural weapons, says Bernstein. Common cures that may assuage certain symptoms include drinking hot water and tea to cleanse the lymph system, taking an antihistamine to relieve sinus pressure and immediately cutting the lights. Here are six integrative remedies to help you treat and prevent the pain.

NATURAL R$_x$
Tools to help you manage and treat headache pain

Researchers are starting to understand that opiates used to treat migraines should be a short-term solution only; scientists Julie Wieseler, Ph.D., and Linda Watkins, Ph.D., at the University of Colorado, Boulder, have found that the opioid pharmacotherapies often used to treat migraine pain, become less effective with repeated use. Try these first:

1. JOURNAL THE JANGLING

Only a lucky few will be able to pinpoint two or three definite signs that a monster migraine is coming on. "People don't realize how many symptoms they're already having," says Audrey Halpern, M.D., a holistic neurologist and founder of the Manhattan Center for Headache and Neurology in New York City.

Start a diary well before symptoms appear so you have a step-by-step plan for when pain hits. For example, Halpern urges sufferers to keep a daily food log leading up to a migraine or to journal headache patterns—anything to narrow down the trigger list. Be sure to jot down the dates of PMS, altitude sickness, work stressors and dietary fluctuations.

2. DETOX YOUR DIGESTIVE SYSTEM

According to ayurveda, India's traditional system of medicine, your digestion is a key factor in chronic headaches, so practitioners emphasize detoxification. "A migraine is a sign that the digestive system isn't removing waste effectively," says John Douillard, D.C., director of the LifeSpa Ayurvedic Retreat Center in Boulder, Colo. He likens the problem to a clogged drain. "If you have too much mucus in your intestinal tract, the drains can get clogged, which creates toxicity in the lymph, resulting in dilated blood vessels—or headache."

To lubricate the intestinal lining, drink tea with demulcent herbs—like slippery elm, marshmallow or licorice—every day, says Douillard. To clean your lymphatic system, take sips of hot water every 15 minutes for two weeks. Toxins that can be removed from the body with teas include caffeine, alcohol, smoke and food additives. Try Traditional Medicinals Throat Coat ($5.50 for 16 tea bags; traditionalmedicinals.com).

3. TAP YOUR TEMPLES

Ignited by muscular stress or biomechanical tension (repetitive stress from raking leaves or baling hay, for example), migraines may be minimized by touch therapy. A small study in the *American Journal of Public Health* found that regular massage greatly reduced the number and duration of migraines. Twice a week for a month, subjects received a 30-minute massage focusing on muscles in the back of the neck, base of the skull and cranium. Afterward, compared with a placebo group, the

Top Migraine Meds (when it's the only thing that works)

If natural solutions aren't working, consider a prescribed medication. "Medications are still the primary approach to effectively treating migraines," says Audrey Halpern, M.D. "Some medications actually treat the underlying disease, and some provide relief from the symptoms. For chronic sufferers, finding relief from pain is most important, so they can go about functioning."

Over-the-counter pain relievers help control mild migraines by inhibiting inflammation. These include aspirin and other nonsteroidal anti-inflammatory drugs like ibuprofen (Advil, Nuprin, Motrin, Medipren) and naproxen (Aleve). Many cause gastrointestinal distress and rebound headaches, warns Halpern.

PREVENTIVES Anti-seizure drugs like Topamax or Depakote, low-dose antidepressants, anti-nausea drugs, anti-inflammatories or heart medications can keep migraines at bay, but finding the right drug is hit-or-miss and side effects can include weight gain, foggy brain and hair loss.

ABORTIVES A class of drugs called triptans (such as Imitrex or Zomig) can halt a migraine in its tracks, but can cost $25 or more per dose.

RESCUERS Opiates (such as Percocet or Vicodin) or short-acting barbiturates (such as Fioricet) can bring short-term relief by masking pain, but may be habit-forming and can cause lightheadedness and other side effects.

massage patients reduced their average number of monthly migraines from seven to two; overall headache duration was halved from eight hours to four. A University of Miami Medical School study published in the *International Journal of Neuroscience* compared two groups of migraine sufferers; one who only took their meds for a month, the other who also got weekly massages; 60% of the massage group had no migraines for the entire month.

TRY AROMATHERAPY MASSAGE. If you're home and feel the warning indications, try combining self-massage with aromatherapy by sitting silently and calmly, says Laurie Binder, M.S., doctor of acupuncture and OB-GYN nurse practitioner. Massage your temples lightly with a few drops of lavender or rosemary essential oils with a carrier like sunflower oil. Lightly move your index fingers in slow, circular motions: Start at the center of your forehead at the hairline and proceed to the temples, then continue behind the ears and finally to the back of the neck. Aim for a minimum of 10 minutes, says Binder. Bodywork and craniosacral therapy massage also help you relax, improve blood flow and correct misalignments that contribute to headaches.

4. GET NEEDLED

Acupuncture—using needles to stimulate certain energy points on the body—may have the same effect as medications like Imitrex and other triptan, anti-migraine drugs. Both release chemicals that cause blood vessels to constrict, according to the American Association of Acupuncture and Oriental Medicine.

A German study published in *Cephalalgia* shows that people who suffer from chronic migraines may benefit from acupuncture to reduce the severity and frequency of headaches. Researchers from Charité University Medical Centre in Berlin followed more than 15,000 adults who had been suffering from either migraine or tension-type headaches at least twice a month for a year or more. Of these patients, 1,613 were assigned to receive acupuncture in 15 sessions over three months in addition to usual care, while 1,569 continued with only the usual care alone. Over six months, acupuncture patients reported significantly greater reductions in headache pain than those who continued with usual care. Headache frequency fell significantly in patients assigned to acupuncture over a three-month span: from 8.4 headache days per month at the start of the study to 4.7 headache days at the end.

TRY ACUPRESSURE. Do-it-yourself digital massage in a dark, quiet room works wonders for some, says Binder, who integrated acupuncture, massage and Traditional Chinese Medicine into a DVD called *Acupressure and Breathing for Childbirth.* To relieve head distress, press the hollow between the front and back neck muscles (just behind the ear at the base of the skull) on the side where the pain is occurring. Press for three minutes, stop for two minutes, then repeat three to five times in a row.

5. CULTIVATE CALMNESS

While directing his first feature film, Ben Affleck was hospitalized with a migraine. "I hardly slept," he said. Stress makes everything worse, says James Gordon, M.D., founder of The Center for Mind-Body Medicine in Washington, D.C. According to Gordon, when you're worried or strained, you're much more likely to suffer migraines, and your hands will grow cold and your heart will beat faster. Consider a few gentle yoga postures to increase your body temperature and decrease your blood pressure and muscle tension, too. "Since stress is such a major contributor to migraines, anything that promotes relaxation is beneficial," says yoga instructor Luciana LoPresto, L.M.T., based in Southern California. "Ease into your gentler yoga poses and do not jump right into poses that may cause strain or trigger an attack."

She suggests doing restorative postures to quiet the nervous system. Keep your head above the heart for most of the poses if the headache is just beginning, she urges. "Keep blood flowing away from the head to reduce pressure that may cause a migraine." Restorative yoga poses such as Savasana, or any comfortable, cross-legged pose, are appropriate. When all else fails, says LoPresto, who suffered migraines after a concussion, try the "Legs up the Wall" pose:

HOW TO DO IT: Lie with legs and tailbone leaning against the wall, your sacrum flat on the floor. Straighten your legs up onto the wall with your shoulders and head also on the floor. Extend your legs straight up the wall and keep your shoulder blades flat on the floor. Rest your arms out to your sides on the floor comfortably, close your eyes and breathe deeply for 10 minutes.

6. HERBAL ESSENCE

One of the best long-term natural strategies is taking supplements to lessen the frequency and severity of migraines. "Most natural strategies that ease migraines can take several weeks or months to show results, so many supplements are unfortunately abandoned prematurely," says Stuart Stark, M.D., medical director of the Neurology & Headache Treatment Center in McLean, Va.

MAGNESIUM: This simple mineral has muscle-relaxing properties and may stave off a migraine by preventing blood vessel spasms, notes Maureen Williams, N.D., a naturopath in private practice in Victoria, B.C.

RESEARCH: In a study published in *Cephalalgia,* patients who took magnesium every day for 12 weeks reported significantly fewer migraine attacks (versus those taking a placebo) after only nine weeks.

DOSAGE: 600 milligrams a day, according to the *Cephalalgia* study

BUTTERBUR: The herb butterbur stabilizes the cells that produce histamine, so it's a good choice for those who also suffer from allergies. Look for products such as Petadolex (migraineaid.com) that are free of pyrrolizidine alkaloids (potentially toxic compounds).

RESEARCH: The herb was shown to significantly reduce migraine frequency in some people, according to the journal *Neurology.*

DOSAGE: 100 milligrams, three to four times a day

FEVERFEW: This herb may work by inhibiting inflammation and stabilizing substance P, the neurotransmitter responsible for the pain response.

RESEARCH: Clinical studies are inconclusive but feverfew has been used as a migraine treatment in folk medicine.

DOSAGE: 100 milligrams, three times a day

COENZYME Q10: It's not clear exactly how the vitamin-like substance known as CoQ10 works, though it might improve the brain's ability to metabolize glucose, Halpern says.

RESEARCH: A study published in the journal *Neurology* found that CoQ10 could reduce migraine frequency by up to 50%.

DOSAGE: 100 milligrams, three times a day

How can I ease motion sickness?

Don't let your Bond-like adventures upset your stomach.

An acupressurist says:

You can experience motion sickness when traveling by water, land or air. When the balance mechanism in your ears tells your brain that you're moving, but your eyes tell your brain that you're stationary, it can result in feelings of nausea.

TREATMENT: If you know you're going to be traveling on a windy road or choppy waters, there's an acupressure point you can press several times an hour before—and many times during—your trip. To find it, draw a line from the middle of your palm down to the center of the inside of your arm; it's three of your own finger-widths below the wrist crease. Place your thumb on the point between your two arm bones and press gradually and firmly; maintain that firm pressure for two to three minutes while taking slow deep breaths. This will start to calm you down and soothe your stomach. Wait one minute and repeat if you continue to feel dizzy.

—Michael Reed Gach, Ph.D.,
author of Acupressure's
Potent Points *and director of*
acupressure.com

An otolaryngologist says:

Motion sickness occurs when the vestibular nerve—which transmits sound and balance information from the inner ear to the brain—senses movement even though the body is still. The brain gets confused by the differing input from the vestibular nerve, the eyes and the rest of the body, resulting in the sensation of nausea.

TREATMENT: If you're on a boat, focusing on the horizon can help because the eyes are able to reassure the brain, "Hey, I'm not really moving." Over-the-counter medications, such as Benadryl and Dramamine (scopolamine) can also be soothing and sedating. These treatments won't directly relieve nausea, per se, but they will slow down the brain and keep it from sensing the signals that trigger nausea. A scopolamine patch placed on the skin behind the ear can also aid in preventing nausea. Eating licorice root or peppermint can help settle the stomach, too.

—Christina M. McAlphin, M.D.,
otolaryngologist at California
Medical Center in Los Angeles

How can I relieve my osteoarthritis pain?

You can treat this common degenerative joint disease naturally—with omega-6s, vitamin D and yoga.

A naturopath says:

Motion sickness is caused by the brain trying to interpret two different signals coming from your eyes and ears. The varying messages trigger feelings of nausea.

THE TREATMENT: If you're prone to motion sickness, take 250 to 500 milligrams of ginger 10 to 20 minutes before your trip. It's really potent in capsule form but you can also chew on a fresh piece. If symptoms continue, take 500 to 1,000 milligrams of ginger every four hours. In one study, ginger worked just as well as Dramamine, but without the common side effects that can include dry mouth and blurred vision. There are two homeopathic remedies that can stop nausea associated with motion sickness: ipecacuanha and tabacum. Adults in good health should take a 200c to 1M dose, one to three times a day, and only when experiencing symptoms of nausea. The formulations available in health food stores don't offer the strongest dosage, so you may want to get these products from a homeopath or naturopath.

—Keith F. Zeitlin, N.D.,
Wallingford, Conn.-based naturopathic physician

A dietitian says:

Osteoarthritis, often referred to as "wear and tear" arthritis (when the breakdown of joint cartilage causes the bones to rub together), is an inflammatory disease, so eating foods known to quiet inflammation—and skipping foods that tend to fan the fire—delivers results for many patients.

TREATMENT: A Mediterranean diet (high in vegetables and fruits, with a moderate amount of whole grains, nuts, seeds and fish) is a good model for an anti-inflammatory approach to eating. Overall, you want to avoid processed foods and make sure you get more omega-3s (healthy fats found in oily fish and flaxseed) than omega-6s (pro-inflammatory fats found in animal products). If you are gluten-intolerant, exposure to foods with gluten, such as wheat and rye, may promote inflammation.

Antioxidants can fight inflammation, so eat one or two servings of dark leafy green vegetables (like kale and spinach) and drink 2 ounces of tart cherry juice a day to help tame osteoarthritis symptoms. In general, though, there are no magic foods— it's the synergy of all the nutrients you get from a whole-foods-based diet that can really have a powerful effect when it comes to osteoarthritis management.

—Sheila Dean, DSc, R.D.,
medical nutritionist in private practice and adjunct nutrition science professor at the University of Tampa in Florida

A *physician says:*

If you're taking nonsteroidal anti-inflammatory drugs (NSAIDs) to deal with your osteoarthritis symptoms, you may be able to control your symptoms—but you're still losing cartilage. By using certain dietary supplements, you can alleviate pain, restore cartilage and curb the inflammation associated with osteoarthritis.

TREATMENT: Natural substances found in healthy cartilage, glucosamine (taken at 1,500 to 3,000 milligrams a day) and chondroitin sulfate (800 to 1,200 milligrams a day) are the supplements with the strongest scientific evidence of effectiveness in treating osteoarthritis. Another solid choice is avocado-soybean unsaponifiables (300 milligrams a day), an avocado-and-soybean-based supplement prescribed for osteoarthritis in France (but only sold as a supplement in the U.S.). Also, make sure to get 2,000 IU of vitamin D daily, because studies show that people with the lowest vitamin D levels have the highest incidence of osteo-arthritis.

When buying supplements, choose ones with the recommended dose of each extract (rather than going with a manufacturer that just sprinkles in small amounts and calls them "complexes"). Give each supplement three to four months to take effect.

—Jason Theodosakis, M.D.,
coauthor of The Arthritis Cure

ASK THE EXPERTS

Q

A yoga therapist says:

Physical activity will strengthen the muscles that support the affected joints, and it also keeps up your mobility and helps prevent weight gain (known to exacerbate osteoarthritis). Yoga may be particularly valuable for people with osteoarthritis, because it reduces stress and often helps patients cope better with their pain.

TREATMENT: Find a physical activity that's easy on your joints, such as swimming, walking or yoga. If you're interested in yoga and have your doctor's OK, call a few studios and ask them to suggest classes that are gentle and appropriate for someone with arthritis. An experienced yoga teacher will be able to help make sure you stay in proper alignment during your practice so you don't injure yourself.

When you get to class, let your instructor know about your osteoarthritis, and stop right away if you feel any pain during a particular pose. Aim for at least three sessions a week, as long as you're not experiencing any joint aggravation.

While the benefits of specific poses vary from patient to patient, Chair pose may be especially helpful for people with osteoarthritis of the knee (the most common type of arthritis): It's great for strengthening the quadriceps (which surround and support the knee), and it can be done with as much or as little knee-bending as feels comfortable for the patient.

—Steffany Haaz, Ph.D.,
registered yoga therapist and health behaviorist currently working with the NIH on investigating the effect of a yoga intervention for underserved individuals with rheumatoid arthritis or osteoarthritis

OSTEOPOROSIS

Everyone's favorite Flying Nun, Sally Field, makes it seem so curable, in those everywhere-commercials for Boniva: After a certain age, your bones need help. They get weaker, and you're at risk for osteoporosis (literally, porous bones); Field herself has it. And after one year on a once-monthly drug (like Boniva, or Fosamax, or Actonel), nine out of 10 women reversed their bone loss, and so can you. Thank goodness, you think: I'll wait till I'm old and pop the pill.

But mounting evidence suggests that taking these kinds of bisphosphonate drugs—until recently considered the holy grail for preventing and treating osteoporosis—longer than five years might actually weaken your bones and *cause* spontaneous fractures, as well as digestive problems. Also, dairy foods are no longer considered the panacea they once were: Study after study shows no decrease in fracture risk with higher consumption. And calcium supplements alone are also losing their status as a cure-all.

The better fix may be to prevent osteoporosis altogether: It's never too late—or too early—to adopt simple lifestyle changes that will strengthen your skeleton and help delay bone breakdown. "How your bones land at post-menopause is hugely dependent on how you take care of your body while you're of childbearing age," explains Amy J. Lanou, Ph.D., senior nutrition scientist for the nonprofit Physicians Committee for Responsible Medicine and coauthor of *Building Bone Vitality*. "Just as with heart disease or type 2 diabetes, it's the daily insults that accumulate over the years into osteoporosis."

SYMPTOMS

It's easy to ignore your bones when you're young, feeling strong and dancing to "Push It" at bachelorette parties. But consider this, Soul Train: Osteoporosis hinges on how much bone mass you accrue in your teens, 20s and early 30s and how quickly you lose it later on, both factors you have some control over.

Bones are living material, constantly building and breaking down in a process called remodeling; physiologists estimate we create 11 skeletons over the course of our lifetime. When we're young, we form new bone faster than we lose old bone, achieving peak density around age 25 to 30, at which point we begin to lose slightly more than we gain. The loss rapidly speeds up post-menopause, when estrogen levels drop sharply (estrogen helps lay down new bone). Half of American women older than 50 will fracture a hip, wrist or vertebra due to weakened bones, and one in five will develop full-blown osteoporosis.

REMEDIES

If you've already been diagnosed with osteoporosis or have several risk factors, it's time to seek medical attention. If not, start building wealth in your bone bank by making frequent deposits based on this expert advice from integrative health experts.

The better-bones diet

AVOID CALCIUM OVERLOAD: Official recommendations encourage women between the ages of 19 and 50 to get 1,000 milligrams of calcium a day and women older than 50 to get 1,200 milligrams. Lanou suggests lowering that to 500 to 800 milligrams, preferably from dairy-free food sources (see below). Lanou explains that a higher calcium intake is unnecessary and, if it comes from supplemental sources, may cause constipation and negatively impact the absorption, production or metabolism of other nutrients. A large Swedish study reported in 2011 in the *British Medical Journal* found that for the average woman, 700 to 800 milligrams of calcium a day is the range beyond which it appears to stop increasing bone density. Recent studies have also linked calcium supplementation of 1,000 milligrams a day and above with increased cardiovascular disease risk in women, and some experts believe that too much calcium can actually make bones brittle.

DON'T DEPEND ON DAIRY: Dairy foods—cheese and ice cream in particular—are highly acidic, but the body prefers a more balanced and slightly alkaline pH; to neutralize the acidity, your body pulls calcium from the bones. Lanou points out that hip fracture rates are highest where calcium intake from dairy foods is highest, including in the U.S. and Northern European countries. Better calcium sources include leafy green vegetables, broccoli, almonds, beans and sesame seeds.

"If you were building a wall, calcium is the bricks, but vitamin D, magnesium and more than a dozen other nutrients are the mortar," Lanou says. An ounce of almonds, a cup of raw kale and a can of salmon (with bones), eaten throughout the day to maximize absorption, will give you 800 milligrams of calcium along with those and other bone-building nutrients.

PILE ON THE PRODUCE: Cultivating a bone-friendly diet also means limiting acidic meat, sugar, sodas, alcohol and packaged products while eating more alkaline foods like fruits and vegetables. Shoot for six to nine daily servings. Calcium is best absorbed from Brussels sprouts, kale, broccoli, and turnip and mustard greens (51% to 64% absorption),

Sticks and Stones

...may break your bones, but these risk factors can *really* hurt you.
- **FEMALE**
- **WHITE OR ASIAN** (black women have heavier bones)
- **PETITE FRAME** (smaller women start out with less bone)
- **LOW WEIGHT OR BMI** < 20 (the thinner you are, the less weight your bones are forced to bear)
- **FAMILY HISTORY** of osteoporosis on your mother's side
- **LATE ONSET OF MENSTRUATION** (after age 15) or early menopause (before age 40); both are linked to fewer years with higher levels of circulating estrogen, which helps lay down bone
- **HISTORY OF AN EATING DISORDER** or skipped periods due to low body fat
- **SMOKING,** past or current
- **ALCOHOL USE** (more than / ounces per week)
- **CERTAIN HEALTH PROBLEMS,** including type 1 diabetes and rheumatoid arthritis, and some medications, can also affect bone health. Celiac disease can inhibit absorption of calcium from the GI tract, and unregulated levels of thyroid hormone can increase bone breakdown. Other drugs that may predispose you to osteoporosis include blood-thinning and seizure medications, steroids like prednisone, acid reflux treatments like Prilosec and Nexium, and Depo-Provera birth control.

then supplements and dairy foods (around 30% each). Besides keeping your blood alkaline, you'll reap extra benefits from the other bone-building compounds in these foods, including magnesium, phosphorus and vitamin K.

SELECT THE RIGHT SOY: According to Beth Reardon, R.D., director of integrative nutrition at Duke Integrative Medicine in Durham, N.C., soy is probably more beneficial for bone building and/or slowing bone loss than for treating osteoporosis. She discourages taking soy supplements because they may impact cancer risk for women with certain tumor receptors and they don't contain the other nutrients and antioxidants found in whole soy foods. Instead, she advises choosing organic, non-GMO soy in the form of ¼ cup of dry roasted edamame or 3 ounces of tempeh daily; these are two of the least processed options and thus retain more health benefits.

STEER CLEAR OF SALT: Sodium increases calcium loss in urine; cap your intake at 2,300 milligrams a day (the equivalent of 1 teaspoon). If you're older than 51 or have high blood pressure, stick to less than 1,500 milligrams a day.

DIG THOSE DRIED PLUMS: A study published in the *British Journal of Nutrition* in 2011 found that women who ate about eight to 10 prunes a day had significantly higher bone mineral density in their forearms and spines, compared with those who ate dried apples. Prunes provide boron and potassium, two elements that help suppress the breakdown of bone.

CAP THE CAFFEINE: Coffee is acidic and caffeine impairs calcium absorption, so limit your intake to no more than two cups per day. Even better, switch to green tea: Reardon notes that it contains flavonoids that help inhibit bone breakdown.

Exercises for a stronger skeleton

GET ON YOUR FEET: Weight-bearing activities—from walking and running to jumping rope and dancing ("What Does the Fox Say"!)—are some of the most efficient ways to build bone density. "They place a higher load on your muscles, tendons and bones, which respond by getting stronger," explains Nicholas DiNubile, M.D., a clinical assistant professor of orthopedic surgery at the University of Pennsylvania.

Weightlessness explains why astronauts lose up to 30% of their bone mass in four to six months. And zero-impact activities like cycling and swimming don't build bone: One study found that competitive male cyclists actually had lower bone density than nonathletes.

PUMP IRON: Strength training is the best kind of weight-bearing exercise. "It gives you the best bang for your buck," DiNubile says. Be sure to log at least two weightlifting sessions per week, each lasting long enough (45 minutes to an hour) to target all of your major muscle groups and core. Moves that utilize your own body weight, like push-ups and lunges, work, too. In a University of Arizona study, women ages 44 to 66 were split into strength-training or nonstrength-training groups; everyone took calcium supplements. After one year, the nonstrength-training group lost .05% of their bone density, while the weightlifters increased theirs by 1% to 2%—and maintained that gain for four years.

TAKE UP TAI CHI: Several studies have demonstrated that tai chi slows bone loss. It's also been shown to decrease production of the inflammatory stress hormone cortisol, a steroid. "High levels of steroids over time can increase the risk of osteoporosis," says David Rakel, M.D., director of the University of Wisconsin-Madison School of Medicine and Public Health's Integrative Medicine Program.

MAXIMIZE EVERYDAY MOVES: Carry your belongings in a backpack (no more than 35 pounds) to load your spine. Take stairs rather than the elevator to strengthen your hips.

Boning up with supplements

CHOOSE THE RIGHT CALCIUM: If you're not getting 500 to 800 milligrams of calcium a day from foods, taking a supplement could be a good idea. But think of it as insurance, not your primary source. Reardon

Assess Yourself

The Fracture Risk Assessment Tool (FRAX) is a simple way to estimate your bone-fracture risk. Enter basic information like your age, height, weight and smoking status, and instantly learn your 10-year risk. Take the test at shef.ac.uk/frax.

suggests choosing a supplement that also includes vitamin K, potassium and boron.

TRY: Jarrow Ultra Bone Up ($32 for 120 tablets; drugstore.com). If you are older than 60, go with calcium citrate over calcium carbonate and take no more than 800 milligrams a day, split into two smaller doses to enhance absorption.

TRY: Pure Encapsulation Calcium Citrate ($18 for 180 capsules; pharmaca.com)

DON'T BE D-FICIENT: Calcium needs vitamin D, which is produced by the body when exposed to sunlight, to function properly. Unfortunately, our indoor lifestyles and sunscreen use have led to a mass D deficiency. Rakel suggests asking your doctor for a blood test (optimum results are 30 ng/mL or higher) and supplementing accordingly.

TRY: Source Naturals D-3 ($5 for 200 tablets; vitaminshoppe.com). Few foods provide vitamin D, but cod, sockeye salmon and UV-B light-boosted mushrooms (from Sun Bella) can help, says Rakel, who advises against relying too heavily on vitamin D-fortified dairy foods because many are high in saturated fat, contain hormones and promote inflammation.

MINERALIZE WITH MAGNESIUM: Legumes, nuts, whole grains and vegetables are rich in this element that enhances bone mineralization, but it can be hard to get all you need from food. Rakel recommends taking 400 to 800 milligrams a day of magnesium glycinate, which is less likely than other forms to cause side effects such as diarrhea. Take your calcium, which can interfere with magnesium absorption, in the morning; and your magnesium, which is a calming mineral, at night.

TRY: Solaray Magnesium Glycinate 400 ($24 for 180 tablets; affordablesolaray.com)

TRY STRONTIUM FOR STRONG BONES: Research presented at the 2011 European Congress on Osteoporosis and Osteoarthritis showed that strontium ranelate, a compound found in trace amounts throughout the skeleton, surpassed Fosamax in bone-forming activity. Other studies show that women who added strontium ranelate to their bone-building program slashed their risk of fracture by 49% in the first year. Its sister compound, strontium citrate, is currently available in the U.S.; Rakel suggests taking 2,000 milligrams a day.

TRY: Nature's Life Strontium ($14 for 60 tablets; iherb.com)

PAIN

If you experience chronic pain, you know how it can occupy your every thought, interfering with even the most mundane tasks, like showering or shopping or struggling through this simple sentence. Or, the opposite: You become so inured to the pain, it becomes just a part of you. The new you. The bitter, defeated, impatient, slightly on-edge you. The you people like less, including... you.

Point is, how you perceive pain is key—and promising research proves it. In a ground-breaking 2008 study, subjects watched their own MRI brain scans and experienced firsthand how learning to control specific brain centers caused the pain to calm down. "It's like turning down the amplifier on a stereo," says Sean Mackey, M.D., Ph.D., chief of the division of pain medicine at Stanford University. "The input is the same, but your experience of pain is turned down."

Ronald Glick, M.D., medical director at the Center for Integrative Medicine at the University of Pittsburgh Medical Center, agrees. "Pain is part of our fight-or-flight response, and mind-body approaches like paced breathing—which is commonly used during childbirth—slow down the heart, lower blood pressure and relax the response to pain." Leslie Davenport, M.S., M.F.T., a San Francisco-based integrative psychotherapist and author of *Healing and Transformation Through Self-Guided Imagery*, urges pain sufferers to adopt relaxing mind-body techniques. "You have nothing to lose but your pain," she says.

SYMPTOMS

More than 100 million Americans suffer chronic pain. Although this book has separate sections on migraines, arthritis, fibromyalgia, lower back pain and the like, this section deals with the discomfort associated with those conditions—the pain that doesn't dissipate after three, four or six months.

REMEDIES

You may have turned to over-the-counter or prescription analgesics—and faced relief, along with side effects like dry mouth, upset stomach and the risk of dependence and addiction. But there's another way—a drug-free path that relieves pain and requires only that your mind and body work together to help you take back your life.

Here, our experts share four cutting-edge techniques that can be used in lieu of medication or—if your doctor recommends it—in conjunction with a traditional medical approach.

1. Guided Imagery

These exercises can help alleviate all kinds of pain by recalibrating the mind, reminding us that the peace that exists outside of pain is still accessible, says Davenport. Advances in neuroscience also confirm that guided imagery can access the brain's "natural pharmacy," releasing opiate-like substances that reduce pain. A 2013 meta-analysis published in the journal *Pain* found that guided imagery was significantly effective for reducing pain, though researchers call for more studies. The practice also helps relax muscles and reduce stress.

"We know that if you're imagining something, your body reacts the same way as if it were actually happening." And while you can work with a certified imagery practitioner (go to academyforguidedimagery.com to find one), it's not necessary. "You can absolutely learn guided imagery on your own," says Davenport.

TRY IT:
1. Sit or lie comfortably. "The key is being a combination of relaxed and alert," says Davenport, who recommends using imagery when the pain is coming on, rather than when it is at peak intensity.
2. Allow an image to form of a relaxing, peaceful place, indoors or out. It might be an open field of flowers, a quiet room, a mountain or even a cloud. The important thing is that the image be a place that you personally find relaxing.
3. Fully engage all of your senses as you imagine this restful spot.

"Notice the sounds that are part of this environment," suggests Davenport. "Feel the temperature. Breathe in the aromas. Observe the quality of the light and the variety of colors." Not only does engaging the senses make the image more real and vivid, but it also engages the more intuitive right hemisphere of the brain, which increases relaxation.

4. Once you have fully imagined your environment, notice how you're feeling. One of Davenport's patients who suffered from fibromyalgia would imagine herself floating in the warm, salty waters of the Caribbean. She imagined the buoyancy of the water taking the pressure off her joints and the warm water providing relief from the constant ache that spread from her spine to her knees. This patient found that if she spent about 20 minutes "floating," she could then spend several hours pain-free. She would also often "float" into sleep at the end of the day.

5. Stay in this soothing place for at least 15 minutes, more if you can.

2. Moving Meditation

In a 2009 study published in *Psychosomatic Medicine*, scientists tested pain perception in a group of people who practiced Zen meditation regularly versus a group of nonmeditators. They found that those who meditated had a much lower sensitivity to pain, even while not meditating.

Because Zen meditation involves sitting still for long periods, it can be a challenge for beginners—especially beginners who are in pain. Instead, try moving meditation, which trains your mind to pay close attention to small movements, says Hugh Byrne, Ph.D., a meditation teacher in Silver Spring, Md. Because your attention is closely focused on the movements, your mind may become calmer, which helps to shift the experience of the pain, he says.

One of Byrne's students was a woman in her 60s in significant pain as the result of treatment for cancer. "At first she found the mindfulness meditation almost impossible because the pain was just too much," says Byrne. "Over time, through the practice of mindfulness meditation, she was able to open up more to her pain and not be so caught up in it. If she could stay with the actual sensations themselves—of pinching or throbbing or heat—she was able to see that some of her suffering came from her resistance to the experience."

TRY IT:
1. Stand with your feet hip-width apart, toes pointed forward, knees slightly bent, and hands relaxed at your sides. "Be aware of the sensations of standing on the ground, of your body breathing, of the weight on the legs," says Byrne.
2. Inhale and slowly raise your arms in front of you, parallel to each other with palms facing down.
3. Exhale while slowly moving your arms out to the sides of your body, then lowering them to the original position on an inhale.
4. Repeat movement for five to 10 minutes, noticing the sensations in your body each time.

3. Autogenic Training

Autogenic training involves speaking (and repeating) positive phrases while focusing on different parts of the body. "Saying these phrases creates images in the brain that stimulate the autonomic nervous system, which is associated with relaxation and a lowered heart rate," says James S. Gordon, M.D., founder and director of The Center for Mind-Body Medicine in Washington, D.C.

"It's really a form of self-hypnosis," Gordon adds. Autogenic training helps you relax into the pain instead of tensing against it, which is what we often do, he says, adding that being able to relax makes all the difference in the world. All the difference in the world. All the difference in the world.

TRY IT:
Sit or lie down quietly, close your eyes and repeat each of the following six phrases—slowly—six times:
1. My arms are warm and heavy. I am at peace.
2. My legs are warm and heavy. I am at peace.

3. My heartbeat is calm and regular. I am at peace.
4. My abdomen radiates warmth. I am at peace.
5. My forehead is cool. I am at peace.
6. My breathing is easy. I am at peace.

4. Soft Belly Breathing

Gordon also recommends soft belly breathing, which he has been using on himself and his patients for more than 40 years. In fact, one of his patients was able to undergo a surgical biopsy using soft belly breathing and forgoing anesthesia—not that Gordon recommended it. "She went into a very deep state of relaxation and was able to not experience the pain," says Gordon. "People have different capacities, but all of us can use these techniques to reduce pain."

TRY IT:
1. Sit in a comfortable chair surrounded by things you find peaceful.
2. Close your eyes.
3. Breathe in slowly through your nose, silently saying the word "soft" as you allow your belly to expand.
4. Breathe out slowly through your mouth, silently saying the word "belly." Relax on the exhale.
5. Bring your attention to the image and feeling of your belly as soft.
6. Do this for five to 10 minutes, once or twice a day.

How can I manage seasonal depression?

To quote Game of Thrones: *"Winter is Coming." Here's how to win the cold war.*

A *psychiatrist says:*

Seasonal affective disorder (SAD) is a form of depression that usually strikes in the fall or winter. Doctors believe people develop SAD when neuro-transmitters—especially the mood regulator serotonin and the "sleep hormone" melatonin—are disrupted by the lack of light, shorter days and cooler temperatures.

TREATMENT: Try phototherapy with a SunBox light box (sunbox.com) or another suitable brand that reaches a luminosity of 10,000 lux (equal in intensity to the sunlight on a clear spring morning) and filters out UV rays. Sit at arm's length from the box for 30 minutes each morning, facing it directly, but protecting your eyes by looking down or reading a book. Also, try walking in the early-morning light for a half hour every day. If symptoms persist, your doctor may recommend supplements such as vitamin D, or an antidepressant if SAD is severe.

—Ronald R. Parks, M.D.,
specialist in integrative psychiatry and medicine in Asheville, N.C.

An ayurvedic physician says:

In ayurveda, SAD is considered an imbalance of the vata dosha, one of the three physiological forces of the body. Dosha is aggravated by cold, dry and changing weather patterns. The imbalance peaks when the days are shortest; this disturbs the neurohormonal system of the body, causing melancholy and depression.

TREATMENT: Daily use of the ayurvedic herb *Bacopa monnieri* helps restore neurohormonal balance by improving concentration and alleviating anxiety. (Find it via the National Institute of Ayurvedic Medicine at niam.com.) Massaging sweet and spicy essential oils like cinnamon, sandalwood and jasmine above your eyebrows and at the crown of your head can also improve circulation of *prana*, or life energy, and brighten your outlook. Finally, try this meditation: Spend five quiet minutes each morning staring at and reflecting on the color gold. The vibration of the color is similar to natural light and can build stability, as its hue is a balance between fire and earth.

—Marc Halpern, D.C.,
*director of the California College of
Ayurveda in Cerritos, Calif., and
author of* Healing Your Life:
Lessons on the Path of Ayurveda

A homeopath says:

The symptoms of SAD vary from person to person and can occur in winter or summer, but generally are caused by your mood, metabolism and other bodily systems being affected by the change in season. While the condition is more prevalent in fall and winter when available light decreases, up to 2% of people may have symptoms of "reverse seasonal affective disorder" or "summer SAD" during spring and summer. These people usually live in hotter climates.

TREATMENT: If you're irritable and tend to isolate yourself from friends and family, try sepia, a remedy made from squid ink. (The standard dosage is 30C three times a day for two days.) If there's no improvement, try *Aurum metallicum*; also known as metallic gold, it can help to calm feelings of depression. Phosphorus is a good choice if you feel worse on cloudy days, while *Rhus tox*, made from poison ivy, relieves the back and joint stiffness often provoked by rain. And if you crave carbohydrates, especially chocolate, you may be deficient in magnesium—a mineral that's involved in the synthesis of serotonin. Take some *Magnesium phosphorica*; it can clear your cravings within days. Note that the key is to treat the dominant symptom—so you may have to change remedies frequently.

—Gayle Eversole, D.Hom.,
Ph.D., M.H., N.P., N.D.,
*founder of the Creating
Health Institute based in the
Pacific Northwest*

How can I treat sciatica?

The nerve pain is debilitating, but drugs and surgery aren't necessarily the best options.

A physical therapist says:

Sciatica is pain that radiates down your back, buttock and leg along your body's longest nerve, the sciatic nerve. Although it can be excruciating, most people who get physical therapy for sciatica can greatly reduce their pain.

TREATMENT: Making sure your sciatica isn't becoming a medical emergency is paramount; a small percentage of people develop cauda equina syndrome (marked by incontinence and numbness in the pelvic region), which requires surgery. But in general, physical therapists can work with you to find positions that can help reduce your pain, such as standing, bending backward, propping yourself on your elbows while on your stomach and sitting with a lumbar-support pillow. These positions, which maintain the natural curve in the lower back, are called "extension" movements, and many people find they help relieve sciatica pain. Bending forward, or "flexion," on the other hand, often aggravates pain; if that's the case, avoid slouching and activities in which you bend at the waist. During acute pain episodes, applying ice for 10 to 20 minutes can minimize inflammation. Studies have shown that staying active is more helpful in easing sciatica pain than bed rest (the reason for this is likely a combination of factors), so work on your endurance and strength (especially back and abdominal) to prevent recurrence.

—Deborah L. Givens, P.T., Ph.D., *orthopedic clinical specialist and director of physical therapy at Ohio State University*

A naturopath says:

It's important to first determine the underlying cause of sciatica symptoms, often a herniated disc or piriformis syndrome. A naturopath will take a history, perform a physical exam and musculoskeletal tests and may recommend consulting a physician. (An X-ray or MRI may be needed.) Then he or she might suggest dietary changes and supplements that can help reduce the inflammation that causes pain.

TREATMENT: Consider a couple of key supplements: magnesium citrate (350 milligrams to 400 milligrams daily) to reduce muscle spasms and 500 milligrams of the enzyme bromelain three times a day between meals to reduce inflammation (when you take bromelain between meals it has a systemic anti-inflammatory effect; this is different from its effect as a digestive enzyme). An anti-inflammatory diet can also help. Cut or limit processed and fried foods, sugar, omega-6 fatty acids (found in soy, sunflower, safflower and corn oils) and saturated fat; eat more veggies, fruits and omega-3-rich foods, such as wild salmon, sardines, walnuts, chia seeds and flax seed. Use ginger, turmeric and garlic liberally in your cooking—these all have powerful anti-inflammatory compounds. For acute pain, try a topical capsaicin cream.

—Cathy Wong, N.D., C.N.S.,
*a Boston-based naturopathic
doctor and certified nutrition
specialist, and the author of*
The Inside-Out Diet

A structural yoga therapist says:

Structural yoga therapists test your range of motion and muscle strength then create tailored pain-reduction programs that involve yoga postures, breathing and relaxation techniques.

TREATMENT: When sciatica pain is severe, stop what you're doing and rest for a week or two. Avoid stretching, especially your hamstrings, as this can aggravate your sciatica. After the pain eases, start a gentle yoga program, ideally restorative yoga, but continue to avoid hamstring stretches and focus on strengthening. A yoga therapist can illuminate how daily activities, stress and relationships can affect your pain. Whether you're working at a computer, doing yoga or arguing with your spouse, ask yourself, "Do I feel steady and comfortable?" If not, make changes until you do.

—Chinnamasta Stiles, R.N.,
*structural and ayurvedic yoga
therapist at the Yoga Therapy Center
in Novato, Calif.*

SEXUAL DYSFUNCTION

Female Sexual Dysfunction

Blame Christian Grey. The trend articles written in the wake of *Fifty Shades* made it sound like every housewife-next-door was chained to the bed, having mind-blowing orgasms. But the fantasy was just that: A Yale School of Medicine study discovered that, in fact, close to 50% of women in the United States are affected by female sexual dysfunction. Rather than getting whipped by a millionaire, they're getting whupped by FSD.

SYMPTOMS

FSD is an umbrella term that covers lack of desire, inability to become aroused or have orgasms, and painful sex. The issues frequently overlap, complicating the matter. For example, if you have trouble becoming aroused, you don't lubricate and then sex hurts. "And you can't be interested in sex if it's painful," says Cathy K. Naughton, M.D., director of the Metropolitan Urological Specialists Center for Sexual Health in St. Louis. "So it's a vicious cycle."

Some women, such as those for whom sex is painful because of certain physical conditions, may require the "big guns" of pharmaceuticals or surgery (see "Three Hidden Causes of Sex Problems" on page 210).

REMEDIES

But most women can find relief from the symptoms of the four most common causes of FSD by trying the natural solutions below. And don't worry, dudes: Although sexual dysfunction "hardly ever happens to me, I swear," we have fixes for you, too.

IF YOU HAVE...
A low libido

After Gail Smith (not her real name) had a hysterectomy at age 52, her desire for sex plummeted. "My husband and I previously had a very active and pleasurable sex life, and we were both devastated," she says. Prescription hormones provided little help. Finally, Smith's doctor suggested the problem was "all in her head." "I'm both a registered nurse and a psychologist. I know my body very well," Smith says. "This was not psychological. I could feel it."

While it's true that stress often causes loss of libido, hormone imbalances that result from antidepressant use, hysterectomy, hormonal birth control, pregnancy, perimenopause or menopause can also be culprits.

"The ovaries' production of hormones actually begins to change in our 30s," explains Genie James, M.M.Sc., executive director of The Natural Hormone Institute of America and coauthor with gynecologist and compounding pharmacist C.W. Randolph, Jr., M.D., of *In the Mood Again: Use the Power of Healthy Hormones to Reboot Your Sex Life—at Any Age*. Starting then, she says, "Progesterone drops 120 times faster than estrogen, and when estrogen is dominant, low libido is a frequent result." We still make testosterone, which helps fuel our sex drive, James adds, but we also make more sexual hormone-binding globulin (SHBG), which prevents it from circulating in the body.

APPLY NONPRESCRIPTION
PROGESTERONE CREAM

Those made with progesterone derived from soy and wild yam and converted into bioidentical progesterone can help mitigate estrogen dominance. Look for brands with 450 milligrams of USP (prescription-grade) progesterone per ounce. Two to try (they're rubbed into the skin) are Emerita Paraben-Free Pro-Gest ($29 for 2 ounces; emerita.com) and Natural Woman Progesterone Cream ($27 for 2 ounces; pronature.com).

Take Femmenessence MacaHarmony, a potent form of maca. The Peruvian root helps stimulate the hypothalamus, pituitary and adrenal glands to support and balance your hormones, including estrogen, progesterone and thyroid ($35 for a one-month supply; naturalhi.com).

TRY TRADITIONAL CHINESE MEDICINE (TCM)

Low libido can be a sign of kidney yang deficiency, says Jamie Koonce, L.Ac., D.O.M., of Phoenix, who recommends consulting a practitioner (find one at nccaom.org) and trying Passion Potion by Sage Solutions or Bu Zhong Yi Qi Tang Jia Wei by Blue Poppy Herbs

Three hidden causes of sex problems

1.
ANTIDEPRESSANTS AND OTHER DRUGS

Female sexual dysfunction symptoms are a common side effect of antidepressants such as Prozac, Paxil and Zoloft. Hormone-based contraceptives and blood pressure medications are other possible culprits. Women with diabetes or who have undergone chemotherapy also may tend to suffer from FSD.

2.
PSYCHOLOGICAL PROBLEMS

"Body issues are huge in female sexual dysfunction," says Cathy K. Naughton, M.D. In fact, studies have shown that societal emphasis on youth and slimness negatively impacts female sexual dysfunction even more than menopause.

3.
HYSTERECTOMY

If the uterus is removed, everything in the pelvis— bladder, small intestine, rectum—can become displaced, and with a partial hysterectomy the cervix can drop down into the vagina. "As you can imagine, that can all cause pain," Naughton says.

($17 for 90 caplets). Her home remedy suggestion is to add fresh lychee and durian fruit to your diet. Acupuncture can also successfully treat a low libido, says Koonce.

CONSIDER BIOIDENTICAL HORMONES

Gail Smith eventually found relief from a personalized regimen that included estrogen, testosterone and DHEA, a precursor to male and female sex hormones secreted by the adrenal glands. She experienced some results immediately, and within a year her sex drive was back to where it had been. "My husband and I are thrilled!" she says. Personalization is the key, according to James. Bioidentical hormones, which have the same molecular structure as naturally produced ones, can restore optimum balance but only when compounded for your particular hormone levels, she says. It's best to start by discussing bioidenticals with your OB-GYN, but if he/she is not familiar or comfortable with them, look for a center that specializes in them, make sure it's staffed with OB-GYNs, M.D.s and N.D.s.

GIVE AROMATHERAPY A SHOT

Aura Cacia Love Potion essential oil could get your juices flowing ($9 for 0.5 ounces; auracacia.com). The massage you get from your partner alone will give you a great start.

GET INTO THERAPY

If body-image or relationship issues have caused you to lose interest in sex, you might want to seek therapy alone or, better yet, with your partner. Find a qualified sex therapist by asking friends, if you have some that you can talk candidly with, or if you're already in marriage counseling, ask that therapist. If you can't find referrals, check the American Association of Sexuality Educators, Counselors and Therapists (aasect.org). Always check on a prospective sex therapist's education and credentials—he/she should have a Ph.D. or PsyC, a marriage and family or social workers license or a masters' in counseling, with a special certificate or training in sex counseling and, of course, lots of experience. Always book a five- to 10-minute interview first (and beware of a therapist who won't), and during your first face-to-face meeting, take a read: Can you relate to her? Do you feel comfortable enough that you can be completely honest, even if she doesn't look like Helen Hunt in *The Sessions*? Then you've got a good start.

IF YOU HAVE...
Difficulty getting aroused

Sometimes, the spirit is willing but the flesh would rather be playing Words with Friends. You try and try and yet your clitoris doesn't swell and become sensitized, and the lubrication never comes. This is the female equivalent of erectile dysfunction.

NATURAL R$_X$
TRY THE AMINO ACID L-ARGININE

Like Viagra, it produces nitric oxide, which helps relax muscles and widen blood vessels. In men, this leads to erections; and in women, to engorgement of the genital area. ArginMax for Women combines it with circulation-enhancing extracts of Korean ginseng, ginkgo and damiana ($25 for a one-month supply; arginmax.com). Dream Cream, an L-arginine-based topical lotion formulated by a doctor, also claims to improve sensation and arousal ($50 for 1 ounce; dreamcream.com).

PLAY AROUND WITH SEX TOYS

A number of manufacturers now produce safe and green versions. Look for those made from silicone (pleasuremenow.com), Pyrex glass (glassfantasy.com), stainless steel (njoytoys.com) or wood (nobessence .com). All can be easily washed, a must after every use. When in doubt about any device, use a condom on it.

SEEK INSPIRATION

Check out adult sex education DVDs (about $30 for a three-disc set; bettersex.com) or female-friendly erotica available at ellorascave.com. Don't be embarrassed: If you're willing to read *Fifty Shades* on the beach, this is your next step.

IF YOU HAVE...
Trouble achieving orgasm

Jennifer Justice, 34, of Doylestown, Pa., who suffered from interstitial cystitis (a painful inflammation of the bladder), also takes medications for vulva pain and chronic neck and back pain. When her soldier husband returned from a year in Afghanistan, she was dismayed to find that while she wanted sex and was able to get aroused, she was no longer able to have orgasms. For many other women, the problem stems less from a medical condition and more from a miscommunication with their partner or misinformation about how their own orgasms occur. Some natural remedies can help.

NATURAL R$_X$
MASSAGE DOWN BELOW

Zestra, a botanical arousal oil that increases warmth, sensitivity and sensation when topically applied to the vaginal area, worked for Justice, who says her ability to climax makes her feel "emotionally and physically better." ($50 for 12 individual packs; zestra.com)

GET HELP FROM EROS

Not the love god, but the NuGyn Eros Therapy device, a small gadget that draws blood to the clitoris, increasing sensation and orgasms. It's available by prescription, FDA approved and covered by some insurance plans ($400; eros-therapy.com).

EXPERIMENT SOLO OR TOGETHER

Masturbating or using a vibrator might help you find your orgasm triggers. "Some women only have orgasms with manual stimulation," says Naughton. See a sex therapist if you want to try to work the problem out together, or ask your partner to wield the sex toys or to touch you in ways and places that work for you.

IF YOU HAVE...
Pain during sex

This is perhaps the most complex FSD. There can be a psychological component in women who have been abused or had a painful first sexual experience, but just as often there's a medical or anatomical reason. The most common is dryness caused by atrophy of the vaginal tissues when estrogen levels drop during perimenopause or menopause. (Breastfeeding can also cause temporary dryness.) Other possible medical causes, says Naughton, are urinary tract or yeast infections, chronic vulva pain, constipation or hysterectomy.

Whatever the cause, once you experience pain, your pelvic muscles can reflexively contract in anticipation when you attempt to have sex, making penetration even more painful and sometimes impossible. A physical exam of all the systems in the pelvic area—reproductive, urinary and digestive—should help identify any medical or anatomical causes.

NATURAL R$_X$
GET A LUBE JOB

Aloe Cadabra is an all-natural, plant-based lubricant made with organic aloe vera ($6 for 2.5 ounces; livewellbrands.com). Yes makes water- and oil-based lubricants with no petroleum products or irritants ($15 for 2.6 ounces; yesyesyes.org).

TRY DO-IT-YOURSELF DILATION

In cases of a painfully tight vagina, if no medical cause is diagnosed, a doctor can gently insert progressively larger dilators to stretch the tissue. You can try the same at home by inserting increasingly larger tampons dipped in a lubricant.

DO YOUR KEGELS

We tend to think of these exercises for tightening the pelvic-floor muscles, but "Kegels help you learn to relax those muscles as well," says Naughton. (See "How to Do a Kegel Correctly" on page 150.)

EAT SOME ROOTS AND BERRIES

Koonce says that vaginal pain caused by dryness can signal a kidney yin deficiency and suggests adding black mulberries to amaranth and cow or goat's milk yogurt, snacking on goji berries and spooning maca root powder into smoothies and cereals.

TRY HOMEOPATHY

Staphysagria, a homeopathic remedy that helps ease pain in the genital region, is recommended for a sore or tender vaginal area; it may help lubrication. Boiron pellets are available at health food stores for about $5.

APHRODISIACS FOR ALL

L-ARGININE

As we just said, this amino acid helps with nitric oxide production, which increases blood flow throughout the body and to the genitals, says Mark Blumenthal, of the American Botanical Council. According to research published in *The Journal of Sex & Marital Therapy* and reviewed in 2013 by Memorial Sloan-Ketting Integrative Medicine Center, an average of 70% of women with low libidos reported that they were more satisfied with sex after taking ArginMax (for perimenopausal women it was 86%!); this contains L-arginine as well as damiana (see below), ginseng and ginkgo, for one month. These women also saw an increase in desire, lubrication, clitoral sensation and orgasms.

DOSAGE: 2,500 milligrams daily

Yes, the skeptical shopper in you might be wary of any sexual-enhancement cures; the ones we recommend contain combinations of the ingredients listed above, which have been shown to improve sexual function. Whether they work better together is your call. It might be worth a try; and remember that the placebo effect can sometimes be quite powerful. But remember also, most herbal remedies require use for at least 12 weeks before real results. Plan ahead—way ahead.

MACA

Ancient Incans consumed this energizing Peruvian plant before battle or a bout of sex, says Chris Kilham, an ethnobotanist at the University of Massachusetts at Amherst. Maca increases sexual appetite, stamina, endurance and even fertility. One 2008 study conducted at the Depression Clinical and Research Program at Massachusetts General Hospital in Boston found that maca helped people with antidepressant-induced sexual dysfunction to regain their libidos.

DOSAGE: 400 milligrams daily

YOHIMBE BARK EXTRACT

This African tree bark extract sends blood flow to the genitals and stimulates the sensitive tissue of the clitoris, says herbalist Ed Smith, a founding member of the American Herbalist Guild, who adds a warning

Just for Her

Here are libido-boosting combinations of the above formulated for women:

ArginMax for Women contains L-arginine and damiana leaf, both proven in clinical setting to boost desire and cut inhibition.
Dosage: Three capsules daily ($40 for 180 capsules; arginmax.com)

Hot Plants for Her contains maca, ashwagandha, *Rhodiola rosea*, *Eleutthero senticosus* root extract and catuaba.
Dosage: One to two tablets daily ($33 for 60 capsules; enzymatictherapy.com)

Intimate Response contains standardized ginkgo leaf extract, ginseng, L-arginine, horny goat weed and yohimbe bark extract.
Dosage: One to two tablets daily, do not use for more than 30 days at a time, take a two-week break in between use ($11 for 30 tablets; sourcenaturals.com)

Women's Libido contains maca, damiana herb and horny goat weed.
Dosage: One capsule, three times daily between meals ($25.99 for 60 capsules; gaiaherbs.com)

Emerita Libido Formula contains damiana leaf extract, muira puama, *Ginkgo biloba* and ginseng.
Dosage: One tablet daily ($16 for 30 tablets; emerita.com)

How can I treat my sinus infection naturally?

A sinus infection occurs when bacteria, fungus or a virus block the airways in your nose and cause infla—infla—infla—sorry, almost sneezed.

An acupuncturist says:

Typically accompanied by yellowish-green nasal discharge, facial pain, headaches and fatigue, a sinus infection can result from exposure to pathogens, allergens, air pollution, weather changes or stress. Antibiotics will help bacterial infections, but not the more common viral variety.

Treatment: Ease pain with acupressure. Using your index finger, massage each side of the nose at the bottom edge of the nasal bones as well as the grooves at the widest point of both nostrils to the count of 10, three times each day. Or try Metagenics Sinuplex, which contains N-acetylcysteine to thin mucus, quercetin to stop your runny nose, vitamin C to reduce swelling of the mucous membranes and bromelain to relieve your headache and facial pressure. Also use an air purifier with a HEPA filter to clean the air of irritants and keep your home dust-free. If your symptoms do not clear up within a week, see an ear, nose and throat doctor.

—Roberta Roberts Mittman, L.Ac.,
owner of Park Avenue
Center for Wellbeing in
New York City

An osteopath says:

Taking antibiotics for a sinus infection significantly reduces the amount of good (as well as bad) bacteria in your respiratory and gastrointestinal (GI) tracts, which allows candida to grow and further inflame the mucous membrane. This can contribute to fungal sinusitis in addition to

that yohimbe can cause nervousness and sleeplessness and raise already-existing high blood pressure (so avoid taking it if you have heart or kidney disease)—and can also negatively interact with antidepressants.

DOSAGE: 200 milligrams of a standardized extract containing 4% yohimbines (the plant's active ingredient) for no longer than six weeks

DAMIANA LEAF (*Turnera diffusa*)

Because it reduces anxiety and inhibitions, this nervous system tonic helps you become more relaxed and amenable to arousal, says registered herbalist Roy Upton, R.H., executive director of the American Herbal Pharmacopoeia. Damiana leaf's aphrodisiac abilities are also linked to a compound it contains, progestin, which is similar to the female sex hormone progesterone (which drops, and dampens libido, as we head toward menopause).

DOSAGE: 1 gram daily

CATUABA (*Rythroxylum catuaba*)

This Amazonian aphrodisiac comes from a tree native to Brazil, where tribes traditionally use it to remedy a lagging libido, impotence and nervousness (a well-known mojo-killer). The plant's active compounds, catuabine A and B, appear to act on the sex centers in the brain, says Kilham, so you may experience erotic dreams when taking catuaba.

DOSAGE: 100 milligrams daily

HORNY GOAT WEED (*epimedium*)

Traditional Chinese Medicine (TCM) views low libido as a deficiency of kidney yang qi, or energy, so Upton advises taking the aptly-named horny goat weed to boost kidney function and—hey now!—your sexual vitality.

DOSAGE: 250 to 500 milligrams daily

MUIRA PUAMA (*Ptychopetalum olacoides*) aka marapuama

A 2000 study conducted at the Institute of Sexology in (where else?) Paris found that muira puama and *Ginkgo biloba*, which is another stimulating sex herb, increased desire, intercourse regularity, sexual fantasies, ability to reach orgasm, intensity of orgasm, and, therefore, satisfaction with their sex lives in women who had been experiencing low libido. Other studies show that this happy-making herb from a tree native to the Brazilian Amazon also counteracts chronic stress, depression and nervous exhaustion.

Dosage: 800 milligrams daily

MALE SEXUAL DYSFUNCTION

We'll just cut to the chase, shall we? The most common male sexual disorder is impotence, sometimes called erectile dysfunction, or ED, and defined as the inability to sustain an erection to satisfactorily perform intercourse or ejaculation. Experts estimate that 18 million to 30 million men in the United States experience impotence in some form. Age is not necessarily a factor in pure impotence, although as a man ages, the force and amount of ejaculation does decrease.

ED can occur as a result of certain medications, fatigue, chronic illness or too much alcohol. Lifestyle factors such as smoking, being overweight, a sedentary lifestyle, poorly managed diabetes (which can impact blood flow to the penis), high cholesterol and stress. Low levels of testosterone and a zinc deficiency also can cause ED.

There also are psychological factors that can cause ED, including fear of intimacy and/or feelings of guilt. Primary impotence is rare, and means a male is completely unable to engage in sexual intercourse. Secondary impotence is much more common—men can only engage in intercourse about 25% of the time—and is situational, usually related to psychological reasons, including less than optimal timing or location, boredom, low self-esteem, performance anxiety and depression. Herbs and supplements that may help:

SAW PALMETTO, which helps oppose the influence of estrogen on prostate tissues

ZINC, which boosts immunity and sexual function

NIACIN, to improve circulation

MANGANESE, which is essential to healthy sexual function

LIPOIC ACID, an antioxidant

PROSTATE PMG AND ORCHEX, which directs nutrients to the prostate and testes

Sexy Combos for Him

Herbal aphrodisiacs have been used in every culture ever since men walked upright. Now there are a number of compounds available that combine stimulants from around the world.

Dr. Schulze's Male "Shot" includes horny goat weed leaf, yohimbe bark, astragalus root, muira puama bark and more to aid with arousal and erections ($66 for a three-pack; herbdoc.com).

ArginMax for Men has shown positive results for maintaining erections in clinical trials. It includes L-arginine, ginseng, ginkgo and zinc ($25 for a one-month supply; arginmax.com).

Steel-Libido for Men contains L-arginine, maca root, ashwagandha root, horny goat weed extract, *Tribulus terrestris* extract and yohimbe bark. It supports sex drive and erections ($28 for 75 gel caps; hormonewell.com).

the infection you were originally trying to cure, making you more susceptible to another infection.

TREATMENT: To stop candida overgrowth, avoid sugar, dairy, wheat and alcohol, and take a daily probiotic (even when you're not sick) with at least two billion CFUs. For the sinus infection, try Allimax (garlic supplement that is also antibacterial, antiviral and antifungal); 200 milligrams of echinacea three times daily; and 1,500 milligrams of the Chinese herb yin chiao three times daily. Also, thin the nasal mucus and flush it out with a steam inhaler and a SinuPulse Elite Nasal Irrigator. Or use a neti pot to rinse out your passages. It also helps to remain hydrated, so drink ½ ounce of water for each pound of body weight daily.

—Robert Ivker, D.O.,
author of Sinus Survival,
cofounder of the American Board of Integrative Holistic Medicine and medical director of Fully Alive Medicine in Boulder, Colo.

An ayurvedic physician says:

Viruses and bacteria may flourish in your nose's mucous membranes and cause a sinus infection. But whether or not you get sick depends on how susceptible your body will be to the germs. An unhealthy diet (think fried foods, red meat and rich desserts), for instance, could make your digestive and immune systems too weak to fight off infection.

TREATMENT: Eat plenty of easy-to-digest foods like warm soups, steamed vegetables, lentils and cooked whole grains, with the exception of wheat if it stuffs up your nose. To clear sinuses and boost digestion, drink warm herbal ginger tea as often as possible and sprinkle stimulating spices like ginger, turmeric, coriander and black pepper on dishes. Avoid cold foods and drinks because they suppress enzymes needed for digestion and toxin removal, plus constrict your already-blocked nasal passages. Also steer clear of congestion-causing dairy foods as well as alcohol, sugar and red meat—all trigger inflammation, which lowers resistance.

—Nancy Lonsdorf, M.D.,
practices ayurvedic medicine in Fairfield, Ia., and is the author of The Ageless Woman: Natural Health and Beauty After Forty

How can I stop snoring?

*This expert advice might just save your night—
and your relationship.*

An integrative sleep specialist says:

Snoring is often considered "normal" because so many of us snore. However, research suggests that, more often that not, it is a very early sign of chronic inflammation, which is associated with weight gain, heart disease and a host of other conditions. We've also discovered that snoring is associated with a lack of muscle tone in the throat. Many of us keep our throat muscles tight during the day and, as a result, those muscles get too lax at night—which then causes snoring.

TREATMENT: If you often feel tightness in your throat that keeps you from saying something you'd like to share, your throat muscles could be the culprits. First, take a look at how well you express yourself. Are you really speaking your truth? Next, sing every day—even if you're just belting out your favorite song in your car. Singing tones the muscles in the throat to help prevent snoring.

—Rubin Naiman, Ph.D.,
clinical assistant professor of medicine at the University of Arizona Center for Integrative Medicine in Tucson and author of Healing Night: The Science and Spirit of Sleeping, Dreaming, and Awakening

A naturopath says:

Allergic rhinitis—an inflammation of the tissue in the nasal passages due to an allergy—is often to blame when it comes to snoring. Common causes of allergic rhinitis include environmental allergens such as dust mites, pet dander, pollen and molds.

TREATMENT: Buy a high-quality air filter, close your bedroom windows and turn the filter on at least one hour before bed. Other crucial moves: Keep pets out of your bedroom (especially off your bed) and choose hypoallergenic bedding and pillows instead of down. You might also have your home checked for mold—especially if you've recently had a leak or plumbing incident. Mold is tough to discover on your own because it grows in the walls. Finally, if your sinuses are congested, use a neti pot before bed every night. The saltwater rinse flushes out allergens and helps ease congestion.

—Nicole Egenberger, N.D.,
clinic director of Remede Naturopathics in New York City

An integrative nutritionist says:

If environmental allergens have been ruled out, a food allergy—often a wheat or dairy sensitivity—might be to blame. To figure out if this is the cause of your nighttime noise, go on an elimination diet: For two weeks, eliminate all wheat products. The following week, slowly add them back into your diet (reintroducing foods you've cut out one at a time, every two to three days). If you notice gas, bloating or other digestive issues, you've got your culprit.

TREATMENT: In addition to cutting out any foods you're sensitive to, eat more anti-inflammatory foods (think wild salmon, fresh fruit, vegetables and other fiber- and nutrient-rich whole foods) and reduce your intake of pro-inflammatory foods (anything processed or containing flours or partially hydrogenated fats). Also, ditch alcohol consumption, as that has been linked to snoring.

—Beth Reardon, R.D.,
director of integrative nutrition at Duke Integrative Medicine in Durham, N.C.

STRESS

At work, on the road, in a marriage, with kids, before a meeting or a deadline, sometimes over the silliest stuff, like a lost sock or a leaky faucet: When the stress hits, every organ in your body winds tighter and tighter. You get irritable. Your bowels contract. What's asked seems impossible. Hopelessness sets in. Fight or flight? You just wanna punch something, or weep, or hide—under a pillow, back in the womb, in an all-day marathon of *Real Housewives...* anywhere but where you are.

Stress is killer. And it's killing us.

SYMPTOMS

The American Psychological Association (APA) reported in 2013 that 77% of us experience stress and its physical symptoms, a Worst Ever list that includes fatigue, dizziness, muscle tension, lack of sex drive and stomach distress. Chronic stress can cause or worsen conditions that include obesity, irritable bowel syndrome, heart disease, Alzheimer's, depression, diabetes, depression and asthma.

If you've experienced any of those, you can probably guess the No. 1 cause of stress is the U.S. It's "work," according to the APA—on-the-job stress which includes coworker tension, work overload and horrible bosses. (Money issues, including job loss and worries over retirement income, come in second.) Thirty percent of Americans say they are "always" or "often" stressed at work, and workers' stress alone costs employers $30 billion a year.

This disastrous effect on your health gives new meaning to the phrase "clocking out." One recent survey of studies found that people in demanding and unrewarding jobs had an 80% higher chance of developing depression than those with more worthwhile positions. Stress can also accelerate aging by up to 17 years. And it gets no easier as you age: A study that looked at elderly who were caring for their spouses found that those stressed-out caregivers had a 63% higher death rate than others their age.

Upshot: Since it's a natural feeling, surely there's a natural cure. For starters, take a deep breath in, counting to five... hold it for four, then slowly let it out to a count of six. 1...2...3...4...5...6....

And read on.

REMEDIES

Stress, the good guy

First, let's get a handle on what stress is—this monster that keeps us driven by day and up all night. For starters, it's not a monster—or at least it's not trying to be. Stress, in the short term, is our defender, says Vancouver, B.C., physician Gabor Maté, M.D., author of *When the Body Says No: Exploring the Stress-Disease Connection*.

"Acute stress is simply a necessary self-protective mechanism," he says. "An emotion like fear may trigger the response, but it's a physiological reaction that you may or may not be aware of."

This fight-or-flight response was at its best for our forebears—think Russell Crowe in *Gladiator*, facing a hungry tiger. A stress episode then was a short—albeit complicated—burst, revving up every body system to win the battle or get away. Gladiator's brain—in particular the frontal cortex, the brain's executive center, sent a red alert to the hypothalamus, the hormonal control center, triggering a flood of the stress hormones adrenaline and cortisol. "The cortisol elevates blood sugar levels, mobilizing energy for a quick escape," says Maté. "The adrenaline provides more energy to fight."

At the same time, this cocktail of stress hormones prompts the heart to quadruple the amount of blood it pumps, from about five quarts to 20 quarts a minute, providing more energy. But the blood travels a different route, away from the skin, gut and kidneys to the muscles, so that energy can be used to fight or flee. Blood pressure, heart rate and breathing rates increase, the lung's airways dilate, and the liver starts converting glycogen—the raw material of body fuel—into glucose, or blood sugar, again for power to battle or retreat.

In modern times, of course, you're not confronting hungry lions. You're facing your a-hole boss, or an urgent e-mail, or a cheating spouse, or the guy who didn't brake. But your body reacts exactly the same way.

Despite these crucial—and yes, sometimes lifesaving—benefits of stress, most of us obsess about it (causing more stress). And so do the media, constantly telling us how stressed out we are or giving us something else to stress about. "Every ad I see is for some illness or disability in the body and spirits," says Judith Orloff, M.D., clinical professor of psychiatry at UCLA. "The media program causes us to be stressed out and sick."

When "good" stress goes bad

Even seemingly innocuous parts of our lives are stressors, says Brad Lichtenstein, N.D., a naturopathic physician and assistant professor at Bastyr University in Seattle. "Stress is any force exerted on the mind and body," says Lichtenstein. "So, by definition, even gravity is stress, exercise is stress, eating is stress."

Unfortunately, our bodies didn't get the e-mail, and they are paying the price, fighting-or-flying from every little situation. The result can be unremitting stress, a modern phenomenon that can be far more destructive than a quick burst of stress that resolves within minutes.

The problem with a chronic stress response is that you produce so much cortisol that your adrenal glands—the factories that produce and regulate our hormone levels—poop out, says Lichtenstein. The result? Constant fatigue, emotional chaos and decreased immunity.

In fact, a number of studies have shown that stress has a direct effect on the immune system. For example, those poor caregivers: Research released in 2008 by Ohio State University found that older caregivers of family members with dementia did not respond well to vaccines, had less control over viruses and more inflammation and accelerated aging of their cells compared with adults who were not caregivers. A UC San Francisco study found that moms with sick kids were so chronically stressed that their telomeres—DNA proteins that are markers of biological aging—were shorter than those of mothers who had healthy children, aging them up about 10 years. Research released in 2009 by the National Institute of Child Health and Human Development saw similar results for fathers and mothers. Studies even show that kids with stressed-out parents are substantially more prone to developing asthma.

And the effect of chronic stress on the immune system is just the start. "Adrenaline increases blood pressure and damages your heart, increasing your risk of stroke," says Maté. "Cortisol gives you ulcers, puts fat on your body in a way that promotes heart disease and gives you diabetes." In fact, Maté believes that chronic stress plays some part in all chronic illnesses.

The psychological ravages are just as brutal. As Judith Orloff notes, long-term stress depletes the body of serotonin, a feel-good neurotransmitter: "That makes you depressed and cloudy, so you can't concentrate. With chronic adrenaline, you're also hyper, more on edge and more irritable. Everything becomes a big deal because it's hard not to sweat the small stuff."

REMEDIES

Trading bad stress for good

What we need, of course, is to get a handle on stress, to ease it back, like Russell did his tiger. For when we're stressed all the time, we become less attuned to our body's alarms, says Kim Turk, L.M.B.T., director of massage services at Duke Integrative Medicine in Durham, N.C. "It's called somatic numbing—when the mind and body are completely disconnected," she says. "Like a mom in a grocery store whose kid is yelling at her but she doesn't hear him anymore, we stop listening to our bodies. Or when you're tight in your neck and shoulders, but you have no idea that you are."

The key is to be aware of that good stress; it's our "on" light, the power behind meeting deadlines, getting the dinner cooked before the guests arrive or exercising instead of reaching for the ice cream. It powers motivation.

Certainly, that's true for Boston's Erin Munroe, 35, a child and adolescent therapist and mother of an 11-month-old: "I used to have a job with summers off, and I didn't know how to function without some stress. I needed to find a way to be productive." But Munroe hit her limit when her son cried nonstop for his first 14 weeks of life. "I was still working full-time, taking care of my child, keeping the house clean and trying to be perfect. I was breast-feeding and I felt really ill and ended up with a breast infection."

Munroe had reached the point, as Maté describes it, when the body says no. If we're "on" all the time, our motor no longer revs. "When we're stressed, our adrenal glands are spent. And then we press the gas when we really need to go, and nothing happens."

So, how to get to our happy place? We know that stress, good and bad, is part of life. So how can we control the worst of it so that good stress can work for us when we need it? Here, the key steps experts insist on.

Run a priority scan

Once you know what's keeping your lights on 24/7, you can figure which ones to turn low.

When her mother became ill and died seven years ago, Rebecca Brooks, 40, a mom of two sons and president of The Brooks Group, a public relations firm in New York City, knew family had to be her focus. "I realized then that I couldn't manage everything myself," she says. "I had to come up with solutions." Brooks learned to delegate and prioritize. She beefed up her staff. And she focused on leaving work at the office. "Now when the kids have something school-related, I'm always there," she says.

LISTEN TO YOUR GUT

"Part of stress reduction is learning to listen to what your gut tells you about your life, about people, about a situation," says Orloff. "Ask, 'Does my energy go up or down around this person? My stress level? How do I feel about this job? Did I leave the job interview feeling sick?' Factor the answers into your decisions."

Your Body, on Stress

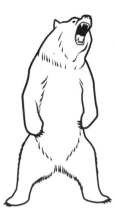

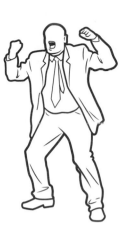

Whether a bear jumps out at you in the woods or your boss disses you at a meeting, your stress circuitry snaps on like soldiers to a drill sergeant's bark. Here, the step-by-step route that stress takes in your body.

1.
Your frontal cortex—the "executive" part of your brain behind your forehead—receives the information about the bear coming toward you.

2.
The frontal cortex sends a blaring message of emergency to the hypothalamus, the brain's hormone control center.

3.
The hypothalamus sets up a chain reaction, triggering stress hormones, adrenaline and cortisol.

4.
The heart starts pumping 18 to 20 quarts of blood a minute, a whopping 400% increase from its normal four to five quarts.

5.
Your blood pressure rises, your breathing quickens, your eyes dilate, your muscles tighten, your airways widen and you become hyperalert.

6.
The blood moves away from the gut (digestion's not important at this moment), the skin (you don't want to bleed too much from the bear bite) and the kidneys (so you don't lose fluids), and heads toward the muscles where the arteries dilate, giving you greater access to energizing nutrients.

7.
The inflammatory part of your immune system revs up, ready to attack any bacteria or foreign body that invades.

8.
Your fat cells release more fat into the blood for quick access to energy.

9.
Your blood platelets turn sticky, the better to clot should that bear slash you.

10.
Your liver converts glycogen, the raw stuff of fuel, into glucose for energy.

You're primed to fight.

Mary Saunders, L.Ac., owner and practitioner, Boulder Community Acupuncture in Boulder, Colo., agrees. "You have to ask yourself, 'What's going on that makes me feel this way—overwhelmed, bitchy, short-tempered,'" she says. In other words, stare down the lion, don't run.

CALM YOUR SYSTEM DOWN

Of course, it may take more than a little introspection, especially if you're a pro at lying to yourself. Candance Reaves tried antidepressants, poetry and physical therapy before hitting on a yoga-meditation class that restored what grief and fatigue had stolen. "The class allows me to have that out-of-body experience when I can look at things differently and really focus," she says. "When I feel stressed now, I sit down and do deep breathing for 10 minutes. At the end I'm focused about what I need to get done first. It gives me energy and peace."

Even three-minute meditations can recenter you, says Orloff. She practices them throughout her day—a way of turning off stress and turning on endorphins, the body's feel-good neurochemicals. "Find a comfortable place," she says. "Close your eyes, take a few deep breaths and begin to quiet your thoughts. Picture yourself breathing in calm, breathing out stress, and find an image that relaxes you—mine is the reflection of the night sky. This quickly turns off the stress response because you're slowing down your system."

DROP STRESSFUL "DE-STRESSORS"

One person's de-stressor is another person's toxin. Driving to a gym, circling for a parking space, changing clothes, pumping iron and returning to a ticketed car, for example, isn't everyone's idea of relaxing.

Erin Munroe had a similar experience: "I was taking hot yoga at 5 a.m. to help me chill out. It was all type-A people and very competitive. The class made me crazy; I would get mad that someone could do a Tree pose better than me. Now I take hatha yoga with people in sweatpants and no makeup, and I've realized I don't need to exercise 9,000 hours a week."

DE-STRESS YOUR DIET

Even if we can't control traffic patterns or TPS reports, we can change habits that make things worse. Try limiting your caffeine. That's an approach Terry Courtney, M.P.H., L.Ac., former dean of the School of Acupuncture and Oriental Medicine at Bastyr University, advises for her frazzled clients. Caffeine stimulates the same stress hormones—cortisol and adrenaline—you're trying to calm. And sugar offers an energy rush, soon followed by fatigue as your blood sugar drops just as swiftly.

"You're left without resources for building energy on your own," says Courtney. "Caffeine also interrupts sleep, so you wake up tired—wanting more caffeine and sugar." But Courtney doesn't recommend going cold turkey, knowing she'd give a coffee lover like you the shakes. "Just look at your patterns and see what's reasonable," she says.

SUPPLEMENT YOUR STRESS

Take a good multivitamin, one that includes a B vitamin complex with folic acid, says Donna Bryant Winston, R.N., an herbalist and nurse based in Bethlehem, Pa. "These vitamins help in the production of serotonin and dopamine in the brain, which relieve anxiety." Vitamin B-rich foods include whole grains, nuts, dried fruits and eggs. Folic acid is vitamin B_9, which helps to stabilize our mood and can be found in dark leafy green vegetables and beans. Turkey contains an amino acid called L-tryptophan, which also helps to increase serotonin levels and help to calm us.

Saunders also recommends magnesium. "It's probably the best supplement for calming the nervous system overall," she says. "It's very alkalizing—and the more alkaline the system, the more resistant the body is to illness and stress. To alkalize the body, limit highly acidic foods (coffee, alcohol, meat, sugar) and load up on highly alkaline foods (vegetables and fruit).

LET THE SUNSHINE IN

Our friendly fireball stimulates the production of vitamin D in our bodies, essential for replenishing the adrenal hormones. Go outside for 20 minutes a day without sunscreen or sunglasses; for those concerned about skin cancer, take 4,000 to 8,000 IU of vitamin D a day.

EXERCISE

"When I'm really stressed, exercise is a big outlet—and I have a better workout," says Brooks, who spins, walks, kickboxes, or does yoga before work five days a week. "It helps me get my aggression out." Saunders also exercises regularly, practicing yoga and taking daily hour-long walks. "In Chinese medicine, we say that the physical movement helps to move the qi, or energy, through the system."

CULTIVATE ACTIVE REST

That's very different from collapsing at the end of the day, says Lichtenstein. "That's just exhaustion," he says. Active rest is spending time relaxing in a way that rejuvenates you—hanging out with friends, listening to music, reading and meditating. "All of these are forms of meditation that give focused attention to the moment."

In a 2009 study conducted at West Virginia University, 35 stressed-out people were taught mindfulness techniques, such as deep breathing and meditation. At the end of three months, they had a 54% drop in psychological distress and a 46% drop in medical symptoms (high blood pressure, and aches and pains among them). The control group had little reduction of stress and an increase in medical symptoms.

USE STRESS TO YOUR ADVANTAGE

"There's a difference between a positive growth response to stress and using stress as a defense," says Saunders. "If it's the kind of stress that promotes growth, I'm all for it." For instance, Saunders sometimes finds long meditation retreats stressful. "But I know that inner work is promoting growth," she says. That's a different stress than forcing herself to do something just because she thinks she should.

"I hear a lot of women say I should do this job or keep this marriage going. We have this idea that it's selfish to say no. But you have to learn to say no, to set boundaries so you have time to do what sustains you.

"All of this stress dissection has been strangely calming," she continues. "With a little attention from me—some slow breathing, a pinch of thankfulness, a no-weekend rule about e-mails—I'm finally realizing that stress doesn't have to be my personal rumba 24/7. I may always have a higher idle than I'd like, but knowing that I can make some stress work for me injects a little pride in my two-step. It helps me relax. And yes, even stress less."

How can I treat a UTI?

And, more importantly, how can I never get one again, ever? Ow.

A urologist says:

Urinary tract infections are commonly caused by E. coli in the bladder (women are anatomically at higher risk), and the only effective treatment for a full-blown infection is antibiotics.

TREATMENT: "I take your medical history (noting symptoms like frequent urges to urinate, burning sensation when urinating, pain above the pubic bone and blood in the urine) and perform a physical exam. I also run lab tests on your urine sample to identify red flags for infection (such as white blood cells) and a urine culture to confirm the UTI and the type of bacteria. In most cases, I prescribe a three-day dose of the antibiotic Macrodantin. Along with antibiotics, take an over-the-counter bladder pain reliever like Uristat. Always urinate after sex, which can push bacteria into the urinary system. After swimming, change out of your bathing suit into dry, loose-fitting clothes."

—Robert Salant, M.D.,
*clinical associate professor,
department of urology,
NYU Langone Medical Center*

A dietician says:

Sugar, caffeine and alcohol exacerbate UTI symptoms and can even invite infection by making the urinary system more acidic— the kind of environment in which E. coli thrives.

TREATMENT: "While you recover from the infection, I recommend avoiding alcohol and caffeine. Instead, drink two ounces of unsweetened cranberry juice diluted in six ounces of water, twice a day. The hippuric acid in cranberries prevents bacteria from adhering to the bladder's lining. Eat five additional daily grams of fiber, which protectively coats the bladder, until your daily fiber intake is 25 grams. While you're on antibiotics— and for at least two months afterward— take a probiotic supplement or eat plain, unsweetened yogurt to get at least five billion CFUs (colony-forming units) of "good" bacteria a day. Drink water with lemon or lime;

both stimulate the release of sodium bicarbonate to neutralize acid in the body."

—Ashley Koff, R.D.,
founder of Ashley Koff Approved,
a nutrition evaluating service

A TCM practitioner says:

According to Traditional Chinese Medicine, most UTIs are caused by damp heat (excess mucus and inflammation in the body) combined with bacteria in the urinary tract.

TREATMENT: "To clear the body of damp heat, I perform 30 minutes of acupuncture on points like Liver 8 (which is just above the knee on the inner leg) and Spleen 9 (just below the knee on the inner calf). I also do tuina massage on the lower back to stimulate blood flow in the pelvic area.

"Take Dianthus Formula (Ba Zheng San) at the very first sign of symptoms; it has anti-inflammatory and antibacterial herbs like rhubarb and licorice that can prevent infection. If you're already on antibiotics for a full-blown infection, supplement with Gentiana Combination (Long Dan Xie Gan Tang) to clear painful heat from the body. Choose pills instead of tinctures, which contain irritating alcohol."

—Jill Blakeway, M.Sc., L.Ac.,
founder and clinic director of the
YinOva Center in New York City

Is there anything I can do about my varicose veins?

Those twisted, bumpy blue lines are more than just unsightly; they might indicate serious circulatory problems.

A yoga therapist says:

Yoga is an effective protocol for preventing and treating varicose veins. The posture that is known to be clinically most effective in both cases is sarvangasana, the shoulder stand, where the legs are inverted and the pressure of gravity is reversed. In this pose, the blood and the lymph drain from the lower extremities back to the heart, thereby reducing the pressure of the pooled blood in the veins.

TREATMENT: Do the shoulder stand pose once daily, with a recommended holding time of about three to five minutes. When you stand up, movement of these fluids in the legs will be greatly improved. People with limited range of motion or high blood pressure should do the modified version of the shoulder stand: Lie on the floor and place your legs in an inverted position against the flat surface of a wall (waterfall pose). If necessary, a small pillow or rolled towel can be placed under your neck for comfort and support.

—Nirmala Heriza,
cardiac yoga therapist at Cedars-Sinai Medical Center in Beverly Hills, Calif., and author of Dr. Yoga

A naturopath says:

Varicose veins can only form if there's weakness in blood-vessel walls, or if there's significant pressure within the vein to overwhelm healthy vessels. By strengthening the vessel walls, which are made of smooth muscle and connective tissue, you decrease the likelihood they will dilate or distend.

TREATMENT: Build up connective tissue and shrink existing varicose veins by taking 2 to 3 grams of vitamin C and 400 to 800 IU of vitamin E daily (if you have a clotting disorder or take blood thinners, check with a doctor about vitamin E dosage). Botanicals such as horse chestnut, bilberry, butcher's broom, and grape-seed extract fortify connective tissue, while fruits like blueberries, elderberries, and cherries contain antioxidants that strengthen vein walls. Varicose veins sometimes lead to clotting, which can reduce the area through which blood flows and force the vessel to dilate even more. To help prevent clotting, eat foods with blood-thinning properties, such as raw onions, garlic, ginger, and cayenne.

—Amy Neuzil, N.D.,
Austin, Tex.

A dermatologist says:

Several factors contribute to varicose veins: genetics, pregnancy, obesity, constipation, taking estrogen and wearing high-heeled shoes and/or restrictive clothing. Everyone with varicose veins should seek medical treatment, since there is a 50% risk of developing leg ulcers or blood clots, especially after a long car or plane trip.

TREATMENT: "One procedure I use to treat varicose veins is endoluminal laser vein closure, which involves using light energy inserted with a fiber into the vein to heat the vein wall and cause it to collapse and seal closed. Bruising from the treatment disappears after a week or two, and patients can return to regular activities right after the procedure. If you have varicose veins, wear lightweight graduated support stockings, especially when you're going to be on your feet for long periods. Avoid crossing your legs while sitting, since it cuts off blood flow and increases pressure in leg veins. Don't wear heels taller than an inch: When you wear high heels, you don't utilize your calf muscles enough while walking, and these muscles are responsible for pumping blood back to the heart. For circulation and vein strength, walk or do another exercise that works your legs for half an hour every day."

—Mitchel P. Goldman, M.D.,
associate clinical professor of dermatology at the University of California, San Diego

WEIGHT MANAGEMENT

The Natural Health Diet

Six easy ways to shred fat fast, with just a few simple changes. You can hear a collective groan each morning, as dieters across the U.S. step onto their scales and discover that, in spite of their best efforts, or the latest fad, the weight simply isn't going anywhere. They're following the conventional wisdom—avoiding fattening foods and getting plenty of exercise—but the pounds are staying put. In fact, according to a recent Pennsylvania State College of Medicine analysis of 14,000 adults, just one in six dieters succeeds at losing 10% or more of his or her body weight and keeps it off for at least a year.

Why is it so hard? "Because it's about a lot more than calories in and calories out," says Pamela Wartian Smith, M.D., codirector of the master's program in medical sciences at the University of South Florida College of Medicine, and author of *Why You Can't Lose Weight*. Indeed, studies suggest that additional culprits—from food sensitivities to stress levels—can sabotage even the best weight-loss efforts. With that in mind, we've developed an exclusive six-step program to help you lose weight fast and keep it off for good—the *Natural Health Diet*.

The key to the *Natural Health Diet* is to consider the possible saboteurs and combat them. Here's a list of the Big Bads.

You're sensitive

Begin by eliminating food sensitivities before dieting—several recent studies suggest a connection between childhood obesity and food allergies. "When you eat things to which you're sensitive or intolerant, you get an increase of the hormones epinephrine and norepinephrine, so you literally get a high," says Smith, who explains that this reaction can result in cravings for the very foods we should avoid. Food sensitivities may also lead to inflammation and water retention. To compound the problem, over-the-counter antihistamines bolster appetite and dull energy, studies show.

TRY: An elimination diet. Start by ditching all of the suspected culprits (dairy, gluten, peanuts and soy are common) for three weeks and add them back one by one. "During this phase you should not be focusing on weight loss, but on identifying the foods that are a problem for you," says Natasha Turner, N.D., a naturopathic doctor in Toronto, and author of *The Hormone Diet.* If medication for seasonal allergies is boosting your appetite, try natural antihistamines like the flavonoid quercetin, vitamin C and the herb butterbur.

You're stressed out and exhausted

CHILLAX. Chronic stress prompts a surge in the "fight or flight" hormone cortisol, which can tear down muscle fiber, impair blood sugar metabolism and boost the brain chemical neuropeptide Y, which sparks cravings, says Smith. Meanwhile, losing just an hour of sleep each night for three days can prompt a surge in the hormone ghrelin, which stimulates appetite, and a slump in the hormone leptin, which tells us when we're full, says Norfolk, Va.-based clinical psychologist Michael J. Breus, Ph.D., coauthor of *The Sleep Doctor's Diet Plan.* Deep sleep, on the other hand, fuels production of the fat-burning human growth hormone (HGH).

TRY: Meditating for 10 to 30 minutes a day. Such calming practices not only normalize cortisol levels but also boost levels of the appetite-suppressing hormone serotonin. To relax your body and keep your digestive system cleansed, try 250 milligrams of magnesium daily. Or take 500 to 1,000 milligrams of gamma aminobutyric acid (GABA) an hour before bed. While studies are scarce, some animal trials and small human trials have shown the amino acid to both ease anxiety and promote fat loss.

You're toxic

Put down that water bottle! A growing body of evidence suggests that exposure to toxins like bisphenol A (BPA), organophosphate pesticides and phthalates may be fueling weight problems. "We are starting to see a lot of human studies showing an association between the presence of chemicals and obesity," says University of California, Irvine, researcher Bruce Blumberg, Ph.D., who coined the term "obesogen" to describe such toxins. A 2011 Harvard study found that adults with the highest concentration of BPA in their urine had significantly larger waists and a 75% greater chance of being obese than those in the lowest quartile. Other research suggests exposure to pesticides and polychlorinated biphenyls (PCBs) may impair metabolism. "They have been shown to poison the mitochondria so it cannot burn fuel," says Walter Crinnion, N.D., chairman of the environmental medicine department at Southwest College of Naturopathic Medicine in Phoenix. "Fuel that is not burned turns to fat."

TRY: Steering clear of products that may contain BPA (including canned goods, which may have BPA in the lining). Be particularly leery of plastics that sport a #7 recycling symbol on them (a good indicator that BPA may be present) and never heat a meal in a plastic container (toxins can be absorbed by the food). Avoid farmed salmon, which may be loaded with PCBs. Also, look for personal-care products that don't contain "fragrance" (often code for phthalates). To hasten elimination of toxins through the digestive tract, take a scoop of brown rice fiber in supplement form three times daily. Also, drink at least two cups of detoxifying, fat-burning green tea daily.

Your thyroid is sluggish

Turner estimates that nearly one third of all men and women have a thyroid that is operating in a suboptimal range, often brought on by stress, a genetic predisposition, working out more than an hour a day or restricting calories too much (less than 1,700 a day for women; 2,000 for men). "The thyroid affects the metabolism of every single cell in the body," Turner says. "You can diet until you are blue in the face, but if your thyroid is out of whack, you will not lose weight." Telltale signs of

Shredding Supplements

The weight's not going to lose itself.
However, several supplements may help burn it off.

GINGER

"Ginger stimulates metabolism by heating the body, which helps us break down fats, digest our food better and burn a few more calories every day," says Sheila Kingsbury, N.D., chairwoman of the botanical medicine department at Bastyr University in Seattle. She recommends taking two 250-milligram capsules twice a day. Try Bluebonnet Herbals Ginger Root Vcaps ($10 for 60 capsules; iherb .com) or Gaia Herbs Ginger Supreme ($22 for 60 capsules; iherb.com).

GREEN TEA

A 2010 meta-analysis published in *The American Journal of Clinical Nutrition* found that green tea extract is associated with reductions in weight, body mass index (BMI) and waist circumference. "Green tea speeds metabolism, and it works really well in tea form," says Gaetano Morello, N.D. Try Tazo Green Ginger Filterbags to reap the benefits of both herbs ($10 for 48 bags; starbucksstore. com).

PRO-BIOTICS

Taking a probiotic supplement may encourage weight loss, according to Cynthia Sass, M.P.H., R.D. "The theory is that having higher levels of beneficial bacteria in the gut can help you burn more calories and may even cause you to absorb fewer calories, she says. Take a supplement with at least five billion live organisms per dose once a day. Sass recommends Primadophilus Bifidus by Nature's Way ($22 for 90 capsules, vitacost.com).

GARCINIA CAMBOGIA

Evidence that garcinia (aka Citrimax) can help suppress appetite is mostly anecdotal, but Elson Haas, M.D., says it might be worth a shot if you just can't stop eating. "It really does help some people feel less hungry," he says. "Plus, it helps the body metabolize fats." Take a 250- to 500-milligram capsule before every meal. We like Natrol Pure CitriMax ($18.50 for 90 300-milligram capsules; natrol. com).

GYMNEMA

This herb has long been used in ayurvedic medicine as a treatment for diabetes. According to ayurvedic physician John Douillard, D.C., it can help with weight loss, too. "Gymnema helps keep blood sugar levels stable so you can stick to eating three meals a days without snacking in between," he says. Take one 500-milligram capsule three times a day with meals; get it in Douillard's formula, LifeSpa Sugar Destroyer ($28 for 90 capsules: lifespa.com).

a sluggish thyroid include eyebrow thinning, constipation, weight gain, dry skin and irregular periods.

TRY: Having your thyroid-stimulating hormone (TSH) levels tested. While 0.4 to 4 ml/UL is considered "normal," a value higher than 2 can slow metabolism and hinder weight loss. Consider taking the herb ashwagandha (believed to jump-start production of thyroid hormones T3 and T4). Also, eat a few Brazil nuts every day (they're rich in the mineral selenium, which is key for proper thyroid gland function).

You've hit a hormonal rut

According to a 2011 study in the *New England Journal of Medicine,* restricting calories and losing body fat can wreak havoc on insulin, leptin, ghrelin and other hormones, prompting a surge in hunger and a slump in metabolism. This typically occurs about 10 weeks into a weight-loss program and can last for more than a year, even after the diet is abandoned. Dieting also prompts dopamine levels to fall, squelching motivation.

TRY: Indulging in one higher carbohydrate "cheat meal" per week to bolster your leptin levels, suggests Turner. Taking a daily omega-3 supplement can also raise leptin levels and promote satiety. Also, make sure you're mixing up the intensity and even the time of day that you're breaking a sweat. You can also try balancing insulin with 300 milligrams daily of alpha lipoic acid. To boost motivating dopamine, take 1,000 milligrams daily of L-tyrosine (which also bolsters thyroid function). Or, have more sex (also known to elevate dopamine levels!).

The latest trend: reprogramming your mind

At only 4'11", 39-year-old Maria Lugo-Perrin was carrying way too much weight—240 pounds—on her tiny frame when a flyer for a weight-loss program at the Beck Institute for Cognitive Therapy was slipped under her office door. Intrigued, Lugo-Perrin went to one of the meetings. "I thought it sounded wacky," admits the self-described veteran of diet pills and grapefruit plans. "But I decided to give it a try." The program, which uses verbal and written exercises to teach its clients how to examine recurring self-sabotaging thoughts and counter them with positive, proactive ones, worked. Lugo-Perrin attended hour-long weekly sessions for 12 months, and she credits the Beck Institute with helping her stick to her goals, even in her darkest hours. By the end of the year, she had lost 65 pounds.

Lugo-Perrin is one of many who are benefiting from the current focus in obesity research on the power of the mind. New studies show that certain "hardwired" thoughts—habitual, subconscious patterns that control what we eat and why—can be reprogrammed with astonishing results. Of course, during any attempt to lose weight, you'll always have to reduce calories and exercise more; but many researchers now believe that changing the way you think about eating and exercise may be the secret to establishing a healthier routine.

Consider Amy Mapes, a 34-year-old high school teacher in Seattle, who lost 18 pounds in 16 weeks after joining a program that stressed mindfulness; or Todd Frank (a pseudonym), 62, an architect based near

How Self-hypnosis Helps

There's only one way to maintain a healthy weight: Adopt a long-term lifestyle that includes new habits. A healthy imagination is useful here, and self-hypnosis can help, says Steven Gurgevich, Ph.D., coauthor of *The Self-Hypnosis Diet: Use the Power of Your Mind to Reach Your Perfect Weight* and cocreator with Andrew Weil, M.D., of the audiobook *Heal Yourself with Medical Hypnosis.* "You have to see a future in which you've learned to love exercise and healthy foods," Gurgevich says. "People can imagine the skinny jeans, but do not see themselves enjoying the lifestyle patterns that will give them the weight they want. Self-hypnosis helps them create healthy eating and exercise habits."

Gurgevich says self-hypnosis is easy—much like daydreaming, only with a focused intention. Here's how: Find a comfortable place and time to let your mind wander to your ideal future. "Imagine yourself in the kitchen, preparing a delicious and healthy meal," he says. Get detailed: Envision you've chosen the best foods, portion sizes and cooking methods. "You've purged your pantry of foods that would interfere with achieving your perfect weight. Get absorbed in the vision of being able to eat anything you want because you're now making the right choices," Gurgevich adds. "Your mind is powerful—if you can imagine it, you can have it."

Boston, who lost 40 pounds in two months and credits his success to hypnosis. Like Lugo-Perrin, they have learned to think themselves into new habits. "Our bodies have powerful instincts—developed when fat and sugar were scarce and the hunt for food could be exhausting—to eat and rest as much as possible," explains Deidre Leigh Barrett, Ph.D., an expert on dreams and hypnosis who teaches at Harvard Medical School and is the author of *Waistland: The (R)evolutionary Science Behind Our Weight and Fitness Crisis.* "But overriding instincts when they've become counterproductive is exactly what our giant brains evolved to do. We have this wonderful capacity to check whether our first impulses and cravings are actually best for us."

Instead of following diets, Lugo-Perrin, Mapes and Frank are now focused on making good decisions. It's not what they eat but how they live that defines their food choices. That difference, many weight-loss experts believe, is what will help take off the pounds and keep them off for good.

Indeed, recent evidence suggests cognitive therapy can have a sig-

Treat Yourself Like a Good Kid

Beating yourself up over food is another knowledge-behavior gap many women fall into. Calling yourself "greedy" or a "fat pig" or "weak-willed" only makes you feel bad about yourself, which often leads to eating more in an attempt to give yourself a boost. It's important to try to stop the negative self-talk, says Freida B. Herron, M.S.S.W., L.C.S.W., a weight-management coach for Women's Way Coaching in Knoxville, Tenn. "I often suggest imagining that your desire to overeat is a lovable 5-year-old child," she says. "You don't want to berate or shame your appetite—that only leads to more dysfunctional eating." Instead, treat yourself with respect,

understanding and affection, as you would that child.

If that doesn't work, try chanting a mantra, suggests Siri Khalsa-Zemel, M.S., R.D., Herron's partner at Women's Way. "It's a good way to interrupt the negative dialogue," she says. You don't have to be a yoga practitioner—or even a spiritual person—to reap the benefits. "We often have a roomful of Baptists chanting a mantra," she says. Any mantra will do, though Khalsa-Zemel often offers this one: Sat nam, wahe guru ("saht-nahm-wah-hey-goo-roo"). It means "Divine truth is my name. That infinite wisdom includes me and goes beyond me."

nificant impact on weight loss. In a 2007 study published in the *International Journal of Behavioral Medicine,* Swedish researchers compared weight loss among women in a cognitive therapy group as opposed to women in a group that received advice on exercise and other behavioral changes. At the end of 10 weeks, the cognitive therapy group had lost an average of 19 pounds, while the other group had lost only 1.5 pounds. Moreover, 18 months down the road, the cognitive therapy participants had maintained an average loss of 13 pounds, while the other group maintained a loss of only half a pound.

The program Lugo-Perrin attended outside Philadelphia was run by Judith Beck, Ph.D., author of *The Beck Diet Solution* and daughter of cognitive therapy pioneer Aaron Beck. The author says many people subconsciously give themselves permission to eat foods they shouldn't. "They might say to themselves, 'It's OK because I'm upset.' Or, 'It's OK because this is a special party,'" says Beck. "We have thousands of these sabotaging thoughts. You need to look at the situation differently and practice alternative responses like, 'I'll feel better about my body and have more energy if I don't overeat.'" She has patients write down compelling reasons why they shouldn't eat and read them at least twice a day.

Lugo-Perrin also keeps a list titled "Advantages to Not Overeating" hanging on her refrigerator. "It's the little things I wanted to accomplish," she says, "like being able to wrap a towel all the way around me, that help me open the refrigerator and take out what I'm supposed to eat, not what I want to eat."

Q

How can I treat a yeast infection naturally?

About 75% of women will suffer from this fungus, which causes an irritation of the vagina and the area around it.

A naturopath says:

There are actually three types of vaginal infections that may appear to be a yeast infection due to their similar symptoms. Bacterial vaginosis is the most common infection, and happens when bacteria replace healthy organisms in the vagina. Candidiasis is a true "yeast infection"—that is, an overgrowth of a strain of yeast called *Candida albicans* as a result of a disruption in the pH balance in the vagina. Finally, trichomoniasis is another type of infection and is considered a sexually transmitted disease. Unless you're absolutely certain it's yeast, you need a doctor to help with the diagnosis.

TREATMENT: While bacterial vaginosis and trichomoniasis often require prescription medications, yeast infections are generally easy to treat with natural remedies. Scientific evidence has shown that boric acid inhibits the grown of *Candida albicans*. Depending on the severity of the infection, I might have a patient insert a boric acid capsule twice a day for three to seven days. Berbarine, tea tree oil [which can be inserted via a tampon], neem oil and goldenseal are also good remedies; talk to your health care provider about the best way to proceed. If your infection doesn't resolve, other health problems may be involved—talk to your doctor about getting tested for diabetes, thyroid dysfunction and HIV virus.

—Tori Hudson, N.D., *author of the* Women's Encyclopedia of Natural Medicine, 2nd Edition

A holistic nutritionist says:

Food plays a role in helping to treat yeast infections and prevent them. A diet rich in sugar and refined carbohydrates can make you more susceptible to yeast infections because yeast feeds on sugar in the body. Excess weight will also increase your predisposition to yeast infections, because extra fat can lead to insulin resistance, which keeps more sugar circulating in the body.

TREATMENT: Reach for yogurt with live active cultures or a probiotic supplement to help repopulate your system with healthy bacteria. Eat a diet rich in vegetables and whole grains to boost your immune system. Reach for every kind of fresh vegetable—particularly immune-boosting powerhouses like sweet potatoes and dark leafy greens. Include whole grains such as quinoa, millet, barley and brown rice. And boost the amount of water you drink to 10 to 12 eight-ounce glasses a day, which will help deliver nutrients to your cells and eliminate waste. You'll also want to scale back on portions when you're fighting a yeast infection. If your body is spending too much time trying to digest large amounts of food, it'll have less energy to spend on other important functions—like working to restore the optimal vaginal pH balance.

—Wendy Bazilian, Dr.P.H., R.D.,
a dietitian in San Diego

A homeopath says:

Homeopathy is based upon the notion that like cures like, so the go-to, first-line therapy for curing yeast infections in homeopathy is a diluted form *Candida albicans*, a key ingredient in many homeopathic yeast tablets and suppositories. That might sound counterintuitive—put more of the stuff in when you're trying to get rid of it? But it works in much the same way allergy shots do. If you're allergic to ragweed, for example, an allergist will give you a shot of diluted ragweed.

TREATMENT: Try the remedy *Candida albicans* first; look for a 30C remedy, and take two to four pellets under your tongue four times a day for three days, or until your symptoms improve. If that doesn't provide enough relief, choose among the following remedies to find the one that most closely matches your symptoms: Kreosotum is good for discharge that's very irritating and has a bad odor, with lots of redness, rawness, and pain during and after urination; pulsatilla works for cases with less pain and bland discharge; sepia is a good choice when there is a yellowish discharge and a bearing-down sensation—as if everything is going to come out; *Calcarea carbonica* is a good remedy for patients who are overweight, flabby, and crave sweet and salty foods; borax is best for cases in which there is a rash in the area, and the discharge is sticky and runny with the consistency of egg whites.

—Timothy Fior, M.D.,
a family practitioner and homeopath practicing in Lombard, Ill.

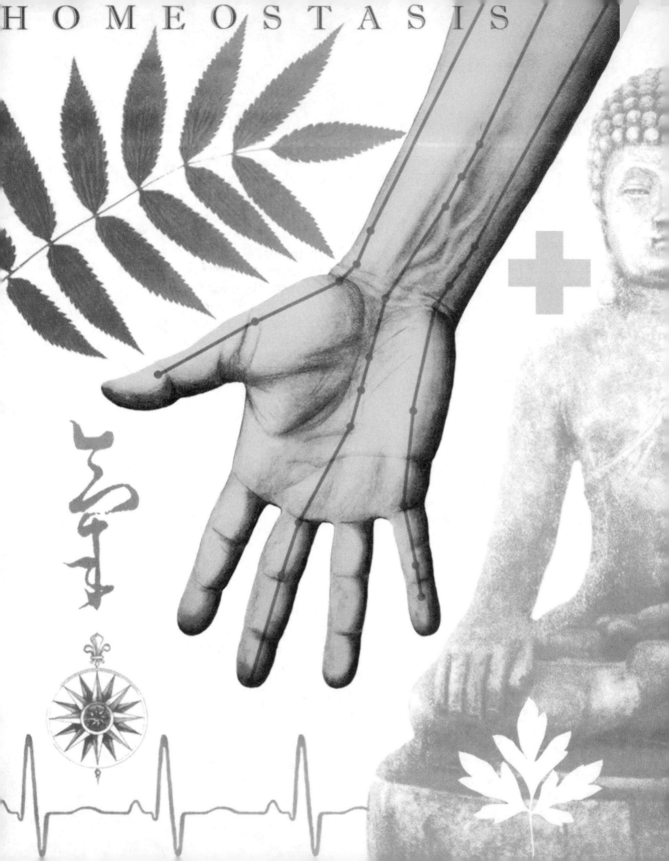

HOMEOSTASIS

Alternative Healing

Thank goodness for modern medicine.
Never thought you'd read that in a book like this? Well, even *Natural Health* is well aware that we can't live without traditional health care (often literally), and we're grateful for the brave doctors and nurses who provide it. Who wants to set his own broken bone? Or perform heart surgery on herself? Or put the lives of their children entirely at the mercy of... wormwood oil? Belief in botanical medicine is one thing. Curing cancer is quite another.

But the future of health care won't be built on one thing or the other. It will involve all kinds of practitioners—Western medicine and alternative therapies alike—working together to provide a sustainable, holistic approach. You've probably already got this happening, albeit in an ad hoc manner. Perhaps you have a trustworthy GP but are also sure to hit the gym three days a week, or never miss a yoga class. Or maybe you get CT scans at the hospital for that bad back, but see a chiropractor afterwards, to get cracking. And after having that baby, did you rely mostly on your OB-GYN, but still sip nettle tea "just in case" it helped with breast milk production?

If so, you're one of the millions already living the future. And this chapter—full of alternative therapies to incorporate into your routine—will ensure that the future looks bright. From how to find a practitioner to what precautions to take, we've got comprehensive sections on the following:

Bodywork
CHIROPRACTIC,
MASSAGE,
OSTEOPATHY

These therapies are touchy-feely, literally. Each involves the manipulation of bones, muscle and tissue to increase circulation and restore balance, but in wildly different ways. Read on to find out how they can relieve anxiety, help premature babies gain weight and lessen the symptoms of PMS.

Chinese Medicine
ACUPRESSURE,
ACUPUNCTURE,
TAI CHI

Before diving into each specific technique, be sure to read our overview of Traditional Chinese Medicine on page 263; it explains the framework behind this ancient yet never-more-relevant system of beliefs.

Mind and Body Purifiers
AROMATHERAPY,
AYURVEDA,
DETOX AND CLEANSING,
ENERGY MEDICINE,
MEDITATION,
YOGA

If this book had a smell, this section's would be—mmm, incense. Each of these therapies, although derived from different philosophies, aims to make you feel at peace with your body, either by how you move it or what you put into it.

Therapies
BIOFEEDBACK,
HOMEOPATHY,
HYPNOTHERAPY,
NATUROPATHY

The most controversial section—if only because there's still research to be done on many of these. Therapies like biofeedback and naturopathy spark the body and mind to heal themselves. Smokers may want to skip directly to hypnotherapy, known for its success with addicts.

In addition to the above, you'll find a series of essential resources, like "The Ultimate Medicine Cabinet" (replace that decades-old calamine lotion with these remedies). Put it all together, and you've got the building blocks for a better you.

BODYWORK
Chiropractic

Whenever **Western doctors** criticize new trends in natural healing, we can't help but think of chiropractic therapy, once condemned by the American Medical Association. Little did they know it'd one day be used by an estimated 23 to 28 million people in the United States, and become the most widely practiced branch of complementary medicine. Its practitioners work in hospitals, sports clinics and private practice, often covered by insurance; some states are designating chiropractors as primary health care providers. The "back-crackers" are comeback kids, and they come with proof.

In 2013, a *Journal of the American Medical Association* study declared it beneficial for low back pain, and a study in the journal *Spine* published in 2012 found that back patients who saw a chiropractor first had a surgery rate of just 1.5%, compared to those who first saw a surgeon, whose surgery rate was 42.7%. A study by Britain's Medical Research Council followed patients who were getting chiropractic treatments for low back pain for two years and found that they were doing better than hospital outpatients. Also, it worked for Joe Montana and Tiger Woods. Condemn that.

Essential Concepts

When there is nerve interference caused by spinal misalignment, known as "subluxation," not only can back pain occur, but also problems throughout the body. Early chiropractors believed that subluxations were the cause of all disease (hence: jail time, see "Science Says" on page 252); today most chiropractors focus on musculoskeletal issues (back, head, neck and joint pain), still believing that spinal adjustments can promote the overall health of the body's nervous system and organs.

Try It Out

A chiropractor (D.C.) will take a medical history, do a physical exam and sometimes order an MRI or X-rays, then manipulate, or adjust, your spine and extremities accordingly. Patients often experience an audible and palpable "click" in the back or extremity being adjusted. This is caused by a gas bubble created by the joint's change in pressure. (We're not gonna lie here—the adjustments take some getting used to.) A chiropractor also will often suggest rehabilitative exercises that you can do at home, as well as better positions for sleeping, sitting and the like, to help ease discomfort.

Note: Chiropractors are not licensed to prescribe drugs, and often employ acupuncture, herbal medicine and homeopathy in their treatments. Electromyography (EMG) is often used in conjunction with spinal manipulation or adjustments.

✻ BEST FOR: Back pain, spine and neck disorders, sciatica, muscle, joint and postural issues, menstrual pain, vertigo and tinnitus, headaches and migraines, asthma (especially for children) and gastrointestinal problems. Many suffering from drug addiction have found that removing subluxations can ease withdrawal and detoxification symptoms, and can improve retention rates, especially since pain is relieved without drugs.

Precautions

Make sure to tell your medical doctor that you are using a chiropractor, especially if you are being treated for a disease, and tell your chiropractor if you are being treated for an illness or condition.

Always seek a licensed, reputable practitioner.

Do not begin a course of complementary medicine, stop using proven conventional methods, without telling your doctor if you are pregnant.

Tell your chiropractor if you have any signs of infection or inflammation, osteoporosis, circulatory problems or a recent break or fracture.

FIND A PRACTITIONER

The best way to find a chiropractor is through a referral from a friend, family member or even another health care provider, especially a physical therapist; medical doctors have also been known to make referrals.

Also: Look for a doctor who will utilize a number of diagnostic tools, such as X-ray and ultrasound, and neurological and orthopedic

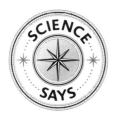

Developed by in the late 19th century by Canadian David D. Palmer (who was jailed in 1906 for illegally practicing medicine), chiropractic medicine was once condemned by the American Medical Association—in the 1960s, the AMA called it an "unscientific cult" and a 12-year legal battle resulted, which the AMA lost. (You can sum up the old-school opinion of chiropractic therapy with a *Family Guy* joke: "And then this one time," says a man at an AA meeting, "I was so drunk, I gave someone a back adjustment. I'm not a chiropractor. You have to go to a *weekend* of school for that.")

Now, thanks to many studies published in peer-reviewed journals, medical opinion is generally positive, especially for treating musculoskeletal issues.

The first time that medical doctors went on record stating that chiropractic treatment is appropriate for some types of lower back pain was in a Rand Corporation study in 1992; and British and Australian research has also found that chiropractic can be twice as effective as conventional back treatments and therefore more cost-effective. A 2008 paper published in *Spine* found that spinal manipulation and mobilization effectively managed patients' chronic low back pain; other research has found it works to ease headaches. Several studies also have found chiropractic safe and effective for children's ear infections and asthma; one study reported that a group of asthmatic children ages 1 to 17 saw a 90.7% improvement after undergoing chiropractic care for 60 days.

tests. Check the chiropractor's record (usually available from your state's chiropractic regulation and licensing board) to see if there are any disciplinary actions.

Make sure the chiropractor's college is accredited by the Council on Chiropractic Education.

Almost every chiropractic visit will involve that infamous adjustment; be wary of any doctor who is not open to questions and concerns.

Do not feel that you must be treated by the first chiropractor you meet; many people interview several before choosing one for long-term treatment.

The American Chiropractic Association (acatoday.org) is a major source for information, and maintains a database of member doctors, as well as information on all chiropractic specialties.

Massage

It has been proven to reduce stress, improve sleep, soothe sore muscles and relieve muscle tension and chronic pain—as well as reduce blood pressure, help preemies gain weight and ease the side effects of cancer treatment. But never has massage been taken as seriously as it will be in 2014. The most recent studies are just too remarkable to ignore. For example:

1. One study, conducted through the Buck Institute for Research on Aging in 2012, found that massage reduced the inflammation of muscle acutely damaged through exercise, on a cellular level. The researchers actually did muscle biopsies, and then compared a subject's massaged tissue to his unmassaged tissue, and found that the massaged leg was *already* healing. The same study showed massage can heal musculoskeletal injuries and maybe even inflammatory disease.

2. New research by the Group Health Research Institute showed massage eases chronic low back pain—subjects had a weekly 60-minute session for 10 weeks (tough gig), and were able to significantly reduce the amount of pain medication they were taking. A month after the study ended, subjects were still reporting better quality of sleep and less anxiety and pain.

3. There are promising studies showing benefits for fibromyalgia patients. And a 2012 Cedars-Sinai study published in *The Journal of Alternative and Complementary Medicine* suggests that massage can alleviate symptoms of depression, anxiety, back pain, asthma, fatigue and even HIV, and that the results are cumulative, meaning the more frequent, the better.

AMERICANS BELIEVE.

According to *The Journal of Alternative and Complementary Medicine* (*JACM*), massage therapy is a multibillion-dollar industry in the United States, with 8.7% of adults receiving at least one massage within the last year. A 2012 report by the American Massage Association says that 75% of those surveyed get massage for medical- (43%) or stress- (32%) related reasons, and 85% view massage as beneficial to overall health and wellness. And 61% said their *physicians* recommended they get a massage.

Before long, health care plans might start to cover it. Plenty of other countries do. The Indian medical system of ayurveda focuses on the healing properties of massage; a Swedish gymnast brought therapeutic massage to popularity in Europe, and Eastern doctors use various types in their own practices.

Essential Concepts

Basically, massage feels good to the skin and to the muscles, releasing endorphins and improving mobility. Manipulation through massage can relax and loosen stiff joints, and deep-tissue massage (along with offshoots like Rolfing and Hellerwork) can restructure the muscles and fascia, the thin tissue enclosing the muscle.

But, since most schools have the basics in common, choosing a "flavor" of massage ain't easy. Until late in the 20th century, "therapeutic" or "relaxing" were your only options (along with the kind that, shall we say, ended happily). When the wellness movement boomed in the 1980s, the rising interest holistic healing also revitalized massage. Now you need a whole new vocabulary. "Swedish massage—or variations on it—used to be the standard," says Anne Williams, L.M.P, C.H.T., a licensed massage practitioner who literally wrote the textbook. "Now you see everything and anything on spa menus: shiatsu, lomi lomi, abhyanga. If you're a massage connoisseur, that's a great thing, because now you don't have to travel the globe to get these services."

Here's a guide to help you make your way onto the padded table that's right for you.

Try It Out

SWEDISH

Warning: more data here. But we can't help ourselves. Recent studies have found Swedish massage—characterized by moderate pressure and long strokes that run along the grain of the muscle—to be not only relaxing, but also deeply healing. At Cedars-Sinai Medical Center, for example, researchers found in 2010 that a single session of Swedish massage had profound effects on subjects' hypothalmus-pituitary-adrenal-immune function—the therapy increased levels of oxytocin and reduced the stress hormone cortisol—findings that may have implications for managing inflammatory and autoimmune conditions. "We've been able to demonstrate that it helps with depression, pain syndromes, immune problems, diabetes, cancer and even HIV," says Tiffany Field, Ph.D., director of the Touch Research Institute at University of Miami Miller School of Medicine. The key to this kind of healing effect? Stress reduction, increased relaxation and, in turn, immunity.

CHOOSE IT IF: you're chronically wound up and need full-body relaxation, or just want to feel deliciously pampered. If you're a beginner or suffering from an autoimmune condition such as MS, start here, says Williams.

DEEP-TISSUE

A results-oriented massage, deep-tissue work incorporates penetrating kneading techniques, cross-grain strokes and trigger-point releases. "Deep-tissue massage really gets into the belly of the muscle and addresses the muscle attachments," says Charlotte Prescott, director of spa and fitness for Canyon Ranch Miami Beach in Florida. "Some people find it painful, but it's very therapeutic." Recent studies have found that deep tissue—aka sports massage in the '80s—heals inflamed muscle at a cellular level, but it also can be relaxing. A 2008 *JACM* study found that deep-tissue massage (accompanied by soothing music) significantly reduced systolic, diastolic and mean arterial blood pressure and heart rate in male and female subjects.

CHOOSE IT IF you have areas of chronic tension or muscular injuries and aren't afraid of a tiny bit of pain.

SHIATSU

This Japanese modality works with the body's energetic meridian system. Therapists use their fingers and hands to apply massage and acupressure, and may incorporate gentle stretching. A 2011 review in the *BMC Complementary and Alternative Medicine* found the strongest evidence for the benefits of shiatsu was for pain (particularly dysmenorrhea, lower back and labor) and postoperative nausea and vomiting, as well as improvements in sleep. At the end of a six-month U.K. study published in the *JACM*, subjects reported feeling significantly less tension or stress and fewer body structure problems, and 80% said they had improved their lifestyles as a result of having regular shiatsu.

CHOOSE IT IF you have chronic stress or areas of tension or muscular injuries.

THAI

You keep your clothes on, lie on the floor and let your therapist work your body through a series of stretches designed to release muscular tension. "It's like lazy man's yoga," says Angie Parris-Raney, R.M.T., a massage therapist in Littleton, Colo. And, like yoga, Thai massage can reduce stiffness and pain. A study published in the *Journal of Bodywork and Movement Therapies* (in 2011) found that Thai massage eased anxiety, muscle tension, pain intensity and pressure pain threshold, and improved flexibility in patients with back pain. And there's a study being conducted to measure the effect of Thai massage on brain-wave activity.

CHOOSE IT IF you want to feel flexible and invigorated. "When my Thai massage clients get done, they're ready to go home and clean the house," says Parris-Raney. "It charges you up."

ABHYANGA

A form of ayurvedic bodywork, abhyanga works to correct imbalances in the doshas (the energies that govern life). Therapists use herb-infused massage oils and apply them with strokes properly paced for your dosha (vata, smooth and slow; pitta, slow and precise; kapha, vigorous). A 2010 German pilot study on the effects of this classic ayurvedic oil massage (published in *JACM* in 2011) found significantly high improvements in stress reduction, blood pressure and heart rate after just one 60-minute session for healthy male and female subjects.

CHOOSE IT IF you're feeling frenzied (vata imbalanced), fried (pitta imbalanced) or sluggish (kapha imbalanced). "It's a good choice to balance mind and body," says Prescott.

REFLEXOLOGY

Reflexology holds the belief that each of the body's organs corresponds with an area on the bottom of the foot. Therapists apply (sometimes intense) pressure to the feet to create changes in the body. The NIH and National Cancer Institute have funded several well-designed studies that show reflexology to be remarkably effective in reducing pain and enhancing relaxation, sleep and the reduction of psychological symptoms such as anxiety and depression. A 2008 summary of 168 studies found the four major benefits of reflexology were: Positive impact on specific organs, especially the kidney and intestines, due to increased blood flow; improvement in symptoms (e.g., positive changes were noted in kidney functioning with kidney dialysis patients); a relaxation effect (blood pressure was decreased, and EEGs measuring alpha and theta waves showed anxiety was lowered); and in pain reduction (27 studies demonstrated a

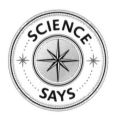

While there is more research done on massage than almost any other complementary treatment, it doesn't occur to many medical doctors to prescribe or refer patients to a massage therapist; while naturopaths, chiropractors and osteopaths have been trained in the efficacy of massage, many M.D.s have not, and so don't feel comfortable prescribing it. Still, the NIH's NCCAM reports that doctors are recommending massage as commonly as deep breathing and meditation to their patients, and a 2009 systematic review published in *Support Care Cancer* critically examined 14 randomized trials that showed the benefit of massage for cancer patients and found across-the-board improvements in such symptoms as pain, anxiety, nausea, fatigue and stress. In other words—quality of life. Massage has been shown to boost immunity, help asthmatics breath more easily, heighten alertness and lower stress. I mean, this whole chapter was basically research: It's this that will encourage M.D.s prescribe it more frequently.

positive outcome for reduction in pain, e.g., AIDS, chest pain, peripheral neuropathy of diabetes mellitus, kidney stones and osteoarthritis).

CHOOSE IT IF you have a health issue. A complement to standard medical care, reflexology can provide relaxation and improve blood flow, which can help reduce pain for a number of ailments.

FIND A PRACTITIONER

• There are no national standards in the U.S.; each state has a different set of licensing and certification rules and requirements, and schools of massage vary widely in their licensing and certification requirements, too. Be sure the therapist has the proper certifications and licenses—L.M.T., N.C.M.T., C.M.T.—these vary so widely that they alone don't guarantee a great massage therapist, but you can look into them. Also find out where he or she went to school.

• If you're paying for a massage (i.e., not going to a student clinic), look for someone with experience (at least five years, if possible) who has a dedicated office or a room in his/her house.

• For most massages you undress completely; Thai massage therapists usually have you put on shorts or loose pants of some kind. So, draping is everything. M.T.s learn how to drape properly so that you can relax and there is no question about their intention.

For information on self-massage or aromatherapy, visit shankara .com or theartofliving.com. The American Massage Therapy Association maintains a national database. Go to amtamassage.org.

Precautions

If you are being treated by a medical doctor, be sure to inform him or her that you are seeing a massage therapist.

Tell your practitioner if you are pregnant; you will probably be propped on your side and avoid lying on your back or belly. If you are pregnant, or have an illness such as cancer, seek a practitioner who has experience with your condition.

Bruises, skin infections, fractures and swollen areas should not be massaged.

Be sure to look for a licensed massage therapist.

Osteotherapy

Osteopaths are a lot like a chiropractors, but they can prescribe drugs and do surgery, so they're a lot like M.D.s. No wonder osteopathy currently seems to be going through an identity crisis; according to a 2008 statement by the Osteopathic Research Center University of North Texas Health Science Center, most evidence in osteopathy is based on expert opinions, case reports, case series and observational studies. Only one systematic review of randomized controlled trials, involving a treatment for low back pain, has been published.

Most people see an osteopath for back, knee and neck pain, but some also claim success in healing asthma, digestive problems and PMS. The best evidence right now is for low back pain, and the National Institutes of Health and Care Excellence (NICE) recommends it for this. Consider it an option, especially if you're the type who'd rather see a "real" doctor than one without a degree.

ESSENTIAL CONCEPTS

Osteopathy is a holistic system based on the principle that the well-being of an individual depends on his or her bones, muscles, ligaments and connective tissue functioning smoothly together. Osteopaths (D.O.s) believe in treating the whole body, not just symptoms, and use touch and physical manipulation to encourage the body to heal itself— osteopathic manipulative treatment (OMT), for example, is thought to align the musculoskeletal system (joints and muscles) so that all the tissues of the body, including the brain and nerves, will be healthy, and the digestive, circulatory and lymphatic system can function properly.

A 2013 NHS review states that plenty of evidence exists that shows osteopathy is beneficial for low back pain, and possibly osteoarthritis, but finds the research lacking for the other conditions osteopaths claim to treat, including stress and depression.

However, osteopaths have been licensed as conventional doctors since 1972, and complete four years of basic medical education, followed by internships and residencies. According to NIH numbers, there are about 39,000 D.O.s currently treating more than 20 million patients in the U.S.; and D.O.s and M.D.s are the only two medical professions in the U.S. with unlimited license to prescribe any recognized health care practice—mainstream or alternative—that might help their patients.

Try It Out

Techniques used include gentle massage and joint movement, articulation (a swift move similar to chiropractic adjustment), myofascial release and cranial manipulation. An osteopath may also make exercise and nutrition recommendations.

✱ BEST FOR: D.O.s believe there are few medical conditions that cannot benefit from osteopathic care, but specifically it has been shown benefits for spinal and joint conditions (including arthritis), back and neck pain, sports injuries and repetitive stress syndrome, sciatica, allergies and other breathing dysfunction, high blood pressure and heart disease, chronic fatigue syndrome and fibromyalgia, headaches, insomnia and

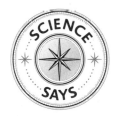

Most existing evidence on the efficacy of osteopathic medicine is anecdotal or not consistently high-quality research. Some research in the United States has shown improvement in hypertension, and studies done in the U.K. and U.S. have shown improvement in low back pain patients. There seems to be much more research published in Europe, and osteopaths themselves generally agree that higher-quality controlled clinical studies must be done worldwide.

Since osteopathy has been integrated into the American mainstream medical community for 20 years now, most medical doctors are accepting of its benefits, although primarily for musculoskeletal issues; but D.O.s provide a full range of health care, and are especially frequented as primary providers in rural areas.

depression, digestive disorders and PMS. Cranial osteopathy has been shown to be very beneficial for children, especially those prone to ear infections, hyperactivity and dizziness.

Precautions

Make sure you tell your medical doctor if you are considering osteopathic treatment, and do not get osteopathy if you have cancer or any bone infections.

- Seek a qualified, licensed and reputable practitioner.
- Avoid vigorous OMT if you have disc problems.
- Consult with your doctor if you are pregnant or being treated for a disease.

FIND A PRACTITIONER

Seeing a D.O. is a lot like seeing an M.D.—in fact, you might have been to one without really knowing it, according to the American Osteopathic Association. As far as finding one, as always, the best place to start is asking for a referral from friends or family, and maybe even your conventional doc. Also:

Check credentials and education. D.O.s should be licensed by the state in which they practice, and certified by the National Board of Osteopathic. Some D.O.s also have medical degrees, and vice versa.

When you're looking for a practitioner, always call ahead for a five- to 10-minute interview. Be wary of one who won't talk to you.

An initial examination involves observation, touch and lots of questions. Use your intuition to judge whether it's working for you or not.

Inquire up-front about costs and find out what your insurance will cover; some health care plans will cover treatments by an osteopath.

Be wary of any practitioner who makes excessive claims and guarantees a cure. Also be wary of one who wants to sign you up immediately for a specified number of treatments.

The American Osteopathic Association (osteopathic.org) provides information for patients and doctors, and maintains a database that's searchable by specialty, state and zip code. Many M.D.s also practice osteopathy, especially integrative doctors.

Traditional Chinese Medicine

In 2011, Chinese scientist Tu Youyou, age 80, won one of the most respected science prizes on Earth for isolating artemisinin, now considered the world's most important malaria drug. She discovered it where? In an ancient Chinese medicine.

We love that story, because it proves how Traditional Chinese Medicine (TCM) bridges the gap between ancient beliefs and real-world 2014.

The practice itself embodies the characteristics of many of the therapies in this book: a strong mind/body component, use of herbs, physical activity, massage, nutrition and lifestyle changes—the usual stuff you'd associate with *Natural Health.*

But TCM also has a very unique—critics and fans both might say "holistic"—view of the human body. We'll outline the complex concepts here, before you dig deeper into our chapters about acupuncture, acupressure and tai chi.

Essential Concepts

TCM is based on the ancient Chinese concept that humans and nature are interconnected, that the body's organs and tissues are interdependent—and that a balance of these organs' energies is essential to health.

The theory of yin and yang is central. In short, practitioners believe that each of our organs, our tissues and our food have a yin or a yang force, and that when one side's more powerful than the other, our bodies are at risk for disease.

Another essential concept is the theory of qi (pronounced "chee"), the vital energy or life force that circulates through your body along pathways called meridians. Qi embraces all energy, from the most material—such as your body, the ground you stand on and your iPhone—to the ethereal, such as heat, light, thought, movement and emotion.

Yin and yang are the opposite qualities of qi. For example, yin qualities are cool, dark, passive, solid, heavy and material. Yang refers to qualities of qi that are bright, aggressive, active, immaterial, expanding, hollow, light and ascending. Everything that is yin has some element of yang; everything that is yang has a little yin. Wellness is achieved when the yin and yang elements of qi are balanced and in harmony with each other. When yin and yang are not in harmony, when there is too much or too little of one aspect of qi relative to another, then there is illness.

TCM uses eight principles to categorize conditions and symptoms: yin/yang, cold/heat, interior/exterior and excess/deficiency. Herbs, therapies and foods are prescribed to help address each. For instance, say you have congestion. Your TCM practitioner might give you herbs called "lung heat" because phlegm is considered an Excessive Hot Interior condition. Then she'd ask about your diet. "Cooling" foods—like cucumber, grapefruit, buckwheat, eggs and green tea—are believed to clear heat and toxins. "Warming" foods—such as mango, greens, walnuts, rice, chicken, cinnamon and many other spices—increase the yang energy to improve circulation and warm the organs. Cold hands and feet, lack of energy and stomach distress are thought to be signs of a deficiency in yang. Since most of qi is extracted from what we eat and the air we breathe, TCM considers good food, herbs, physical comfort, clean air, mental stimulation, social interaction and love very important.

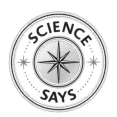

The principles of TCM are difficult for Westerners to understand, and it's especially difficult for medical doctors and skeptical researchers to accept the theory of qi, which cannot be measured. A number of studies have suggested that the therapeutic actions of acupuncture can be attributed to the release of endorphins at the points where needles are inserted. Most studies on TCM have been done in China, and while medical doctors might believe in TCM's efficacy, they have a tough time understanding all of the principles, and again, believing in that qi.

Try It Out

A visit to a TCM practitioner starts with observation and information gathering. He/she will talk to you, listen and observe your demeanor, movements, voice and complexion. She also will look at your tongue and feel your skin, muscle tone and internal organs. She is looking for disharmony and imbalance; with this information she'll make a diagnosis.

Then, she will employ any number of treatments, including herbal medicines, acupuncture, massage/acupressure, cupping and lifestyle counseling, and will give you some things to practice at home, such as meditation, dietary changes, stretching and other physical activities.

If any of this sounds too "out there," remember you'll hardly be alone: The National Health Survey estimates that about 3.1 million American adults use acupuncture each year, and 17% use Chinese herbs and other products. Thousands practice tai chi and qigong, and studies have found that tai chi can reduce the symptoms of prenatal depression, improve neuromuscular function in the elderly and help curb cocaine addicts' cravings. Research in China recently found that an herbal formula compared favorably with an anti-hypertension drug, and acupuncture has been showing promise in boosting the success of IVF and reducing symptoms of menopause. A small study in the U.K. found that acupuncture during labor enhanced women's birth experience.

✱ **BEST FOR:** TCM is used with success for chronic and degenerative conditions, and complex diseases with multiple causes. TCM herbal medicines are used widely to treat asthma, allergies and respiratory illness, including colds. Acupuncture is used to treat low back pain, addictions and emotional disorders such as depression and anxiety, digestive issues (such as GERD and IBS), fibromyalgia, migraines and arthritis. Acupuncture is very effective for treating pain, is showing promise for Parkinson's disease and is being used to boost IVF success for pregnancy. Moxibustion is used to turn a baby who's in a breech position. Trials are ongoing to test the efficacy of herbal medicine and acupuncture to treat HIV/AIDS. Acupressure is also a part of TCM, and is being used for pain, relief from nausea and weight loss.

Precautions

- Always tell your doctor if you are seeing a TCM practitioner, and list any herbs you are prescribed.
- Make sure to tell your TCM doctor about any prescription and OTC medications, herbs and supplements you are taking.

FIND A PRACTITIONER

Word-of-mouth is a good place to start, and you can always ask a school of Oriental medicine for referrals. Practitioners of acupuncture and TCM come with myriad different licenses, and the Accreditation Commission for Acupuncture and Oriental Medicine accredits TCM schools and colleges that teach it. Only six states in the U.S. do not regulate the licensing of the practice of TCM. Titles include D.O.M. (doctor of Oriental medicine) L.Ac (licensed acupuncturist), but since an NCCAOM certification is a prerequisite of licensure in most states, it's a good place to start. Also:

- Check education and certificates.
- Try to set up a pre-appointment phone call, to check out how you might get along with the practitioner.
- Look for a TCM practitioner with a wide range of therapies, not only acupuncture and herbs.
- Also, stay open: You are going to be learning some very different concepts about health and the human body, so ask questions and listen carefully.

The National Certification Commission of Acupuncture and Oriental Medicine (NCCAOM) maintains a database of nationally certified TCM practitioners.

Acupressure

Just like acupuncture—but without the pricking sticks— acupressure is based on the theory that for your body to cure itself, your life energy, or qi (pronounced "chee"), must be balanced and free-flowing. To kick-start this healing, pressure is applied to the body's trigger points—those supersensitive hot spots in your muscles that hurt if you prod them too hard. A practitioner will use his hands, elbows, even feet to treat you. It's bodywork, in other words, but this highly precise massage technique is grounded in ancient theory: Acupressure was developed more than 5,000 years ago in Asia and is rooted in Traditional Chinese Medicine (TCM). Acupuncturists often use acupressure as part of their treatments, and it's also something you can do in the comfort of your own home, given proper guidance.

And studies are showing it works, especially for pain and allergies: A 2013 study by Chao Hsing Yeh at the University of Pittsburgh School of Nursing found that auricular point acupressure (APA, or ear acupressure), which is done with small objects, such as pellets applied to the ear with waterproof tape, reduced chronic low back pain (CLBP) by as much as 75%. The study was published in *Evidence-Based Complementary and Alternative Medicine,* and controlled for the placebo effect, to which conventional medicine continues to attribute much of the success of acupressure and acupuncture (many even call it "sham" APA instead of placebo).

This was one of the first randomized controlled studies on acupressure for CLBP, and of course, many more need to be conducted. APA was shown to ease menstrual pain and dysmenorrhea (excessive menstrual pain) in a randomized 2013 Taiwanese study and APA does appear to be the most promising form of acupressure; an ongoing randomized study at the University of Mississippi Medical Center will examine whether ear acupressure can ease seasonal allergy symptoms.

It works, in a pinch.

Essential Concepts

Acupressure is used to reduce muscular tension and stress, boost circulation and encourage deep relaxation, which in turn promotes health and resistance to disease. TCM holds that acupoints, which are used in both acupressure and acupuncture, lie along 12 meridians—invisible channels through which vital energy, or qi, flows. These meridians begin at your fingertips and connect to your organs. When a meridian is blocked or imbalanced, illness can occur. And by stimulating these points, one can ease pain, cure illness and promote harmony.

Try It Out

An acupressure session starts with an evaluation of your condition, and acupressure is usually done with you lying on a massage table, fully clothed, while the practitioner gently presses on acupressure points, sometimes stretching you or massaging the points as well. The acupressure points related to your condition are often tender. A session will last about an hour, and you may require several treatment

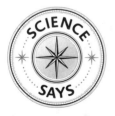

Many Western medics find it hard to believe that pressure on the body can have an effect on internal organs, and attribute any healing effect from acupuncture or acupressure sessions to increased blood flow and other physical effects of massage, including endorphin and cortisol release.

And yet: Acupressure has been extensively studied for its prevention of nausea, both during pregnancy and after surgery and chemotherapy, and found to be very useful. Research has also found it effective in treating anxiety, pain, stress, sleep apnea, sexual dysfunction, addiction and other conditions; but further high-quality research is needed.

sessions. If you are getting APA, you will be sent home with beads or seeds taped to acupressure points in your ears; this technique has also been used for weight loss.

Although it's best to consult an acupuncturist for proper instruction, if you can persuade your partner to learn, he'd have the tools at hand: Acupressure is generally done by using the thumb, finger or knuckle (or even a pencil eraser) to apply gentle but firm pressure to an acupoint. The pressure is steadily increased for about 30 seconds, held for 30 seconds to two minutes and then gradually released, and is usually repeated three to five times.

✱ BEST FOR: Relieving pain, stress, anxiety, depression, fatigue and insomnia, headaches and migraines, musculoskeletal issues, including arthritis, nausea and morning sickness, digestive disorders and women's health issues. Some practitioners use acupressure as a beauty treatment, to enhance sexual energy, to heal emotional issues and to treat addictions. It's also used to induce labor, which is why certain points in the legs and abdomen should not be pressed during pregnancy.

Precautions

Certain acupressure points should not be stimulated during pregnancy, except to induce labor.

Make sure your medical doctor knows you are seeing an acupressure or acupuncture practitioner, especially if you're being treated for an illness.

Be cautious if you're taking blood thinners, and be sure to tell your practitioner about these and any other medications you're taking.

See also "Acupuncture" on page 271.

FIND A PRACTITIONER

Acupressure is often practiced by an acupuncturist or a shiatsu massage therapist. The best place to start is to ask for a referral from friends or family, or even your conventional doc. Also:

Check credentials and education. While there is no governing body that accredits acupressure practitioners, some states require a license in another area, such as nursing or massage therapy, to practice. Some massage schools offer a certificate in acupressure or shiatsu as well.

When you're looking for a practitioner, always call ahead for a five- to 10-minute interview. You'll be spending lots of time with this doctor, and you need to have a sense that you can be comfortable with and trust him/her. Be wary of one who won't talk to you.

An initial examination involves observation, touch and lots of questions. Use your intuition to judge whether it's working for you or not.

Inquire up front about costs, and find out what your insurance will cover; some health care plans will cover treatments by an M.D. but not a yoga or massage therapist.

Be wary of any practitioner who makes excessive claims and guarantees a cure. Also be wary of one who wants to sign you up immediately for a specified number of treatments.

Acupuncture

I f you're in physical or emotional pain, the thought of someone sticking needles into you might seem like the best idea since never. But such is the widely reported success of acupuncture, that this ancient Traditional Chinese Medicine (TCM) technique is now being practiced by medical doctors in the West as a way of treating such diverse conditions as migraine, smoking addiction and impotence. And let's get one thing clear from the get-go: The needles are tiny, and while you may feel a little discomfort during treatment, it really doesn't hurt.

Acupuncture became well known in the United States in the 1970s when its powers of pain relief were first publicized. Its goal is to alleviate illness by balancing the body's vital energy (qi, pronounced "chee"), which flows through meridians, or pathways, that run through the body; you can think of these meridians as the body's energetic highways, and the stagnation that builds up as traffic jams. Practitioners place very fine needles along these meridians to unblock qi, and this triggers the body to release pain-killing endorphins, stimulates the nervous system, and boosts circulation; this in turn means that healing signals are relayed faster.

Acupuncture has been researched well and widely, and a 2012 review of 29 randomized trials published in the *Annals of Internal Medicine* confirmed its efficacy for many kinds of pain, including chronic headaches, neck and back pain and arthritis. New research in the journal *CNS Neuroscience & Therapeutics* shows it also may be effective for chronic obstructive pulmonary disease, Parkinson's disease and weight loss. Acupuncture also has been shown to help cancer patients' side effects.

The NIH estimates that 6.5% of Americans use acupuncture, most commonly for pain or fibromyalgia (in China, 25% report using it). When you think of alternative medicine, it's often acupuncture that most associate with CAM (complementary and alternative medicine).

Acupuncture practitioners often use complimentary therapies like herbal remedies, massage and cupping—a detoxifying "reverse" massage using suction on the back. Cupping generally feels great, but can leave blotchy patches on the skin for a few hours after treatment. You may have seen these oversize hickey marks on red carpet photos of Gwyneth Paltrow and Jennifer Aniston. If it's good enough for those natural health cheerleaders...

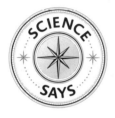

The amount of positive scientific research associated with acupuncture is pretty staggering. Studies have shown that acupuncture is very effective for certain conditions, including eliminating nausea during pregnancy and following chemotherapy. American studies have shown that it relieved neck and back pain. A 2012 study published in the *Archives of Internal Medicine* found rigorous evidence that acupuncture may be helpful for chronic pain. A 2012 Swedish study found that acupuncture relieved post-surgical pain; and other recent Swedish studies have found it can aid fertility treatments and ease polycystic ovary syndrome (PCOS). *The Lancet* reported in the early 2000s that alcoholism responded well to acupuncture; it's estimated that more than 2,000 drug and alcohol treatment programs in the U.S. and 40 other countries are using auricular (ear) acupuncture in addition to other therapies in their protocol. A landmark study in the *Journal of the American Medical Association* found that up to 75% of women suffering from breech presentations before childbirth had fetuses that rotated to the normal position after receiving moxibustion, a TCM practice that involves burning a small, cone-shaped amount of moxa (aka mugwort) on top of an acupuncture point. A 2012 review of eight trials (and a total of 1,346 women) confirmed its efficacy, and recent studies also have found acupuncture (particularly moxibustion) effective for knee osteoarthritis, insomnia and infertility.

Essential Concepts

Acupuncture is a key part of TCM, which also includes acupressure, herbs, exercise (such as qigong) and nutritional know-how. The concept of yin and yang—opposite forces whose balance is essential to well being—is fundamental to TCM. The five elements of fire, water, earth, metal and wood are considered to be inherent in all things, including the organs of the body, and each element is assigned a yin organ and a yang organ. Acupuncture is used to unblock and balance the energy so that your organs are able to work in harmony, and any deficiencies or excesses are addressed. Let's take our spleen as an example. This blood-filtering yin organ is associated with the earth element, and if it's diagnosed as deficient, a TCM practitioner might prescribe herbs that are also associated with the earth.

Try It Out

At a typical treatment, you'll start by talking with your acupuncturist about what ails you—this could be a physical injury or an emotional issue, as both are equally valid in acupuncture. Your practitioner will decide where to place the needles on your body to really maximize the benefit, and she'll explain to you which meridians she's setting out to unblock. You'll lie on a comfy massage table while she pops in the tiny needles, then after making sure you're comfortable, she'll leave the treatment room for a half hour or so while the needles do their work. Acupuncturists like to play soothing music during sessions, so if you're nervous about the treatment, why not bring in some music that will put you at your ease? (Nine Inch Nails, maybe?)

Most needling doesn't hurt. You might feel a little tenderness at the spots, though; some people experience a bit of nausea when the needles are removed, and some feel totally exhilarated. Everyone is different. You might take home a bunch of herbs specific to your condition; most are in capsule form.

＊ **BEST FOR:** Pain relief, anesthesia, addictions, musculoskeletal problems, arthritis, hay fever, asthma, depression and anxiety, migraines and other headaches, digestive disorders, nausea, high blood pressure, general health, women's health, erectile dysfunction, infertility and reproductive health.

Precautions

- Seek only a qualified, licensed practitioner
- Make sure your practitioner sterilizes, or uses disposable, needles
- Tell your practitioner if you are pregnant or have an STD, AIDS or hepatitis

FIND A PRACTITIONER

Acupuncture is most often practiced by licensed acupuncturists who are schooled in TCM, but many integrative medical doctors have learned the techniques and received certifications. The best place to start is to ask for a referral from friends or family, or even your conventional doc. You can also ask for referrals from TCM schools in your area, and might find a low-cost clinic, too. Also:

Check credentials and education. In most states, practitioners must have an L.Ac. (licensed acupuncturist) certification.

When you're looking for a practitioner, always call ahead for a five- to 10-minute interview. You'll be spending lots of time with this doctor, and you need to have a sense that you can be comfortable with and trust him/her. Be wary of one who won't talk to you.

An initial examination involves observation, touch and lots of questions. Use your intuition to judge whether it's working for you or not; an acupuncturist with great test scores and education might have a lousy "bedside manner," so pay attention to whether it feels like a good fit.

Inquire up front about costs and find out what your insurance will cover; many health care plans will cover acupuncture treatments, especially if done by an M.D.—but check first.

Be wary of any practitioner who makes excessive claims and guarantees a cure. Also be wary of one who wants to sign you up immediately for a specified number of treatments.

The American Association of Acupuncture and Oriental Medicine maintains a national database of practitioners. Learn more: aaaomonline.org.

Tai Chi and Qigong

You've seen those oh-so-serene groups of people in the park, slowly performing vaguely martial-art arm-circles—unrushed, considered, precise, at one with nature. They look so at peace. You wish you could achieve such nirvana, and exhibit such self-control. It's OK to watch—we've all been a little tai-curious.

Often described as "meditation in motion," tai chi might well be called "*medication* in motion," according to a Harvard Medical School 2009 report. Studies show that tai chi strengthens upper- and lower-body muscle, even though weights are not used. It's popular partly because it can be done by anyone, anywhere, because movements are gentle, muscles are relaxed and joints are not taxed.

The benefits are proven: It reduced pain and improved mood and physical functioning for people with arthritis, a 2008 Tufts University study found; it significantly lowered blood pressure and improved symptoms—including cholesterol and insulin levels—in people at high risk for heart disease, says *The Journal of Alternative and Complementary Medicine.* And the quality of life and functional capacity improved in women with breast cancer who did 12 weeks of tai chi, according to *Medicine and Sport Science.* Next time you're in the park, join in.

Essential Concepts

Practitioners of Traditional Chinese Medicine (TCM) believe that illness is caused by an imbalance of the life force called qi (pronounced—all together now—"chee"). Tai chi (a subcategory of qigong) strives to promote the smooth flow of qi through the body's meridians, a theory that is shared with the systems of acupuncture and acupressure. Tai chi and qigong usually use a rhythmic cycle of moves, involving forms of hand

and body movements, including "Pushing Hands," "Standing Like Tree," "Snake Creeps Down to Water" and other movements that often are based in nature. The exercises are ideally done outside, so that the qi of the body and the qi of the earth can be united. And practicing with a group of people of all ages enhances the feeling of a united community. Repetition and refinement of the movements through practice are crucial.

Try It Out

Tai chi and qigong classes can be found at local YMCAs, recreation centers, martial arts studios and community centers. Ask around for referrals, or simply observe that group in the park, and, once you join, give it some time. The slow pace might be weird to you at first; but be patient. Also, here are a few tips on how to tell you're in a good class (meaning—learning from a good teacher):

LOOK FOR AN INSTRUCTOR WITH AT LEAST FIVE YEARS OF EXPERIENCE

Yes, everyone needs to start somewhere, but if you're a beginner, you need a teacher who knows how to teach.

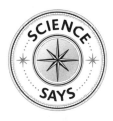

Tai chi and qigong studies have consistently pointed out their benefits for treating stress- and age-related diseases. Many studies have shown that tai chi relaxes the muscles and nervous system and improves posture, flexibility and joint health. Studies also have shown that it can improve the health and vitality of the elderly, easing pain and anxiety and improving balance. Research on qigong, much of it based in China and Taiwan, has shown it useful for reducing hypertension due to its ability to raise blood levels of HDL ("good") cholesterol and lower LDL ("bad") cholesterol. Qigong has been shown in studies to be useful in regulating stress hormones and reducing stress, easing asthma symptoms and even decrease blood glucose levels in diabetics.

However, while most medical doctors accept tai chi and qigong as a powerful relaxation tool, many are skeptical of the theories of energy meridians and qi.

GAUGE HIS/HER ENERGY

If the teacher is pale and listless, he's not going to inspire you.

LOOK AT THE OTHER STUDENTS

There should be some who also seem healthy and energetic. And if you notice a lot of injuries (or you experience more than normal muscle achiness), high-tail it out.

ASK QUESTIONS

Your teacher should be able to answer intelligently. She also should be well-versed in TCM, since that's what tai chi and qigong are based on.

LOOK FOR KINDNESS...

...patience and tolerance.

For more information, go to the National Qigong Association (NQA) website (nqa.org) and the International Integral Qigong and Tai Chi Training Institute, overseen by Roger Jahnke, OMD, chairperson of the NQA (healerwithin.com).

✴ **BEST FOR:** Tai chi is excellent for improving and maintaining mental clarity and reducing stress, so the practice is often recommended for tension, depression and anxiety, as well as for conditions of old age. Any condition caused or worsened by stress can be improved with tai chi and qigong. They also can enhance physical and mental control and general health.

Precautions

As long as you have no physical restrictions, tai chi and qigong are safe practices.

A Simple Qigong Routine

Stressed out? Slow your roll, and join the thousands of people increasingly turning to qigong, a traditional Chinese wellness practice similar to, but even older than, tai chi. A 2010 *American Journal of Health Promotion* review of 77 studies found that anxiety decreased significantly for participants practicing qigong compared to an active exercise group. That's largely because, as the review authors noted, qigong—like tai chi and yoga—is a unique type of exercise known as "meditative movement." And with meditation, of course, comes calm; in fact, meditating is one of the best ways to manage stress and the ailments that come with it.

Among the additional benefits of qigong discovered in the aforementioned review: improved bone health, cardiopulmonary fitness, physical function, balance, general quality of life and immunity. Plus, qigong allows you to mix and match exercises in whatever order you like. Although it may take a few tries to get accustomed to moving in such a slow and relaxed manner, the more you practice, the calmer—and yet more energized—you'll feel.

The plan

Perform these six popular qigong moves daily or even twice a day (morning and evening) as an individual practice or precursor to other activities. Repeat each move six to eight times; the set should take about 15 minutes to complete. Due to the gentle and flowing nature of the exercises, you don't need a formal warm-up or cool-down. There's no equipment required, and you don't even need to change your clothes. As you move, place the tip of your tongue against the roof of your mouth; this helps to induce calmness and focus. Also, breathe rhythmically and deeply. (Unlike yoga or Pilates, the breath is not connected to each part of the movement.) To enhance your practice, inhale through your nose, expanding your rib cage and belly; exhale through pursed lips, gently pulling your belly in.

1.

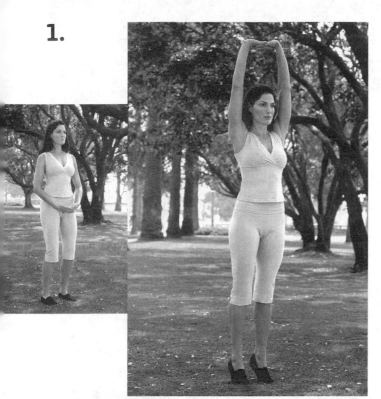

Pressing the Heavens with Two Hands

Stand with your feet separated slightly and knees gently bent. Interlace your fingers, turning the palms up, with your arms hanging in front of you, elbows slightly bent. Draw your tailbone down and pull in your belly (far left). Raise your arms slowly overhead, keeping them straight. Turn the palms back up as you rise on the balls of your feet. Circle the arms down, lowering your heels (near left). Return to starting position and repeat.

Stretches the entire body; may help balance metabolism and enhance lung, stomach and spleen function.

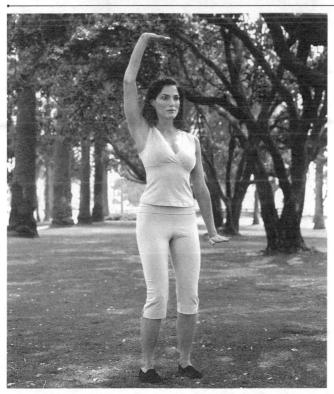

2.

Separating Heaven and Earth

Standing with feet hip-width apart, knees bent and arms at your sides, raise your right arm overhead, keeping the palm up and fingers pointing to the left. At the same time, press the left hand down, wrist flexed and fingers pointing forward (left). Press both palms away, lengthening the arms. Circle the arms back to starting position and repeat, switching arm positions.

Stimulates internal organs, helps prevent gastrointestinal disorders, balances brain function and stretches arms and shoulders.

3.

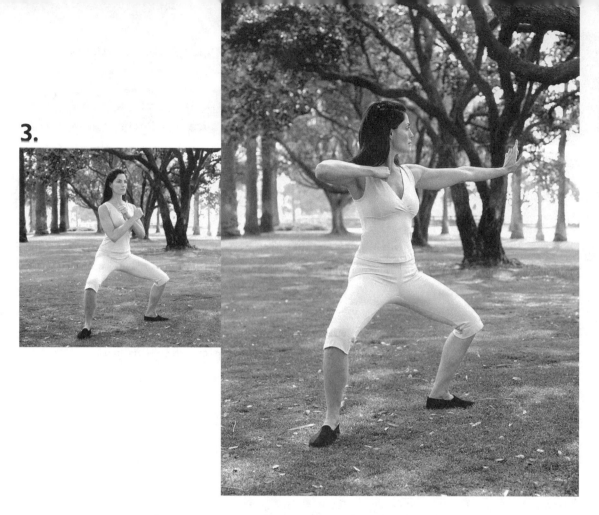

Drawing a Bow and
Letting the Arrow Fly

Take a step to your left so your legs are slightly more than hip-width apart. Bend your knees, lowering your hips into "horse stance," toes and knees aligned. Cross wrists in front of your chest, with your right arm on the outside, palms facing out (above left). Maintain "horse stance" and extend your left arm in line with the shoulder, forefinger pointing up, thumb stretched back and other fingers bent. At the same time, make a fist with the right hand and lift the right arm to shoulder height as if drawing a bow; look at your left hand (above right). Return to starting position and repeat, alternating sides.

Expands the chest to stimulate lungs, loosens up shoulders and arms, improves spine function and strengthens legs.

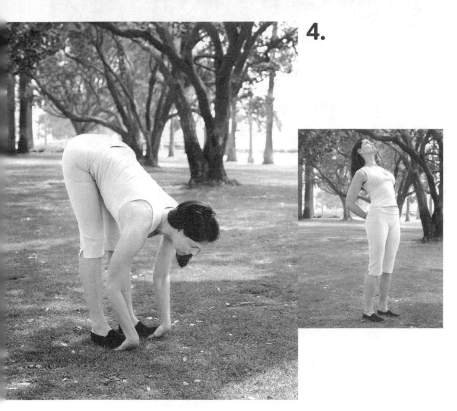

4.

Pulling Toes

With your feet slightly separated, bend forward from your hips, keeping the legs straight but not locked. (If you need to, bend your knees.) Grasp under your feet with both hands. Keep your spine straight and rib cage pulled in, and look slightly ahead (far left). Stand upright, grasping your right wrist at the base of your spine with your left hand, and extend into a slight back-bend (near left). Straighten to stand tall, then repeat both moves.

Strengthens back muscles, may improve adrenal and kidney functions.

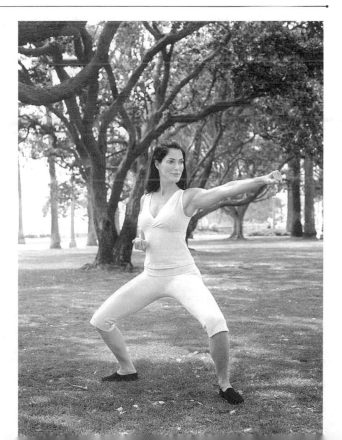

5. Punching with Angry Gaze

Separating your feet slightly more than hip-width apart, bend your knees into "horse stance." Bend both elbows close to your sides at waist level, fists clenched, palms up. Maintaining "horse stance," extend your right arm up and out to shoulder height, rotating the palm down; look at your right hand (right). Bend the right elbow to return to starting position and repeat, alternating arms.

Stimulates the autonomic nervous system, boosts circulation and increases muscular strength and stamina.

6.

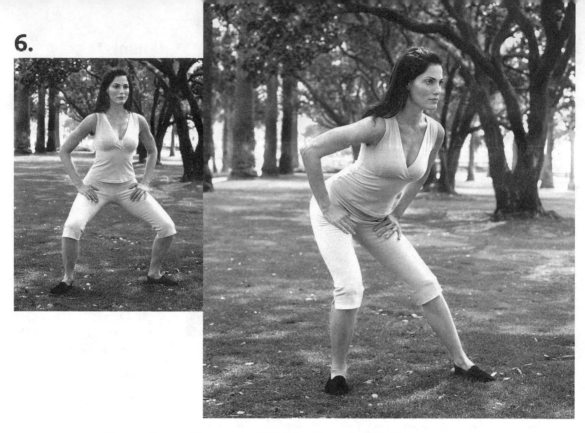

Drawing a Bow and Wagging the Tail

Separating your feet slightly more than hip-width apart, bend your knees into "horse stance," and place your hands on your thighs (above left). Bend the torso forward from the hips and sway to the left. At the same time, sway your hips and buttocks to the right, stretching out your left leg and straightening your back (above right). Return to starting position and repeat, alternating sides so your body moves like a pendulum.

Reduces stress and balances the heart and nervous systems.

Make your qigong practice more purposeful with these tips:

Minimize your motion. If you think you can move more slowly, you probably can.

Relax with every exercise. This is a moving meditation, so if you feel tense, you've lost the purpose.

Stay low. Many exercises in qigong are based on "horse stance." So always try to "ride your horse" and lower your center of gravity.

Aromatherapy

The proof that aromatherapy is beneficial, beyond a shadow of a doubt, isn't found in some Harvard study or at the Mayo Clinic. It's in a food court, near the Cinnabon. That distinctive, seductive smell—of the icing dripping down a hot, sugary roll—makes most people feel, at worst, warm inside, and at best, strangely alive. The company's sales are proof.

Smell is one of our most forceful, evocative senses. Aromatherapy builds on that power; it uses essential plant oils for healing, and has been used for centuries around the world to promote wellness and treat disease.

Modern aromatherapy is based largely in France, created by a chemist who discovered the healing properties of lavender; doctors in France often prescribe essential oils instead of conventional medicine. OK, it might not cure the big C, but aromatherapy does make cancer patients feel better, and can help you relax, feel calmer and even sleep. It definitely can improve your mood. Just think of how sexy you feel when you wear Chanel Coco Mademoiselle—and see if men pick up the scent.

Essential Concepts

The theory of aromatherapy holds that essential oils are absorbed by the body either by inhalation (via bath or diffuser) or during massage, and enter the nervous system, altering a person's emotion state or health. Chemically, this is true: It stimulates smell receptors in the nose, which then send messages through the nervous system to the limbic system—the part of the brain that controls mood and emotion. While limited scientific research has been done on it, studies have shown that aromatherapy can relieve anxiety and depression, and an NIH 2012 overview found that using essential oils can improve quality of life for people with chronic health issues such as cancer. Sleep studies have found improvement as well. Essential oils are extracted from plants, and therefore you should look for oils from organic sources.

Also according to the NIH overview, lab and animal studies have shown that certain essential oils have antibacterial, antiviral, antifungal, calming, or energizing effects. Some of the most popular essential oils for healing are: clary sage, lavender, chamomile, rosemary, peppermint and tea tree oil.

Try It Out

IMMUNE-BOOSTING AROMATHERAPY SHOWER

With one bottle of essential oil, a body brush and 15 minutes to spare, you can transform your shower into an all-over aromatherapy treatment that will keep you feeling energized all day.

By using aromatherapy in the shower, you'll aid stress relief, prevent dry skin, invigorate your lymph and circulatory systems and increase overall vitality, says Valerie Cooksley, R.N., founder of Flora Medica Integrative Aromatherapy (floramedica.com). Try her at-home regimen three or four times a week:

1. Start by selecting a skin-friendly essential oil such as mandarin, grapefruit, lavender, ylang-ylang or bergamot. These are the most stress-fighting and uplifting oils, Cooksley says.

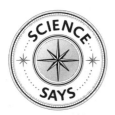

While the psychological effects of smell have been well-researched, not much has been done on claims for the effects of essential oils on medical conditions. Most doctors do not feel it is any more beneficial than a massage. However, doctors do accept that deep relaxation and a feeling of well-being associated with a certain smell can help patients feel calmer, which in turn has a healing effect. Doctors do hope to see more quality research into the specific qualities of essential oils.

2. Add several drops of oil to a dry skin brush, then exfoliate head-to-toe to stimulate circulation.

3. Close the drain, pour a few drops of oil onto the shower floor, and run the water as hot as you can tolerate for a minute or two. This will create a steam-like experience and foot soak, Cooksley explains. Focus on taking slow, long, deep breaths.

4. Stay in the hot water for at least two minutes, then turn down the water temperature to get a blast of cold. Ending a shower with cold water can strengthen circulation and close the skin pores, says Cooksley. Alternate between hot and cold water several times; the greater the difference between the two temperatures, the greater the health benefits.

"When you begin your morning with intention, pleasure and natural body care, you can reap health-giving benefits for body and mind," says Cooksley.

∗ BEST FOR: Digestive disorders, stress-related conditions such as headache and insomnia, skin conditions, insomnia, asthma, colds, cystitis, general good health, menstrual problems and pregnancy and labor.

Precautions

Many essential oils should not be used during pregnancy, such as clary sage, German chamomile and rosemary.

Some essential oils may interact negatively with drugs and homeopathy, and some should not be used if you suffer from high blood pressure or epilepsy.

When used on the skin, essential oils should be diluted; for people with sensitive skin, some may cause a rash.

Make sure your doctor knows you are using aromatherapy, especially if you are being treated for an illness.

Seek only qualified practitioners.

Use inhalation with care if you have asthma.

FIND A PRACTITIONER

Aromatherapy can be used for self-treatment for stress release, colds and other respiratory conditions, but an aromatherapist is trained to answer any questions you might have about dosage, purity, application methods, contraindications and possible interactions between essential oils and other medications you may be taking. A good rule of thumb is, if you are in doubt, contact a knowledgeable aromatherapist or work with a health care provider you trust who is willing to investigate with you and help you devise your plan. As with any other kind of service provider, the best way to find a good aromatherapist is through referrals from your health care providers, family, colleagues and friends. Also:

When choosing a practitioner, it is important to consider his/her education and training, experience, and philosophy of care.

Inquire up front about costs and find out what your insurance will cover; it's doubtful that your health care plan will cover treatments unless your are referred by an M.D., but you can try.

Be wary of any practitioner who makes excessive claims and guarantees a cure. Also be wary of one who wants to sign you up immediately for a specified number of treatments.

The Aromatherapy and Allied Practitioners' Association (aapa.org.uk) can supply more information; and you can find a U.S. practitioner at aromaweb.com. Lists of aromatherapists are also available online (see the Aromatherapy Registration Council).

Ayurveda

Can you be an overnight sensation when you're more than 5,000 years old? If you're holding this book, chances are you'll also have at least heard of ayurveda, the sister science of yoga. The ancient Indian tradition has become the latest craze in the alternative cure movement: shorthand for clean living and balanced healing, with the attractive benefit of possibly getting a sweet, sesame oil head massage during treatments. But ayurveda isn't some fad. It aims to do nothing less than balance and integrate the entirety of you: mind, body and spirit.

It works for many. According to the most recent NIH National Health Interview Survey, which included a comprehensive survey of complementary and alternative medicine (CAM) use by Americans, more than 200,000 adults use ayurvedic medicine every year.

Essential Concepts

Ayurveda philosophy centers on the five elements—ether, air, fire and water—and simplifies them into the three basic body types or doshas: vata, pitta and kapha.

Know your type, and you'll be able to make smart lifestyle changes—whether that's sharpening your focus at work, clearing up your IBS or boosting your fertility. Energetic, creative vata types tend to be thin and wiry, running on nervous energy and prone to anxiety. Pittas have a medium or athletic build and tend to be what we'd call "type-A's"—ambitious, driven high-achievers who get wound up and are prone to anger. And mellow, stable kapha types are slow metabolizers with large bodies and loving hearts, prone to stagnation and depression.

Centered around digestion of all kinds, ayurvedas consider it vital to rid the body of toxins, so diet and detoxification are key principles, as are herbal remedies, yoga, meditation and massage. As far as healing systems go, this is among the most mellow.

Try It Out

Your ayurveda practitioner will determine your dosha at your first consultation. On meeting, you'll discuss what you're seeking treatment for, and she'll look at your tongue, nails and lips, and take a detailed reading of your pulse—known as *Nadi Pariksha.* This is more than just counting the beats: By carefully placing her fingers on your wrist, she can assess the balance of your doshas, as well as the flow of your prana, or essential life force. You may be surprised at just how much information your practitioner is able to uncover about what's going on in your physical body from this seemingly simple exam. (There's no hiding that Chick-fil-A you had for lunch.)

Once she has an idea of what's going on, the two of you will look at your lifestyle as it is—what, when and how you're eating, how you're spending your time—and together you'll work out what changes can be built into your daily routine to cure what ails you. Your practitioner will likely also recommend a course of ayurvedic herbs for you to take, and recommend—or even teach you—some yoga routines.

For those of you who are simply curious about ayurveda, take our quiz on page 290 to discover your dosha. Working out your ayurvedic type means you can customize your pathway to health by working out the biggest challenges your type has, and choosing the best lifestyle, diet and exercise program for you. No wonder it's getting so popular.

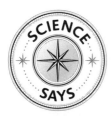

Most research on ayurvedic medicine has been done in India; the studies have been small, and have had other issues that have rendered findings less than significant, so more evidence is needed. That said, a 2011 study found that patients with rheumatoid arthritis improved after using *Boswellia serrate,* an herb used in ayurveda.

Ongoing trials by the National Center for Complementary and Alternative Medicine (NCCAM), a division of the National Institutes of Health, are exploring the use of ginger, boswellia and turmeric to treat inflammatory disorders such as arthritis, plus herbal therapies such as curcumin for cardiovascular conditions and gotu kola to treat and prevent Alzheimer's.

✱ BEST FOR: Heart disease, digestive problems, anti-aging, allergies and asthma, anxiety and insomnia, rheumatoid arthritis, skin conditions, viral infections (especially hepatitis), wound healing, women's reproductive issues and general overall health.

Precautions

Make sure your practitioner is qualified to prescribe herbal remedies; go to an M.D. who practices ayurvedic medicine, if possible.

Before using an ayurvedic remedy, find out if any rigorous scientific studies have been done.

Before embarking on any alternative plan, consult with your conventional doctor if you are pregnant or trying to conceive.

Avoid enemas and other purgative treatments if you are pregnant or elderly or if you have heart disease. Enemas should not be used on the very young.

Tell your medical doctor about any complementary remedies you are taking and do not stop taking any prescription medication without consulting your doctor first.

FIND A PRACTITIONER

You have to be your best advocate when seeking the most qualified ayurvedic doctor for you, which means committing to some research. The best place to start, of course, is asking for a referral from friends or family, including your yoga teacher, or even your conventional doc. Also:

Check credentials and education. The International Society for Ayurveda and Health recommends partnering with a practitioner who holds a doctoral degree (e.g., M.D., Ph.D. or Phys.D.) and has completed training at a recognized ayurvedic medical school in addition to these qualifications.

When you're looking for a practitioner, always call ahead for a five- to 10-minute interview. You'll be spending lots of time with this doctor, and you need to have a sense that you can be comfortable with and trust him/her. Be wary of one who won't talk to you.

An initial examination involves observation, touch and lots of questions. Use your intuition to judge whether it's working for you or not, and of course whether any inappropriate behavior occurs.

Inquire up front about costs and find out what your insurance will cover; some health care plans will cover treatments by an M.D. but not a yoga or massage therapist.

Be wary of any practitioner who makes excessive claims and guar-

QUIZ:

Discover Your Dosha

Understanding your ayurvedic dosha can help you chart a course toward a healthier and more balanced lifestyle. Doshas are our mind-body tendencies, and each of the doshas has a propensity to react to the world in a more or less patterned and predicable way. Know your dosha, in other words, and you can get a pretty good handle on what's coming up—and know how to balance yourself to handle it with grace and ease. Think of this as a personality quiz. To discover your predominant mind-body-spirit type—or dosha—put a check next to the statements in each column that you can relate to. Then turn the page for helpful advice.

COLUMN 1

○ I'm an ectomorph—long and lean.

○ My energy comes and goes in quick bursts.

○ I'm prone to constipation or gas.

○ I love cold, dry, windy weather.

○ When stress gets the best of me, I feel anxious and fearful—as if I might freak out.

○ I have a hard time falling or staying asleep.

○ My skin is dry, thin and prone to fine lines.

○ I sometimes forget to eat.

antees a cure. Also be wary of one who wants to sign you up immediately for a specified number of treatments.

The International Society for Ayurveda and Health (ISAH); ayurvedahealth.org) maintains a database of local practitioners along with their credentials and education.

COLUMN 2

○ I'm a mesomorph—medium build with good musculature.

○ My energy is intense, and I am driven to accomplish my goals.

○ I often get heartburn or even ulcers.

○ I don't do well with hot or muggy conditions.

○ When stress gets the best of me, I feel angry and impatient.

○ I sleep pretty well.

○ My skin is oily or reddish, and prone to rashes or irritation.

○ I'm the life of the party. I like a lot of change and excitement around me.

○ I'm career- or goal-oriented. I'm the kind of person who likes to focus and get things done.

○ My appetite is strong. I have a hard time missing meals.

COLUMN 3

○ I'm an endomorph—big-boned, with a tendency to put on weight.

○ My energy is never super-high, but it's always steady.

○ I've got a sluggish metabolism.

○ I don't like cold and rainy days.

○ When stress gets the best of me, I feel withdrawn—I want to hide out.

○ My sleep is long, deep and heavy—I never want to get up.

○ My skin is thick, smooth and cool—though prone to cystic acne.

○ I'm caring and devoted. Whether it's a job or a relationship, I tend to be in it for the long haul.

○ I'm a little bit hungry most of the time; I like to graze.

If you've got the most check marks in the first column, you're primarily a **VATA**—creative, flighty and prone to nervousness and irregularity.

If you've got the most check marks in the second column, you're primarily a **PITTA**—driven, forceful and ambitious, with a tendency toward inflammation and irritability.

If you've got the most check marks in the third column, you're primarily a **KAPHA**—earthy, stable and loving, but also highly susceptible to stagnation and weight gain.

FIND YOUR DOSHA

The Creative Type: VATA

For artistic vata types, every moment is a new adventure. These expressive individuals are always on the move, traveling through life from one pursuit to another. They tend to be thin, have trouble putting on weight and are prone to anxiety and fear.

BODY TYPE: Ectomorph, thin, long and lean
EMOTIONAL TENDENCY: Anxiety
BIGGEST HEALTH RISKS: Heart conditions such as arrhythmias, palpitations, tachycardia and vascular spasm
HEALTH FOCUS: Stress reduction

Vata's motion-driven, high-strung nature has direct consequences for health. Research published in the *Journal of the American College of Cardiology* in 2008 found a direct link between anxiety and heart disease—men who tested high (in the top 15% of study participants) on four separate scales for anxiety had a 30% to 40% increase of risk for heart attack. Less is known about how anxious women fare, though the problem is likely to be as prevalent if not more so, since it's well-documented that women are more likely to suffer from anxiety than men. Indeed, many female heart attacks are misdiagnosed as panic attacks, and women are far more likely than men to suffer from palpitations, arrhythmias and the kind of vascular spasm that can lead to Takotsubo cardiomyopathy—or broken heart syndrome, a condition brought on by a surge of stress hormones.

The key to keeping these creative types healthy is to focus on creating calm. "The vata mind is like a pinball machine," says John Douillard,

D.C., Ph.D., ayurvedic practitioner and founder of LifeSpa in Boulder, Colo. "Vatas love to be stimulated—but then it's easy for them to get completely overwhelmed. The most important thing vatas can do for themselves is get on a good quality routine and stick with it to create a little more regularity in their lives."

FOCUS ON... STRESSING LESS

Ayurvedic experts agree: The single most important thing a vata type can do is to adopt a stress-reduction program. Learning new ways to deal with anxiety when it does come up can help a vata type take it in stride. But don't bother telling a vata to sit still and calm down—their restless nature will often resist, say, seated meditation. Better to give them something to *do* with all that nervous energy. Slow and gentle breathing exercises are perfect, because they calm the nervous system.

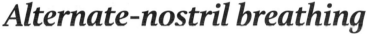

Alternate-nostril breathing

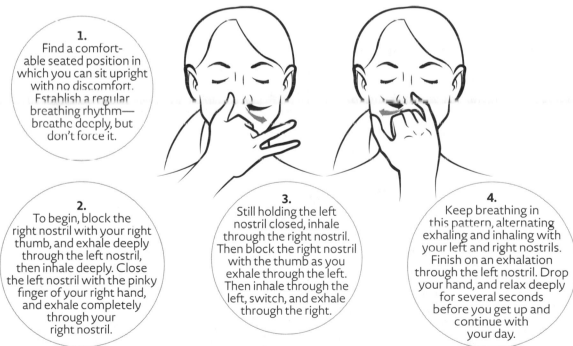

1.
Find a comfortable seated position in which you can sit upright with no discomfort. Establish a regular breathing rhythm—breathe deeply, but don't force it.

2.
To begin, block the right nostril with your right thumb, and exhale deeply through the left nostril, then inhale deeply. Close the left nostril with the pinky finger of your right hand, and exhale completely through your right nostril.

3.
Still holding the left nostril closed, inhale through the right nostril. Then block the right nostril with the thumb as you exhale through the left. Then inhale through the left, switch, and exhale through the right.

4.
Keep breathing in this pattern, alternating exhaling and inhaling with your left and right nostrils. Finish on an exhalation through the left nostril. Drop your hand, and relax deeply for several seconds before you get up and continue with your day.

Fitness Fix
GET CREATIVE WITH YOUR WORKOUTS

Instead of hitting the gym five days a week, try mixing up your exercise routine by dancing. A vata likes to be creative, emotionally expressive and spiritually uplifted. Dance is perfect. Inwardly, vatas always know they need to dance, but sometimes you have to give them permission to do it. Sign up for salsa or ballroom dancing lessons, find a NIA or Zumba class, or join a local dance circle. Vatas will make a beeline for vigorous, athletic yoga practices like ashtanga yoga, but what they really need on a regular basis is a slow, soothing restorative yoga class.

REACH FOR HEALTHY FATS

Wispy vata types need food that can help weigh them down a little. In contrast with other types, they can benefit from adding more fats into their diet (choose healthy monounsaturated fats, such as olive or flax-seed oils, or use ghee, clarified butter). They should choose foods that are warm, soupy or heavy; root vegetables are especially grounding. Avoid the salad bar, especially when stressed, as those cold, dry, rough foods can make a vata feel unbalanced.

VATA SEASON: FALL

Fall is a transitional season, and with its erratic shifts in temperature and chilly winds, this can be a tough time of year for already flighty vatas. Air types should find a steady routine, wrap up well and eat warm, nourishing foods. Thinking of going on a cleanse? Opt for mineral soups rather than cold juices.

The Type A: PITTA

Bright and perceptive, pittas are the go-getters of the world, harnessing their fiery energy to achieve their goals. They usually have an athletic, muscular build and reddish hair. Pitta types have a strong ambition, and drive themselves incredibly hard—it's not about being good enough, it's about being the best.

BODY TYPE: Mesomorph, medium-build with good musculature
EMOTIONAL TENDENCY: Anger
BIGGEST HEALTH RISKS: Inflammation, high blood pressure and
sudden heart attack
HEALTH FOCUS: An anti-inflammatory diet

While these type-A go-getters can set their sights on an ambitious goal and marshal their will to achieve it, all this focus and intensity can lead to burnout and to anger—the emotional default-setting for an out-of-balance pitta. And anger can be devastating to health, says cardiologist Mimi Guarneri, M.D., medical director of Scripps Center for Integrative Medicine in San Diego and author of *The Heart Speaks: A Cardiologist Reveals the Secret Language of Healing.* "When you get angry, your blood pressure goes up, your platelets get sticky, your immune system gets suppressed," she explains. "Anger is a lethal emotion; for instance, your risk of suffering a heart attack goes up by 230% after an angry outburst."

Driven pittas might not feel the effects of their anger until it's too late. They tend to have a high pain threshold, and can keep pushing themselves even when they are not well.

Another pitta-related risk factor is inflammation—a side effect of all that inner heat. Pitta types are the most likely to have elevated levels of C-reactive protein (CRP), which indicates inflammation in the body. The key to good health for pittas, then, is to chill out—from the inside out.

FOCUS ON... YOUR DIET

An anti-inflammatory diet is essential for imbalanced pittas. That means emphasizing a plant-based diet that includes lots of dark leafy greens, beans, fresh herbs, whole grains and cruciferous vegetables like broccoli and cauliflower. Sweet seasonal fruits also help dampen the fire of inflammation—but should not be eaten in excess. The American Heart Association recently revised its dietary recommendations to limit sugar intake, in part because of the link between sugar consumption and inflammation.

Just as important for pitta types is what *not* to eat: Anything with too much caffeine, alcohol, "flesh foods" (such as fish, chicken and red meat) can aggravate pitta. And spicy foods can be a highway to hell for those around you—not to mention your own digestive tract after years of hot curries. But limiting these foods can be a hard sell for aggressive pittas. "Pittas often have voracious appetites, and will leverage their intensity with food," says Scott Blossom, L.Ac., a certified yoga therapist and ayurvedic consultant based in Berkeley, Calif. "They love the thrill of a triple macchiato, the intoxication of a 16-ounce steak, the cocktails they drink while they're trying to play as hard as they work. But this will only lead to more inflammation." Instead, reach for these cooling, pitta power foods: apples, pears, coconut water, kale, cucumbers, sweet potatoes and cooling spices such as cilantro, fennel or coriander.

Fitness Fix
QUIET YOUR COMPETITIVE STREAK

Pittas naturally gravitate toward competitive pursuits, which can be a good source of exercise if not taken to the extreme. But if you stop having fun—or the people around you stop having fun because of you—you need to reconsider what would be fun for everyone. Tennis and golf are good; pittas will also like anything that has a quantified result, such as a 10K race. Yoga is a great option, though pitta types should avoid sweaty Bikram and ashtanga classes, and opt instead for calming viniyoga or Iyengar classes where their attention to detail will be appreciated. Swimming is even better, as the water is inherently cooling.

CALM YOUR ANGER BALL

Since pittas are typically headstrong and can lose their temper easily, mantra-based meditation can be an effective tool for immediate—and ongoing—stress relief. Choose a mantra that helps you calm down and use it not only during meditation, but whenever anger or frustration becomes an issue—when you're standing in line, stuck in traffic or waiting on someone who's late. Transcendental meditation is great for this.

Another quick stress reliever is a *shitali pranayama*, or cooling breath. Curl your tongue as you extend it and inhale fully through your mouth; then close your mouth and exhale through your nose, gulping the air into your throat and feeling the coolness radiate throughout your body.

PITTA SEASON: SUMMER

If you sleep next to a pitta type, you'll notice they seem to emanate heat. Suffice to say, the summer can draw out pitta's most fiery qualities. As the temperature soars, pittas are likely to be more irritable and aggressive. Now is the time to up your intake of cooling foods like cucumber, coconut and cilantro, and go take some quiet time in a shady place. Please.

The Earthy Type: KAPHA

Kapha types tend to be the "rocks" that pittas and vatas lean on for support and stability. They resist change, even when it is badly needed. They are slower by nature, and don't like to do anything without having a clear methodology. They are typically larger-boned and tend to put on weight easily.

BODY TYPE: Endomorph, large-boned and slightly overweight
EMOTIONAL TENDENCY: Depression
BIGGEST HEALTH RISKS: Obesity, high cholesterol and congestive heart failure
HEALTH FOCUS: Regular vigorous exercise

The gifts of a kapha type's nature are many: Kaphas are loving, strong, stable, nurturing, supportive, capable, accepting and have great endurance and stamina. But the cost of a kapha's nature is that they're also prone to inertia and depression and the accumulation of fat, weight, phlegm, water and cholesterol. This excess creates a taxation on the organs, which have to work harder to work against all that weight.

What's worse, that excess weight tends to accumulate around a kapha's midsection—called central obesity—the weight gain pattern most closely associated with poor health. The National Institutes of Health defines central obesity as having a waist measurement higher than 35 inches for women and 40 inches for men. It's a clear marker for the development of diabetes, high triglycerides and high blood pressure, which are risk factors for heart disease.

As kaphas gain weight, they become ever more stagnant—in the best of times, they don't like to move; in the worst of times, it gets harder and harder to do so. The emotional consequence is often depression, a risk factor for heart disease that ranks right up there with smoking. In a 2008 study published in the *Journal of the American Medical Association,* researchers found that depressed people are 31% more likely to have a cardiovascular event. Yes, we said event. Add depression to a propensity to build up arterial plaque to inaction, and you can see why imbalanced kaphas are poster children for disease. Sorry, guys.

FOCUS ON... GETTING OUT THERE

Running, kickboxing, cycling, rowing and circuit training are all good choices—the more challenging the better. Kaphas should push themselves to get the blood pumping, says John Zamarra, M.D., a cardiologist and ayurvedic practitioner based in Fullerton, Calif. He also recommends lots of cardio and weight training, so that they work up a sweat every day. While kaphas will tend to prefer a slow, snoozy restorative yoga class, they'll thrive on challenging forms of yoga, such as Bikram, ashtanga and power yoga.

Since kapha is the most other-centered of the doshas, Yarema recommends team sports: "Kaphas thrive in a situation where there's activity and social interaction. They love to laugh and have fun. When they play team sports, they'll laugh and laugh—if only at their own performance."

One caveat: Kaphas who have been sedentary for a long time may need to take baby steps toward a new, active lifestyle. Exercise-related injuries will only lead them back to the couch. So move slowly (start with a daily 15-minute walk), but move—inactivity will only lead to more weight gain and stiffness.

LIGHTEN UP YOUR DIET

American dietary staples like burgers and processed convenience foods are especially bad for the earthy kapha type. Why? Kaphas often use sweet, rich, heavy, greasy foods to sedate themselves and to cope with stress. They don't mind that stagnant feeling that junk food creates—it may even factor into the appeal of that gooey dessert. Whole fruits and vegetables—foods that literally come from the ground—are most grounding and balancing to kapha types. Vegetables are the best choice, especially cruciferous and crunchy ones, like broccoli.

Spicy foods will also boost a kapha's slow metabolism. Go crazy with the black pepper, garlic, ginger and cumin. Whole grains should be light in nature—barley, buckwheat, millet and quinoa are among the best choices. And we'll say it again: fried, processed, salty, sour and excessively sugary foods should be avoided. "When kaphas overload on carbs, bad fat and processed foods, their bodies don't know what to do with all that junk," says Welch. "It gets packed away in the vessels, and the vessels get lined with plaque." Not so tasty now, huh?

MOVE THROUGH STRESS

Mellow kapha types don't wear stress on their sleeve. But since their stress response is to freeze (whereas vatas flee and pittas fight), it pays to develop an active practice of releasing worry and keeping depression at bay. Emphasis on *active*: Walking meditation is an ideal choice to focus the mind even as the body keeps moving.

Regular trips to the spa can also be beneficial in helping kaphas relax without inviting stasis. Saunas, steams and herbal wraps can help congested kapha types sweat out toxins and release excess water. Body brushing or exfoliation treatments help stimulate the skin and open clogged pores. Massage can be helpful if it involves movement (such as Thai massage or shiatsu), vigorous strokes (such as lymphatic drainage) or deep-tissue work (such as Rolfing).

KAPHA SEASON: WINTER

With its long, cold nights, winter is the perfect time for staying home and snuggling—which can seem like bliss for kaphas. But beware of turning into a couch potato. To ward off depression (as well as too many extra pounds) kaphas need to get out and socialize—and yes, you can help yourself to those spicy peanuts at the bar.

Detox and Cleanses

Your world is toxic. Every second, you breathe chemicals—
or eat them, drink them, rub them, absorb them. Mercury, lead,
pesticides, food additives, plastics... they're there from day one:
Studies have shown that even babies carry thousands of toxic chemicals in their tissues and blood. Fortunately, our bodies—primarily our
livers—are designed to eliminate toxins regularly. But today's overload
from the toxic soup we live in is too much for them to handle, and the waste
accumulates faster than they can be eliminated. Throw in the junk we
ingest voluntarily—alcohol, cigarettes, caffeine, prescription and less-
legal highs—and our bodies don't stand a chance.

Linked to all this: decreased immunity, autoimmune diseases,
reproductive and hormonal malfunctions, mood disorders, allergies and
skin conditions. Even cancer.

The interest in detox diets has recently exploded, especially among
those interested in alternative medicine, with at least 25 books on
Amazon's best seller list alone. And cold-pressed juice shops and delivery services such as Organic Alley, Blueprint and ReJuice are popping
up all over towns despite costing upwards of $9 a bottle. Detoxification
therapy—detoxing, cleansing, fasting—done in a safe, well-planned
manner, can help the body eliminate toxins and waste products
efficiently and help restore vitality and energy. Some believe it can cure
diseases, even cancer.

Essential Concepts

Champions of the detox believe that by doing cleanses on a regular basis—some people follow three- or five-day juice fasts and cleanses,

some undergo 21-day cleanses—our bodies can devote more energy to elimination than to digestion and battling inflammation; our liver's workload is lightened, and our bodies can more efficiently push toxins out. What's required is a cleaning up of the diet and a kind of emptying, paired with the fiber needed to allow our bodies to gather, process and eliminate toxins. During the first three to four days of a cleanse, participants may experience headache (especially if one is going through caffeine withdrawal) and fuzziness, possibly irritability. But as the weeks go by, skin and eyes become clearer and digestion markedly more efficient, and energy levels may soar.

Try It Out

There are many different types of detox, including juice cleanses, fasting, mono diets and vitamin C therapy; all have proved useful. Acupuncturist Christopher Hobbs espouses a periodic liver flush during which citrus, ginger and olive oil concoctions are used. The most sustainable, we find, is the type that Elson Hass, M.D., and others support, in which acidic, inflammatory foods and drink are eliminated from your diet, and as many toxins as possible from your surroundings. Haas

Are You a Candidate for Detox?

YES: Do you suffer from constipation, bloating, gas, fatigue, poor skin quality, breakouts, muscle pain, bad breath or PMS? Do you wake up tired, crave sweet foods, always feel hungry, feel irritable or have difficulty concentrating?

NO: Are you pregnant or nursing? Do you have an eating disorder? Are you anemic? If so, now's not the time to detox. If you have cancer or have any kind of chronic health condition, including diabetes or liver, heart, kidney or autoimmune disease, you should only try a detox program under the supervision of a health care provider.

calls it The Detox Diet, and many experts, including medical doctors Mark Hyman, Frank Lippman and Neal Barnard, and author Kris Carr, have based their programs on it. We call it The Doable Detox, and what follows is the guide to a 21-day program.

✱ BEST FOR: Anyone experiencing fatigue who feels in need of a reboot. Cleansing can help jump-start a weight-loss program (although one should have additional motivation to detox). The healthier eating habits often stick, leading to reduced inflammation and the benefits associated with that: reduced blood pressure and risk of heart disease; improved immunity; and reduction in allergies and asthma. Some practitioners have even found improved results in fights against cancer.

Precautions

See "Are You a Candidate for Detox?" on the previous page.

Make sure you tell your medical doctor that you are doing a cleanse, especially if you are being treated for a disease such as diabetes, cancer or heart disease.

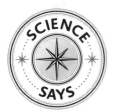

Most medical doctors hate the idea of a detox diet or juice cleanse being effective for anything but robbing you blind. While many medical doctors recommend detox diets for therapeutic and health reasons, and countless people have shown that it works, scientific evidence based on controlled studies is scarce. Any change in unhealthy eating habits can make us feel better, but the theory that a cleanse helps the body get rid of an overload of toxins is disputed. And most doctors do not recommend a cleanse or detox for weight loss, because once regular eating is resumed, the weight will come back.

THE DOABLE DETOX

Think you need a yoga retreat to cleanse the toxins from your body? Think again. Follow this simple, step-by-step plan to feel happier and healthier—this week, right now.

Detox. One little word with a lot of appeal. Sure, it's not the easiest of endeavors (good-bye coffee, hello, uhh, herbal tea!), but the promise is huge: Just a week into a detox and you're likely to experience a boost in energy, clearer skin, less gas and bloating, fewer aches and pain and even less congestion.

What's behind this seemingly miraculous transformation? Elimination. Since humans are at the top of the food chain, we're most likely to be exposed to an accumulation of toxic substances in the food supply and beyond. Even if you take good care of your body, you're still bombarded with toxins—constantly. They're in the food you eat, the water you drink and the air you breathe. Eating fewer animal products during a detox, for instance, means consuming fewer toxins, additives and saturated fats from the get-go. Your body naturally produces toxins, too. It's up to your digestive system—especially the hardworking liver, the body's main detoxifier—to send those toxins packing.

In an ideal world, our bodies would eliminate these toxins with ease. However, as our exposure to toxins increases, our ability to deal with them decreases, experts say. The solution? Give your weary detoxifying organs a rest (read: Go on a cleanse) so they become more efficient.

But before you drastically alter your diet, listen up: To detox safely and effectively, you'll need to prep your body for elimination, eat lots of fresh, whole foods (detoxing doesn't mean you have to fast!) and learn how to transition back into the "real world" when your detox is finished. "Just going back to your same old habits after you detox is more violent on your body than not detoxing at all," says Mary Saunders, L.Ac., the founder and director of Boulder Community Acupuncture in Colorado. For a safe, do-it-yourself detox plan, read on.

One Week Before You Detox...

Many practitioners will tell you not to go cold turkey on sugar, caffeine and all of the other foods you'll be forgoing during your cleanse. "If you jump right into a detox, you're more likely to have unpleasant symptoms early on," says integrated medicine physician Elson M. Haas, M.D., *Natural Health* advisory board member; founder and director of Preventive Medical Center of Marin in San Rafael, Calif.; and the author of *The New Detox Diet*. Instead, take a week to gear up for your detox, slowly eliminating off-limits foods and drinks. This not only prepares your body physically, but also emotionally and practically. "People have strong attachments to food, and it's less emotional if you slowly let those things go," says Saunders. Here's how to prepare for a successful detox:

CHOOSE A D-DAY: During the first couple of detox days, it's common to feel fatigued or experience an increase in the exact same symptoms that led you to want to detox in the first place. So, it can be helpful to start on the weekend, or another day when your schedule is a little lighter. Also, don't start at a time when you have a lot of social commitments coming up, such as weddings or birthday parties.

Get Ready to Cleanse

Ideally, take a week to wean yourself off the foods, drinks and other substances that you will eliminate during your cleanse: animal products (including dairy), alcohol, coffee, sugar, gluten and processed foods.

Cut back on alcohol—try to drink only organic red wine and limit it to two each week.

Slowly eliminate coffee by drinking just one cup a day, then ½ cup a day—it's not just the caffeine, but also the acid in coffee that is inflammatory.

Reduce consumption of dairy and other animal products, including butter.

Cut down your servings of gluten (wheat and other processed grains—read the labels) to three servings a week.

Try to eat only whole, unprocessed foods.

Of course, any unnecessary or recreational drugs should be tapered and eliminated.

WEAN YOURSELF OFF YOUR VICES: Spend the week transitioning off what Haas calls the Big Five: caffeine, alcohol, sugar, wheat and dairy. Caffeine tends to be the most difficult for people, as quitting outright can result in the notorious caffeine withdrawal headache. If you're a coffee drinker, wean yourself off by drinking part caffeinated/part decaf one day, then decaf the next, then black tea, green tea and finally herbal teas.

LEARN LABEL LINGO: You'll want to start reading ingredient lists—not just the Nutrition Fact labels—if you don't already. Sugar is often a surprise, because it's in everything: bread, soup, salad dressing, sauces. Also beware of sugar by another name. Aliases include high-fructose corn syrup, sucrose, fructose, dextrose, maltose, as well as molasses, honey and maple syrup. Look for labels that specify foods are gluten-free and not processed in plants that also process products that are not gluten free.

EAT MORE GREENS: Organic vegetables will be the mainstay of your diet during a detox, so get a head start by incorporating them into your meals now. No. 1 on the list? Cruciferous vegetables like broccoli, kale, collard greens, brussels sprouts, bok choy, Chinese cabbage and artichokes. "They have powerful sulphur compounds that enhance the detoxifying enzymes and boost the liver's ability to detoxify," says Beth Reardon, M.S., R.D., L.D.N., an integrative nutritionist at Duke Integrative Medicine in Durham, N.C. Cook them very lightly with garlic and onions, which help boost the body's production of glutathione, a protein that serves as a powerful antioxidant. "Over 60% of the toxins that go to the liver are detoxified by glutathione," says Cathy Wong, N.D., C.N.S., a Boston-based naturopath and the author of *The Inside-Out Diet: 4 Weeks to Natural Weight Loss, Total Body Health, and Radiance.* For a quick list of detoxifying foods, see "7 Great Detox Foods" on page 309.

FILL UP ON FIBER: Your bowel is a major route of elimination, and if it isn't working well, you will feel terrible when you detox. Ideally, before your detox you want to be having at least one well-formed bowel movement a day (and these smooth moves will become quite a focus). If you need help getting things moving, add one to two tablespoons of ground flaxseed to your diet daily.

DRINK MORE WATER: During a detox you'll need to consume at least eight glasses of filtered water (tap water and even bottled water may contain chemicals and toxins) or herbal tea each day to keep your body hydrated and help speed elimination. "If you increase fiber and you aren't drinking enough water, you'll end up with constipation," says Wong.

PUT ON YOUR APRON: Few, if any, convenience or processed-prepared foods are going to fit the bill for foods allowed on a detox diet, so break out the pots, pans and cookbooks, and check out the end of the chapter for what to eat.

START TAKING A HIGH-QUALITY MULTIVITAMIN, IF YOU'RE NOT ALREADY: "A daily multivitamin ensures that you are getting the nutritional support your liver needs to do its job," says Wong. She recommends taking a multi that offers at least 100% of the daily value of these liver-friendly nutrients: vitamins B_1 (thiamin), B_2 (riboflavin), B_3 (niacin), B_6 (no more than 100 milligrams per day), B_{12}, D, C and E (no more than 200 IU per day), along with chromium, zinc and selenium. But too much vitamin A in the form of retinol (which may be listed as "retinol," "retinyl palmitate" or "retinyl acetate") can be toxic to the liver, Wong cautions, so don't exceed 5,000 IUs a day. And, there should be no artificial colors or flavors. Vitamins we like: Rainbow Light's Just Once Naturals Women's One Multivitamin and New Chapter's Every Woman's One Daily.

ADD AN OMEGA FATTY ACID SUPPLEMENT: "Not having enough omega-3s in your diet can lead to excess inflammation, which disrupts cell membranes and allows toxins to leak in," says Wong. She recommends Nordic Naturals ProEFA because the fish oil is filtered to remove toxins and has the ideal ratio of omega-3 (EPA and DHA) to omega-6 (GLA) fatty acids, which is five-to-one. Take one capsule three times per day with meals for maximum absorption. (If you're a vegetarian, try Spectrum Organics Vegetarian DHA, one capsule three times a day.)

DUST OFF YOUR YOGA MAT: Daily exercise is crucial to detoxification because it stimulates the circulation of the blood and lymph, boosting your body's ability to eliminate, says naturopath Peter Bennett, N.D., R.Ac., the director of the Meditrine Naturopathic Medical Clinic in Langley, British Columbia, Canada, and the coauthor of the *7-Day Detox Miracle.* Still, this is no time for boot camp. "You're trying to rejuvenate your body; exercise should be moderate so you don't wear it out," Bennett says. "When detoxing, nothing beats a gentle yoga program." Walking is another great option.

On Birth-Control Pills?

Take extra precautions to prevent pregnancy when detoxing, especially if you're taking herbs to enhance detoxification of the liver (which can speed up drug clearance in the body).

Reach for These Supplements

Take these daily in addition to your daily multi:

FIBER: Getting enough fiber (25 to 40 milligrams per day) during a detox is essential. Fiber is food for the beneficial bacteria in the gut, and it helps with elimination. Even though the liver has packaged the toxins up for elimination, the body still wants to recycle them. Fiber helps to escort that package out before it gets reabsorbed. Psyllium husk powder is a traditional fiber supplement, but many practitioners say a better option is to add one to two tablespoons of ground flaxseed to a bowl of oatmeal, soup or a smoothie.

PROBIOTICS: "Probiotics help strengthen the intestinal wall," says Cathy Wong. N.D. "If that barrier isn't working, it allows toxins to get into the bloodstream. They're then sent back to the liver, adding to its burden." Try Metagenics UltraFlora Plus DF, because it's dairy free. Take one capsule twice a day.

MILK THISTLE: "A compound called silymarin in the seeds of milk thistle enhances detoxification and increases the synthesis of glutathione, a powerful antioxidant," says Wong. She advises looking for extracts that have been standardized to 70% to 80% silymarin. Try Nature's Way Thisilyn or Puritan's Pride Silymarin (both are 175 milligrams per capsule). Take one capsule two to three times per day. But, steer clear of this herb if you're allergic to daisies, kiwi, artichokes or plants in the aster family, as you may have an allergic reaction to milk thistle as well.

VITAMIN C: Extra vitamin C helps the body recycle glutathione and protects the detoxification pathways in the liver. Take at least 500 milligrams twice a day and up to 2,000 milligrams two or three times a day.

MAGNESIUM: Magnesium relaxes the bowel and speeds up transit time, and supplementing is especially important if your bowel is sluggish. Try Complete H20 Minerals Magnesium Concentrate and take 400 milligrams to 800 milligrams divided up throughout the day. Start taking 100 milligrams to 200 milligrams throughout the day and increase the dose as tolerated. If you experience loose stools, take less.

During Your Detox ...

Now that you've prepped your body, you're ready to detox. Most experts recommend that a detox diet last a minimum of one week, and—to get the most benefit—up to three weeks. "You need three weeks to eliminate all the toxins and reeducate yourself to have a healthy relationship with food," says Saunders. Here, expert-approved guidelines:

THINK FRESH, WHOLE, ORGANIC FOODS: Eat plenty of vegetables (choose sweet potatoes instead of white potatoes), fresh fruits, nongluten grains, beans, legumes, small amounts of nuts, seeds, nut butters, lean, organic poultry and wild fish. Steam vegetables very lightly to keep nutrients and enzymes intact.

SIP WISELY: In addition to drinking lots of filtered, mineral or sparkling water, reach for fresh, organic vegetable juice and herbal teas. Good news for caffeine addicts: Small amounts of green and white tea are OK. "The catechins in green tea increase the production of enzymes that help the liver detoxify chemicals," says Wong. Steer clear of caffeine, alcohol, soda, red meat, sugar, flour, processed and refined foods and anything artificial. Also, avoid wheat and anything with gluten, dairy, soy and eggs. These are common food allergens, and if you're even slightly intolerant, it'll make your system work harder to digest them—the opposite of what you want to do during a detox.

What to Expect When You're Detoxing

SMOOTH MOVES: You may find yourself spending more time in the ladies' room than before the detox, and that's a good thing. It's optimal to have a bowel movement two to three times a day, but one is fine.

THINGS MAY GET WORSE BEFORE THEY GET BETTER: "You may feel irritable, tired and headachy at the end of the first day, especially if you haven't given up caffeine before this point," says Haas. "Sometimes Day 2 is the hardest day; but by the end of day 2 or 3, people generally start feeling better." You also might find yourself getting a cold. "A lot of the things we call problems in Western medicine—colds, flu, sinus congestion, allergies—are the body's attempt to make itself better by getting rid of the mucus, the congestion, from accumulated acidity," says Haas.

7 Great Detox Foods

Reach for these during and after your detox to give your body the best shot at getting rid of the toxins you're exposed to every day, says Jonny Bowden, Ph.D., C.N.S., author of *The Most Effective Ways to Live Longer*

DRIED PLUMS (aka prunes) are high in fiber and antioxidants, helping to both keep your digestive system moving toxins efficiently and reduce oxidative stress on cell membranes, which eases inflammation along the way.

GARLIC is loaded with allicin, a phytonutrient that helps remove environmental toxins from the body.

DARK LEAFY GREENS like kale, chard, spinach and collard greens are packed with chlorophyll, which supports the liver in filtering toxins out of the body. Greens are also a rich source of iron, crucial to a healthy circulatory system.

LEAN MEATS AND COLD-WATER FISH are the best sources of complete proteins. Protein deficiency causes the body to burn protein for energy instead of using it to maintain the liver and kidney functions necessary to remove toxins.

FRUITS like pomegranates and acai are loaded with antioxidants, which help keep the gastrointestinal tract functioning by reducing inflammation.

WHOLE GRAINS are great sources of water-soluble fiber, which helps regulate cholesterol.

YOGURT with live active cultures is the easiest—and tastiest—way to supplement your gastrointestinal tract's natural store of probiotics, the "good" bacteria it needs to properly digest nutrients and fight infection and irritable bowel syndrome. To limit consumption of animal products, look for a vegan yogurt made from coconut or soy.

DAILY DOs

Try to do the following each day while you're on the detox:

MOVE YOUR BODY: If you have the energy, exercise will increase circulation and get the lymph moving. Try to get at least a half-hour a day of gentle yoga or easy walking.

GIVE YOUR BODY THE BRUSH-OFF: In addition to getting your lymph moving, dry-brushing your skin daily (with a natural-bristle brush) stimulates the circulation of blood in the tiny blood vessels that are within body tissues, helping to flush them out. Brush dry skin—before a shower is ideal—and always brush toward your heart, experts say. Before a shower, brush from your feet up to your hips and from your hands toward your shoulders, from your abdomen toward your chest, and from your lower back to your shoulders.

How to Eat

Crazy Sexy Diet author Kris Carr teaches that during your cleanse, you'll eat foods that reduce inflammation and eliminate those that cause it—trading acidic foods (meat, coffee, diary) for alkaline ones such as organic vegetables and juices. Her tips:

Breakfast: When you wake up, drink a glass of purified water with lemon, then herbal tea. Make a green juice from cucumber, kale, romaine lettuce, ginger, carrots and half an apple. If you are still hungry, make a smoothie with bananas, greens and a green, vegan supplement powder.

Lunch: Pile your plate with brightly colored, organic vegetables, healthy fats and protein: kale, carrots, tempeh, nuts, beans and raw vegetable "pastas." For a more filling plate, also have a steamed sweet potato or other vegetable, some soup, or some gluten-free whole grains and/or nori rolls.

Snacks: Have green juice, raw almonds or brown rice cakes with hummus or guacamole.

Dinner: For dinner, have salad, steamed veggies, tempeh, quinoa—be inventive and use colorful and unusual ingredients and experiment with dressing made with sunflower butter, lemon and olive oil. If you are feeling deprived, have a small square of dark chocolate.

TURN HOT AND COLD: Shower daily to remove toxins from your skin and open pores for further elimination, says Haas. To boost circulation and pep yourself up, get the water as hot as you can stand for three minutes, followed by as cold as you can stand for 30 seconds. Repeat this three times, then dry off quickly and get warm again to replenish your body heat.

SWEAT IT OUT: Like the bowels and the urinary tract, the skin is a route of elimination. Sweating in a sauna or steam room a few times a week during a detox can help promote the release of chemicals. But it's critical to slowly increase the time you spend in a sauna, get out if you feel dizzy or nauseous and replace electrolytes right after you come out (coconut water is great for this).

CHILL OUT: Relaxation doesn't just give you a break, it gives your liver one, too. Stress has a real physiological effect. Mindfulness meditation and journaling are not only relaxing, they can help you get in tune with the signals that your body gives you. A massage is well-earned, too.

SNAG EXTRA SHUT-EYE: "Getting adequate rest is especially important when you're trying to rid your body of toxins," says Saunders. Try to get at least eight hours a night to give your body time to heal and recharge.

AFTER YOU DETOX

Congratulations! You finished the detox. But don't celebrate with a caramel macchiato. "The transition back into the right diet for you is the most important part of the whole process," says Haas. "The No. 1 reason for doing a detox is to improve your health and create more healthful habits. So it's important to figure out what your best diet is and not just jump right back into consuming coffee, sugar and wheat." Ideally, you'll think of this 21-day cleanse as a new way of eating and living. "If you do go back to your old ways, drinking coffee and eating processed foods, keep them to a minimum," says Carr, "and stick to your daily juicing and smoothies; just remember you now have a home-base healthy diet to come back to."

When to Call It Quits

Stop your detox if you feel weak, extremely tired, nauseous or dizzy. If it is anything beyond a mild headache or sluggishness, see advice from a health care professional experienced in detoxification.

THE NATURAL MEDICINE CABINET

Restock your old medicine shelves at home
with The Essentials—for aches and pains,
colds and flus and more

S ome people have attics, basements or storage units;
others have a medicine cabinet filled with old bottles, vials, tubes,
small boxes and a thing of Bayer from 1985. It might be pretty funny, in a *Hoarders* kind of way, if it weren't for the fact that storing expired
medications means you're not making room for the things you really
need. (Not only that, but you should toss those old meds anyway—check
with your pharmacy for safe disposal.)

So what should you always have stocked on hand? What are the absolute must-haves? The solutions are simpler than you think. "You don't
usually need the big guns," says Karen Koffler, M.D., medical director
of Canyon Ranch Hotel and Spa in Miami Beach, Fla. "For day-to-day
ailments, home remedies like arnica for sprains, aloe for burns, cayenne
pepper to gargle with warm water for sore throats, ginger tea for nausea
and witch hazel for itchy, inflamed skin are often still adequate." Koffler
and other experts offer the following suggestions for a more natural,
well-rounded medicine cabinet.

General Aches and Pains

MUST-HAVE: Magnesium oil, Epsom salts, lavender essential oil, an ice pack, a bandage

For everyday strains or mild muscle pain from a too-tough workout or a twisted ankle, always stock a portable ice pack. According to the American College of Sports Medicine (ACSM), during the first 24 hours of muscle strain, apply ice to lessen swelling and reduce stiffness several times per day. Bruising occurs when blood vessels break, spilling blood into the tissues and turning them a purplish or other dark color. If you can see bruising, the ACSM recommends resting, icing, compressing (with a taut bandage) and elevating the affected limb or joint for up to 72 hours.

Magnesium effectively helps relax muscles, which in turn relieves muscular aches and pains and helps you sleep, says Carolyn Dean, M.D., N.D., author of *The Magnesium Miracle.* Take 400 milligrams twice daily—or, to avoid the side effect of loose stools—spray Ancient Minerals Magnesium Oil ($29; ancient-minerals.com) on sore spots three to four times a day. Natural Vitality's Natural Calm magnesium citrate powder ($24 for 8 ounces; shop.naturalvitality.com) can be dissolved in warm water and sipped through the day. And for no laxative effect and 100% cellular absorption, choose Pico-Ionic ReMag liquid ($135; rnadrops.info), which provides support during high-stress periods.

ALSO TRY: Soak in a warm bath (not hot, which may exacerbate swelling) with two cups of Epsom salts, the household name for magnesium sulfate. Add a few drops of lavender or rose essential oil to relax further, and stay put for 20 minutes.

Cuts and Scrapes

MUST-HAVE: Cotton balls and swabs, hydrogen peroxide, Neosporin or other antibacterial ointment, calendula cream

To prevent infection, rinse the scrape with a cotton ball soaked in hydrogen peroxide, says Woodson C. Merrell, M.D., executive director of The Continuum Center for Health and Healing in New York City and author of *Power Up: Unleash Your Natural Energy, Revitalize Your Health, and Feel 10 Years Younger.* If the cut looks nasty, follow the rinse with a dab of Neosporin, an over-the-counter antibiotic ointment, applied with a cotton swab.

Dean recommends calendula, a yellow flower with anti-inflammatory, antibacterial and antiviral properties. Apply a calendula cream (2% to 5% strength) liberally to cuts and scrapes three or four times a day, and cover with a bandage. "Homeopathic antibacterial creams work well on minor scrapes," she says.

ALSO TRY: "Silver-infused bandages block the growth of bacteria without any danger of germs building resistance," Dean advises. "When you apply an antibiotic bandage, you may contribute to germ resistance by using them when they're not necessary."

Colds and Flu

MUST-HAVE: Echinacea (tincture or pills), sea salt, neti pot, Esberitox

Echinacea is one of the most commonly used herbal products, but controversy exists about its true benefit in the treatment of the common cold. A meta-analysis evaluating 14 different studies on the effect of echinacea supports its benefit in decreasing the incidence and duration of a cold. In one study published by *The Lancet,* echinacea decreased the odds of developing the common cold by 58%.

Naturopathic doctor Stephanie Ogura, N.D., of Montreal, Quebec, prescribes a dose of up to 1,500 milligrams of a good-quality *Echinacea angustifolia* and purpurea root per day. "However, if you are not better within a week, consult a doctor," Ogura says. She advises checking with your health professional to find a reputable manufacturer who uses standardized formulations.

To use a neti pot, says Keri Glassman, M.S., R.D., best-selling author of *The New You (and Improved!) Diet,* fill it with ¼ teaspoon salt and 8 ounces lukewarm filtered water, lean forward, tilt your head to one side, and insert the spout gently into the raised nostril and pour. Breathe through your mouth as the salt water flows through your sinus and out the other nostril. (If it drains out of your mouth, lower your forehead in relation to your chin.) When the neti pot is empty, face the sink and exhale vigorously to clear the nasal passages. Refill the neti pot, tilt your head the other way and repeat through the other nostril. Use daily, and remember to take your vitamins, Glassman urges.

ALSO TRY: Merrell recommends Esberitox ($16 for 200 chewables; vitacost.com), a mixed-herbal tablet with more modest amounts of echinacea. Take three tablets three times a day. New Chapter LifeShield Immunity uses mushrooms for those with a reaction to Echinacea ($24; vitacost.com).

Hot Flashes and Mood Swings

MUST-HAVE: Black cohosh, primrose oil, CoQ10

To counter common menopausal hot flashes and irritability, try black cohosh, an estrogen-less remedy that Native Americans and Europeans have used for decades. "Research from Germany shows it works, although scientists aren't sure exactly why," says Mary Jane Minkin, M.D., clinical professor of obstetrics and gynecology at Yale University School of Medicine in New Haven, Conn. "It probably acts on the hypothalamus, the part of the brain that controls temperature."

Minkin recommends taking 20 milligrams twice daily of over-the-counter Remifemin, a vegan black cohosh supplement in pill form, each morning and evening, to minimize these premenopausal and menopausal symptoms. You can buy it at most drugstores along with high-potency primrose oil ($21 for 120 tabs; drugstore.com). Evening primrose oil has been shown to ease symptoms of menopause such as hot flashes.

Since new research indicates a vitamin D deficiency can also cause mood swings and exacerbate PMS symptoms, Glassman says, "It makes sense to get regular sunshine; and although we don't have exact recommendations yet, it's suggested that people get anywhere from five to 30 minutes of sun exposure to the face, arms, back or legs two to three times per week. Based on research and what feels reasonable to me, I recommend getting sunshine for 15 minutes a few times a week, and I try to get out after the strongest sun. My moisturizer has sunscreen in it, and I recommend that my clients always use moisturizer that contains sunscreen, too."

ALSO TRY: Ubiquinol, a natural active antioxidant form of CoQ10, the substance produced in the human body up until around age 30, that fights free radicals. Glassman says, "While young, healthy people in their 20s easily produce CoQ10 and convert it into ubiquinol, after 40 the body has a more difficult time with this conversion process." She recommends supplementing with CoQ10 or Solgar ubiquinol ($35 for 50 softgels; vitacost.com).

Stings/Itches/Burns

MUST-HAVE: Po Sum On oil, calendula ointment, pure aloe gel, witch hazel astringent, calamine lotion

For stings and itching, a Chinese tea-based herbal oil called Po Sum On ($3–$9; solsticemed.com) comes highly recommended. It reduces inflammation with a combination of menthol and cinnamon that cools, then warms, the affected area. "Po Sum On facilitates blood flow and healing, and it's miraculous for relieving itching from minor rashes and bites," says herbalist and acupuncturist Kristen Burris, L.Ac., an anti-aging expert in Eagle, Idaho. "Don't put it on broken skin or burns, and wear gloves or wash your hands afterward to avoid accidentally irritating your eyes." Apply the oil up to five times a day as needed.

Dean recommends calendula ointment (see "Cuts and Scrapes" on page 313) in a 2% to 5% strength, applied three to four times daily, for insect bites and minor stings.

ALSO TRY: Pure aloe gel or a witch hazel astringent for skin irritations. Glassman says, "Apply with a cotton ball as needed. And if you live near poison ivy, stock a healthy supply of calamine lotion."

Allergy and Sinus Problems

MUST-HAVE: Neti pot, stinging nettle

A neti pot (see "Colds and Flu" on page 314) is highly effective for sinus problems. According to studies at the University of Wisconsin-Madison, a saline wash for those with chronic sinus problems decreased congestion and sinus headaches, as well as the need for nasal sprays and antibiotics. "Anytime I feel sniffles, I head to the neti pot with filtered water and flush twice a day," says Glassman. She coaxes her young children to do the same when they have cold symptoms.

ALSO TRY: For hardcore allergy symptoms like itching eyes, runny nose and congested sinuses, Burris recommends stinging nettle, a plant containing compounds that inhibit histamines. Dosages vary, so carefully follow the directions on every label, says Burris.

Earache

MUST-HAVE: Garlic-infused olive oil, mullein oil, herbal tinctures

Koffler suggests steeping ½ clove of garlic in 1 tablespoon of olive oil overnight, then using an eyedropper to squeeze four drops into infected ears twice daily. Garlic contains a compound called allicin, thought to be effective against bacteria. Be sure the eardrum hasn't burst, which is signaled by pus: "I only recommend antibiotics when the ear contains pus," says Koffler. You can store the garlic-infused oil in the refrigerator for weeks. Or try mullein oil, which comes from a flower that combats inflammation and viruses; use two to five drops in the affected ear one to three times a day.

ALSO TRY: Tap 100% natural eardrops as an alternative to antibiotic treatment for ear infections, and to treat viral and fungal infections of the ear.

Try Rainbow Light's Pain-Eze ($10 for 30 tabs; pharmaca.com) or Native Remedies Ear-Heal ($32; nativeremedies.com) to ease ear inflammation.

Indigestion and Stomachache

MUST-HAVE: Fresh ginger, probiotics, yogurt, chamomile and peppermint teas, DGL

Consider opening a branch office of your medicine cabinet in your kitchen. Along with garlic-infused olive oil (see "Earache," this page), that's where you'll find help for a troubled stomach. Ginger is particularly helpful for pregnancy-related nausea and vomiting. For any kind of nausea, slice three or four pieces the size of a quarter and steep them in mint tea; drink a cupful as often as needed. Or use up to three droppers of tincture per day (containing a total of 3,000 milligrams of ginger extract) as needed. To rebalance your gut during bouts of diarrhea, Koffler advises taking probiotic supplements such as Metagenics Ultra Flora Plus ($37 for 60 capsules; pureformulas.com) and New Chapter Organics Probiotic All-Flora ($25 for 120 capsules; iherb.com), also found in most health food stores. "They have a mix of organisms that can support the mix in our bowels," she says. While it's less effective than probiotics, you can also consume one to two cups daily of yogurt with live active cultures to generally keep the bowel flora healthy. Look for the National Yogurt Association Live & Active Cultures (LAC) seal, which guarantees 100 million live cultures per gram. Chamomile and peppermint teas also calm a gassy, bloated bowel and ease muscle spasms—and if you have diarrhea, they're rehydrating. Try Traditional Medicinals Organic Smooth Move Chamomile and Peppermint teas ($5; traditional-medicinals.com).

ALSO TRY: For both heartburn and constipation, Koffler prefers DGL, a form of licorice that soothes the inflamed mucous lining of the gastrointestinal tract and loosens the stools. Chew one or two 380-milligram tablets (but not the sugar-free ones) 20 minutes before meals as needed. ($9 for 200 chewables; puritan.com)

Headache

MUST-HAVE: MigraSpray, butterbur, magnesium glycinate

For headaches and migraines, Koffler likes the homeopathic remedy MigraSpray ($40 for a 20-day supply; migraspray.com); spray 10 times under the tongue and hold for 30 seconds before swallowing. A key ingredient is feverfew, an herb that may reduce the inflammation that results when the brain's blood vessels dilate, a possible cause of migraines. It may also prevent blood platelets from clumping, just as aspirin does. Koffler also suggests the herb butterbur: Take the herb in 75-milligram tablets twice a day with food to sidestep headache pain. Butterbur's ingredients may inhibit histamines and leukotriene, a substance that inflames blood vessels. Acupuncture has also been very effective in the acute treatment of migraines, as well as for preventing their recurrence.

ALSO TRY: Magnesium's muscle-relaxing powers (see "General Aches and Pains" on page 313) may also help prevent headaches and migraines. Take 400 milligrams of magnesium glycinate at bedtime, says Koffler. It can also keep bowels moving regularly and help with leg cramps ($16 for 180 tablets; vitaminshoppe.com). You can also try good old Tylenol Extra Strength Pain Reliever ($12 for one hundred 500-milligram caplets; drugstore.com).

What to toss and when to toss it

Before you add new essentials to your more natural medicine cabinet, you'll have to make room for them. Here's what to save and what to purge:

Honor the expiration date. "Never buy anything without an expiration date or that doesn't list the active ingredients," says Woodson C. Merrell, M.D., executive director of The Continuum Center for Health and Healing in New York City and author of *Power Up: Unleash Your Natural Energy, Revitalize Your Health, and Feel 10 Years Younger.* Throw out natural products within six months of opening. Keep oils like vitamin E and fish oil supplements in the refrigerator so they won't turn rancid.

Know your sources. Alternative remedies don't yet have a federal agency overseeing quality control, so buy from reputable suppliers. Ask your integrative physician, homeopath or naturopath to suggest specific items. Merrell recommends Willner Chemists (willner.com) and Whole Foods (wholefoodsmarket.com) for their reliable brands. Product reports are available at consumerlab.com.

Use a toxic waste service. To keep chemicals from getting into the water supply, dispose of expired medicines as you would toxic or medical waste. Or ask your pharmacist or doctor to dispose of medicines for you or to recommend services that will. Most natural medicines can safely go in the regular trash.

Energy Medicine

We live, now, on wireless connections. They allow us to plug into a world of information, connect with people and, when we're not watching "What Does the Fox Say?" for the 100th time, make an impact worldwide. A similar invisible connectivity is in place in our bodies—a wireless energy matrix whose circuits flow in and around us. This energy field has a significant impact on our health, and getting it up to speed can help us feel rejuvenated, invigorated, stronger—like we've given ourselves a reboot. The field of energy medicine harnesses this—it's a blend of healing touch and heightened consciousness whose practitioners define health as an unimpeded energy flow, with illness occurring when that energy gets blocked.

This type of work "can make an amazing, astonishing difference in healing," says Santa Fe, N.M.-based holistic physician Larry Dossey, M.D., author of *The Extraordinary Healing Power of Ordinary Things* and other books on healing.

Essential Concepts

Unlike more vigorous, anatomically oriented treatments, energy healing is usually done with a light touch while the patient lies on a table fully clothed. "The components of compassion, caring and love are a very important part of what happens," Dossey says.

The ephemeral nature of these kinds of treatments means no one knows exactly how they work, and scientific, double-blind, randomized studies have been hard pressed to explain or effectively prove how they do—but a surprising amount of anecdotal research supports their efficacy, particularly their ability to reduce pain and anxiety. A 2008 University of Cincinnati study found that Healing Touch, an energy therapy often used in conjunction with other traditional medical treatments, reduced anxiety and improved the efficacy of sedation for surgical patients. Thousands of doctors, nurses and other health professionals use Therapeutic Touch (probably the most researched) in their practices. Renowned integrative physician Andrew Weil recommends cranial sacral therapy for babies' ear infections. Like many mind-body therapies, conditions with a mind-body component stand the best chance of benefiting from energy medicine healing techniques; some of the most popular are profiled here.

Try It Out

REIKI

A Reiki session typically involves the practitioner lightly touching the patient's head and torso in a specific order. "Reiki doesn't aim to diagnose or treat, but simply to bump up one's own ability to self-heal," says New York City Reiki master Pamela Miles, the author of *Reiki: A Comprehensive Guide;* she calls it "a gateway to wellness." The *Journal of American Cardiology* recently published a study showing that Reiki had a positive effect on people suffering from acute coronary syndrome (severe chest pains or heart-muscle damage). Reiki is available in about 15% of hospitals nationwide as a standard part of care, and there are plenty of private practitioners as well. Roughly 200,000 Reiki masters practice worldwide.

✱ BEST FOR: According to Miles, a number of small studies show that Reiki treatment can improve blood pressure, heart rate and heart rate variability, and reduce anxiety and pain. Research also suggests it might be useful for fibromyalgia, cancer and depression.

THERAPEUTIC TOUCH (TT) AND HEALING TOUCH (HT)

TT is a certificate program used widely by nurses and doctors (an estimated 40,000 worldwide) to ease pain and anxiety, both pre- and post-op. With her hands hovering just above the client's body but not actually touching it, the TT therapist "reads" cues in the person's energy field. Then, based upon those cues, the therapist uses sweeping movements that begin at the head and move toward the feet, modulating or directing energy to smooth out the "energetic knots." "You extend your personal energy field toward a person, get in sync, and begin to pick up on what is not in balance with that individual," explains TT co-developer Dolores Krieger, Ph.D., R.N. Studies have shown that patients report a wide range of benefits, from increased energy levels to decreased anxiety.

HEALING TOUCH, an offshoot of TT, involves light touch on the body and around its energy field. The therapist's role "is to act as a conduit to self-healing, similar to the way a midwife assists and encourages a mother in labor," says Barbara Welcer, R.N., a certified holistic nurse and certified Healing Touch practitioner and instructor in Albuquerque, N.M. HT is on its way to being the first energy medicine program to receive national accreditation by the American Nurses Credentialing Center.

✱ BEST FOR: Like Reiki, TT and HT are widely used in hospitals; measurable effects include improved oxygen levels and heart rates; decreased pain and anxiety; and improved quality of life during chemo-

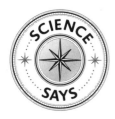

There has been limited scientific research on Reiki and other energy therapies, although the NCCAM continues to urge further study. Heat-sensitive photographs of a Reiki practitioner's hand before and after treatment reportedly show an intensification of heat during the session. A growing number of nurses are using Therapeutic Touch (TT) in hospitals with great success, although the medical establishment is skeptical. A U.S. study found that TT was effective in reducing anxiety, and most subsequent research has found that to be its best use; a 2012 *Cochrane Summaries* review declares that evidence does support the use of touch therapy for pain relief, and that no statistically significant placebo effect is evident. No adverse effects have been discovered. Many of the positive effects of energy healing are thought by the medical community to be a placebo effect.

therapy and radiation. Both therapies work for a range of conditions, especially those with a psychosomatic element, but are also used pre- and postoperatively to speed recovery.

POLARITY THERAPY

This approach is based on the idea that electromagnetic energy currents flow in channels throughout the body. "When the channels flow more efficiently, things work better," says John Chitty, a cofounder of the Colorado School of Energy Studies in Boulder, Colo. "What makes polarity therapy so unique, however, is its comprehensive approach, which always looks at the larger picture." As such, it encompasses a variety of touches and techniques, including pressure points, stretches, breath work and rocking movements, as well as nutritional advice and emotional counseling.

✴ **BEST FOR:** If you suffer from conditions such as anxiety or depression, polarity therapy can work well because of its "talk therapy" component, Chitty says.

CRANIAL SACRAL THERAPY (CST)

CST is based on the cranial sacral rhythm, a wavelike pattern of expansion and contraction that undulates throughout the body. Using a very sensitive touch, the practitioner palpates this wave at points on the head, spine and tailbone, looking for an abnormal rhythm that may signal injury, and then removing any impediments to the flow.

While CST is the most physically oriented of all the techniques described here, it still relies heavily on an energetic model of health and illness. "During a session, the body turns off the fight-or-flight response and accesses its natural ability to restore itself," says Lee "Ganesh" Veal, a cranial sacral instructor and practitioner in Kansas City, Mo.

✴ **BEST FOR:** CST can be very effective for many conditions, including anxiety/depression, whiplash, sports and impact injuries, dental problems, temporomandibular joint disorder (TMJ) and headaches, It also has been found to be effective in treating and preventing ear infections in children, especially those younger than 1 year old.

Precautions

No adverse effects have been reported, but if you like your medicine steeped in science, the energy healing route might *not* be for you.

FIND A PRACTITIONER

Many people are first introduced to energy healing—especially TT and HT—in the hospital; Reiki practitioners often are also trained massage therapists who utilize Reiki in their practice. So, the best referrals come from friends, family and other health care providers. Each of the modalities has its own certifying body, so make sure your therapist is, indeed, certified. Also:

When looking for a practitioner, always call ahead for a five to 10 minute interview. A sense that you can be comfortable with and trust him/her is very important. Be wary of one who won't talk to you.

Inquire up front about costs and find out what your insurance will cover; some health care plans will cover treatments by an M.D., but not a yoga or massage therapist.

Be wary of any practitioner who makes excessive claims and guarantees a cure. Also be wary of one who wants to sign you up immediately for a specified number of treatments.

Meditation

Your brain is the world's noisiest apartment building, filled with a cacophony of neighboring thoughts. Tell one to shut up (let's call him guilt), and the twins get louder (let's call them hopes and dreams). Try to sleep, and the guy downstairs (desire) rings your bell (again). Soon, the entire third floor is throwing a party, inviting stress, thrills, distraction, nostalgia, wonderment, despair. This is life. This is self-awareness. This is feeling—and what makes us human.

Yet meditation is about quieting the neighbors, and reclaiming some space for yourself. You start by trying to think of... nothing, no one at all.

It's a 5,000-year-old practice (or maybe timeless, since cavemen stared into fire)—and was made popular in the U.S. in the 1960s and '70s by the Beatles, among others. But it couldn't be more current. Research in 2013 at UC Santa Barbara showed meditation improved memory. In 2012, a UCLA study found that long-time meditators showed higher levels of gyrification, a fold of the cerebral cortex associated with faster information processing. Another study, published by the University of Washington, asked subjects who had taken eight weeks of mindfulness meditation to perform a stressful chore, alongside subjects who hadn't. The meditators reported less stress.

Probably the most-often studied type of meditation is transcendental meditation (TM)—which is what John, George, Paul and Ringo went to India to learn from Maharishi Mahesh Yogi. More than 350 studies on

TM have been conducted at universities and medical schools in the past 40 years. One of the most recent, published in the journal *Circulation: Cardiovascular Quality and Outcomes* in 2012, studied people with heart disease and compared the effects of a health education class promoting better diet and exercise to one in which they learned TM. The researchers followed up the participants for the next five years and found that those who took the meditation class had a 48% reduction in heart attack, stroke and death.

Modern TM fans include Russell Brand, David Duchovny, Ellen DeGeneres, Katy Perry and—still sticking with it—Paul McCartney. And Google employees in Silicon Valley are taking classes in meditation to help them focus, manage their emotions and get ahead. Something from nothing means something.

Essential Concepts

The goal of most meditation practices is simple enough: Bring your attention to one thing in order to deepen your awareness of the present moment. For people accustomed to multitasking, doing this can be a challenge. Vary it up: If sitting and breathing is not your thing, perform a simple walking meditation. If you're not comfortable focusing on the noise inside your head, listen to the sounds outside it. If silence seems scary, repeat a mantra.

Your work will pay off holistically. Mounting medical evidence shows that the practice can boost the immune system, improve circulation, lower cholesterol, ease chronic pain, end insomnia, counter anxiety, relieve gastrointestinal distress and actually extend your lifespan. "Meditation is a wonderful way to reduce stress," says Timothy McCall, M.D., author of *Yoga As Medicine.* "Stress not only makes people miserable in their day-to-day lives, it also undermines their health."

✷ BEST FOR: Research has shown benefits for any condition that can be eased through reduction of stress and anxiety, including addiction, allergies, PMS, menopause, insomnia, anxiety, obsessive-compulsive disorder, sexual dysfunction, eczema and other skin disorders, hypertension, cardiovascular disease and depression. Studies have shown the conditions are eased by a reduction in markers such as blood pressure, heart rate and cortisol release, and by a relaxation of brain waves.

Try It Out

Here, we offer a guide to five beginner-friendly techniques, with advice from some of the world's leading meditation instructors. Try each style on for size, and when you find one that fits, stick with it. "It's like exercising a muscle," says Richard Rosen, author of *The Yoga of Breath* and a cofounder—with Rodney Yee and Clare Finn—of Piedmont Yoga in Oakland, Calif.; With each workout it gets stronger. Soon you'll carry the centered awareness gained from meditation into the rest of your daily activities, making everything more satisfying. As Rosen says, "First it's a chore, eventually it's a pleasure."

You can sit in the Lotus position (see drawing on page 329) if you want to—but any comfortable cross-legged position will do, and you can just as easily be seated on a chair or sofa, lying on the floor or even standing up and walking around. Don't get too hung up on form; the best position is the one that helps you stay focused.

What's your meditation style?
One of these is right for you.

Basic Breathing Meditation

WHAT IS IT? The cornerstone of all meditation techniques, this practice centers on something we always do but rarely notice: breathing. "You do not have to do anything with your breath but observe it," says yoga and meditation teacher Rosen. Eventually, you can work on changing your breath, and sending it into new areas of your torso. But at first, just become aware of each inhalation and exhalation; let your mind track how the breath moves, mapping where it goes to develop an understanding of your own unique "breathing identity."

WHAT'S IT GOOD FOR? Use this meditation to get centered anytime and anywhere. "Breath is with us always," says Rosen. "You can retreat into your breath whenever you're feeling dull, tired or stressed out."

HOW LONG DOES IT TAKE? Start with 10 minutes at first, then work your way up to 15 and finally 20 minutes. You can do this practice any time of day, but do it regularly, five to seven days a week.

HOW DO I DO IT?

1. Sit in a comfortable position with your legs crossed. Or lie on your back with a firm pillow or rolled-up towel under your knees to provide comfort and support and to open your pelvis; place another pillow or towel under your neck and head to help release tension in your throat. Your body should be more or less straight, and your arms should rest about 45 degrees from your torso.

2. Breathe in and out through your nose. Feel each breath as it moves through your torso, and quietly observe it. Feel where the breath is moving and where it is not. Notice what it sounds like.

3. Begin to notice how your breath changes as you focus on it, and how your awareness changes in turn. (Rosen likens this process to a feedback loop between the breath and "the witness," or self, observing it.)

4. When your mind drifts, gently bring it back to focusing on your breath.

5. After you've practiced for a week, begin to bring your breath into areas of your body that feel dull or "un-breathed." Imagine your torso as a container, and try actively sending breath into the places it's not reaching, such as your pelvis or the small of your back. Don't force the breath, just allow it to follow your consciousness as you breathe into those dull areas.

6. At the end of your session, wiggle your fingers and toes, then stretch your legs and arms. If you're lying down, roll over to one side and pause before pushing up to a seated position. Roll up slowly, leading with your torso and raising your head last.

TIP: Try wearing earplugs to amplify the internal sound of your breath (they help give the breath "an ocean sound," according to Rosen) and to block out distracting noises.

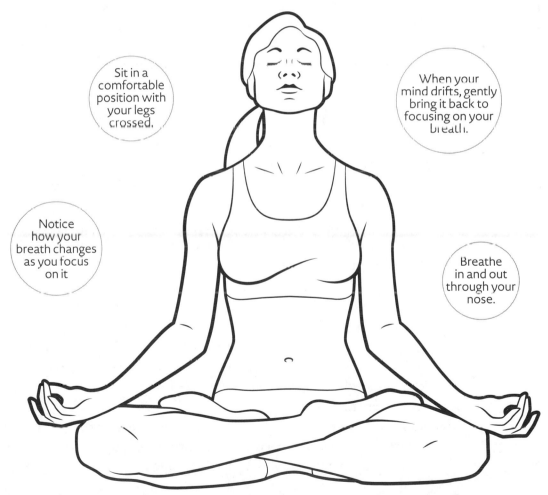

Sit in a comfortable position with your legs crossed.

When your mind drifts, gently bring it back to focusing on your breath.

Notice how your breath changes as you focus on it

Breathe in and out through your nose.

Mindfulness Meditation

WHAT IS IT? "Mindfulness meditation is about insight," explains Sharon Salzberg, cofounder of the Insight Meditation Society (dharma.org) in Barre, Mass., and author of *Lovingkindness: The Revolutionary Art of Happiness,* among other books. "It's not about achieving bliss or tranquility. Its aim is to see things more clearly."

WHAT'S IT GOOD FOR? Mindfulness meditation is a form of "mind training," says Salzberg. Bringing direct awareness to drinking a cup of tea, for instance, means that you really feel the warmth of the cup in your hands, and really taste the sweetness or the bitterness in your mouth. This applies to our emotional states, too—you can observe with awareness and perceive more accurately what your experience really is.

HOW LONG DOES IT TAKE? Start with five minutes daily. Gradually add a few minutes to your session each day until you can sit for 20 minutes.

HOW DO I DO IT?

1. Sit in a comfortable position on a pillow, chair, couch or floor.
2. Listen to the sounds around you while you relax. Practice letting the sounds come and go without chasing them, holding on to them or pushing them away.
3. Now shift your awareness to your body, starting with your breath. As you inhale, think "in"; as you exhale, think "out." Let this action be a kind of home base.
4. When your mind drifts, pay attention to where it goes. It may wander to a pain in your shoulder, for instance, or to a mental image of an argument from the night before. Acknowledge this thought or feeling, spend a moment with it, and then bring your awareness gently back to your home base. Rather than rushing past the new sensations you experience, bring your full awareness to them.
5. If you find yourself getting stuck in an emotion or sensation, it may help to put a mental label on it, to identify it as "anger" or "pain." Then bring your awareness back to your breath.

6. The traditional way to end this meditation is to acknowledge the positive energy you've created and to dedicate it to others. Try saying: "May the merit of this practice be dedicated to all beings everywhere." Stand, and continue to practice mindfulness as much as you can throughout the day.

TIP: Make sure your back is straight and supported as you settle into a comfortable seated position. This helps your breath flow in and out, and also helps keep you awake!

Listening Meditation

WHAT IS IT? While many meditation techniques require solitude and silence, this one has you engage with sounds all around you; it invites you to work with and use the noise instead of fighting it. Listening meditation also encourages you to harmonize with your surroundings, and, by extension, the universe. The intent is to experience sound as vibration, rather than information. "The listening practice is a way of interacting with the environment that allows you to take in the whole energy of the present moment," says Sally Kempton, a spiritual guide who teaches yoga and meditation at her Carmel, Calif.-based Awakened Heart Meditation, and author of *Meditation for the Love of It.* She wrote *The Heart of Meditation: Pathways to a Deeper Experience* under her monastic name, Swami Durgananda.

WHAT'S IT GOOD FOR? Especially adaptable and portable, listening meditation can be practiced in crowded, noisy situations—on a bus, at the office—that would hinder other styles. (Kempton once led a listening meditation workshop in the middle of a busy Whole Foods store!) People with particularly chattering minds may need to couple this practice with a mantra or breathing meditation. However, many people welcome the chance to focus outward rather than inward and find that listening meditation is one of the easier techniques to undertake. "You'll come away from it feeling refreshed, expanded and at ease with your environment," declares Kempton.

HOW LONG DOES IT TAKE? Try for five minutes at first, then add a minute or two at a time until you can do it for 15 or 20 minutes at a time.

HOW DO I DO IT?

1. Sit in a comfortable position and close (or half-close) your eyes.

2. To get centered and quiet your mind, first bring your awareness to your breath, noticing but not trying to change it.

3. Now "open" your ears and bring your awareness to the sounds around you. The goal is to listen to the whole range of sounds, without favoring one over another and without identifying them. Hear the quiet sounds and the silences as well as the dominant sounds.

4. When you find yourself identifying sounds ("There's a fire engine"; "That's a dog barking"; "That's my neighbor's TV"), gently redirect your attention from listening to a specific noise back to hearing the whole spectrum of sounds.

5. To end, slowly open your eyes, stand and carry this heightened awareness with you for as long as you can.

TIP: Do a one-minute mini-listening meditation while standing in line or sitting at your desk, or any time you feel frazzled: Close your eyes, breathe and listen to the sounds around you. Like the practice of counting to 10 when you're in the heat of an argument, this will help you pause, center and regroup.

Walking Meditation

WHAT IS IT? This component of numerous meditation traditions slows the walking process with the intention of bringing into awareness its most basic parts—lifting the foot, swinging it, placing it down—in order to bring a greater consciousness to daily life. When we break down the motion of walking, we realize how each action is actually a collection of sub-actions, and how the mind and body work together to create

Binaural Bliss Out

Feel you're too scattered, smothered or fried to meditate on your own? Try tuning in to a high-tech solution: binaural beat technology. Binaural beats are sub-audio sounds that create resonance between the right and left hemispheres of the brain, naturally inducing a theta state (the brainwave pattern associated with deep meditation). There are plenty of CDs, downloads and smartphone apps out there—most of which use ambient sounds or New Age music to create a pleasant listening experience. "They really work," notes meditation teacher Sally Kempton. Here are a few worth trying—just remember to use your earphones; binaural beats won't have their intended effect if you play them on stereo speakers.

HOLOSYNC

Though relatively expensive ($179 for the introductory kit), this program—Kempton's favorite—makes meditation accessible and beneficial for both beginners and the most advanced practitioners. At the most advanced levels, the company offers the opportunity to record your own positive affirmations to accompany the binaural beats. (Find out more at centerpointe.com.)

HEMI-SYNC

If you want more than meditation—to heal your body, enhance your creativity or stoke your energy—try Hemi-Sync, which offers a broad array of binaural programs aimed at creating specific effects. Of course, there are plenty of choices for relaxation and stress relief, too. (Find out more at hemi-sync.com.)

EQUISYNC

With programs titled "Enlightenment" and "Ascension," it's clear that EquiSync's focus is on spiritual development. (Find out more at eocinstitute.org.)

BINAURAL BEATS APP

Download this app for your iPhone, and choose one of seven short programs—including headache killer, memory helper and deep meditation. (Find out more at iTunes.)

physical movement. "This is not walking for transportation, it's walking as a tool for developing mindfulness in the present moment," says John LeMunyon, L.M.T., co-owner of Heartwood Yoga in Birmingham, Ala., and a meditator for more than 30 years.

You can practice walking meditation by itself, or combine it with one of the seated styles. Used as an interlude, the walking technique is a good way to embody the insights gained during seated practice and to heighten their relevance in daily life.

Walking meditation shows clearly the Buddhist precept that "all action is preceded by intention," says LeMunyon. "There's always an intention, and when we are present to the moment there is always a choice. It's at the level of intention that we make our choices of how skillfully we want to live our lives."

WHAT'S IT GOOD FOR? When you find yourself feeling restless or agitated, a physical practice like walking is a great way to quiet your mind and find grounding in your body. It can also help ease your transition from sitting meditation to the motion of "real life," and vice versa.

HOW LONG DOES IT TAKE? To begin, try walking for about 15 steps in two directions, about five minutes total. Beginners can also try interspersing this with five minutes of sitting meditation.

HOW DO I DO IT?

1. Find a private place indoors or out with level ground and at least 20 feet of space.

2. Stand in a relaxed position with your feet parallel, shoulders loose, arms draped at your sides or clasped lightly in front of or behind you. Focus your eyes softly on the ground about 6 to 8 feet ahead (looking right at your feet can be distracting).

3. Breathe in as you lift your right heel. Pause and breathe out, leaving your toes resting on the ground.

4. Breathe in again as you slowly swing your right foot forward. Place the heel of your right foot on the ground as you exhale and roll the rest of the foot down, transferring your weight so it's balanced equally between both feet. Pause for a full breath.

5. Repeat with your left foot, matching each movement with an inhalation or exhalation, alternating for 15 steps. The goal is to keep your mind fully focused on your bodily sensations; it may help to think or softly say, "Lift, pause, swing, place, transfer, pause," as you perform these movements.

6. When you've completed your paces in one direction, come to a stop with your feet parallel and pause for a few breaths. Then turn slowly, using the same movement pattern and match each movement of your turn with an inhalation or exhalation. Pause again, facing the path you just walked. End by retracing your steps back to where you started.

TIP: You may feel self-conscious walking this way, so try it in your hall or backyard rather than a park where onlookers may distract you. (Also see the breathwalking meditation on page 50.)

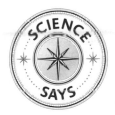

Meditation has been studied for its mind/body benefits since the 1960s by psychologists, physicians, psychiatrists and other health care researchers, and as a result is widely recommended. Studies have shown that conditions that may benefit from a reduction of stress biomarkers, such as cardiovascular disease, depression, anxiety, Alzheimer's, arthritis and sexual dysfunction are eased by a reduction in markers such as blood pressure, heart rate and cortisol release and by a relaxation of brain waves. Because of the wide body of research conducted by such mind/body researchers as James Gordon, M.D., director for the Center for Mind/Body Studies and Harvard professor Joan Borysenko, Ph.D., author of *Minding the Body, Mending the Mind,* many practitioners across fields now prescribe meditation to their patients.

Mantra Meditation

WHAT IS IT? Mantra meditation utilizes the power of sound and vibration to create stillness, calm the nervous system and ultimately transform the mind. The words typically come from ancient spiritual languages, such as Sanskrit or Gurmukhi. The sacred meanings of the words enable you to establish a connection to profound truths that have been spoken for thousands of years, explains Krishna Kaur, a kundalini yoga teacher since 1970 and founding member of the International Association of Black Yoga Teachers (krishnakaur.org).

WHAT'S IT GOOD FOR? Because each mantra differs in its meaning and vibrations produced, you can select mantras to create specific effects—such as increasing mental clarity, developing intuition, or reducing anger and stress. Kaur suggests starting with the simple mantra "sat nam" because it's easy to say and remember, yet offers profound effects. Sat translates as "truth," and nam as "identity." This mantra helps you identify with a universal spiritual truth in which such transient emotional states as fear, anger and doubt fall away.

HOW LONG DOES IT TAKE? Start with three to five minutes, increasing by a minute at a time until you can sit and chant for a full 11 minutes.

HOW DO I DO IT?

1. Sit comfortably in a chair or on the floor with your spine straight to help the sound and breath flow smoothly. Close your eyes and bring your attention to your breath for a moment to get centered.

2. Take a long, deep inhalation through your nose. As you exhale, utter an extended "sat" (pronounced "sut") to almost the end of your breath, followed by a short burst of "nam" ("nom"). Together, the mantra will sound like "saaaaaaaaaaat nam."

3. Inhale slowly and evenly, then repeat the mantra as you exhale. Continue this pattern for as long as desired.

4. At the end of your session, inhale and hold the breath for a few seconds, then exhale through your nose. Do this three times, then sit quietly for a moment and feel the energy flow through your body.

Open your eyes, stand slowly, and carry your sense of calm and clarity with you.

TIP: Try doing mantra meditation with other people. "Group energy is powerful and heightens the individual experience," says Kaur.

Precautions

Meditation is perfectly safe for anyone.

Learn More

Meditation is being taught at health clubs, churches, schools, fitness and yoga studios and just about everywhere else. Find out more about meditation through the Insight Meditation Society (dharma.org), the Mindfulness Awareness Research Center (marc.ucla.edu). Transcendental Mediation is done with a teacher and requires seven steps of introduction; the first three are free, the next—during which you get a personalized mantra, which seems to be the key—cost $1,500 total. TM is being taught (gratis) in schools and to veterans with great success. For more, go to the TM website (tm.org), or check local listings.

13 WAYS TO BOOST YOUR BRAIN POWER

The nation's top integrative experts share tactics to help you keep your memory strong, your faculties clear and your head in the game.

You walk into the room, scissors in hand, then stop and wonder: What am I doing here? You look into the face of a co-worker—the same one you've seen every day for six years—and draw a blank. You call up an old friend to tell her... What were you going to tell her again? It seemed important a second ago...

There's a scientific term for this kind of memory failure: "brain fart."

As we grow older, circulation to our brains may decrease, our brain cells burn energy less efficiently, messages between those cells can get muddled and the brain may even begin to shrink. That leads to impaired memory, inability to focus clearly and an overall sense that we're just not as quick as we once were.

This sort of cognitive decline is happening to many of us earlier and earlier. "'Senior moments' are now dipping down into the 30s and 40s," says Dharma Singh Khalsa, M.D., author of *Brain Longevity*. "I attribute this to the stress associated with our modern lifestyles. Stress leads to higher levels of the hormone cortisol in our blood, which leads to memory problems and depression." Which in turn leads us to... um um um um ummmm. Oh, right: Optimizing brain function.

Khalsa says that there's plenty you can do to stop the process of decline, or even reverse it. We asked her and the nation's top brain-savvy experts to share their thoughts. Here are their finest ideas, as far as we remember.

1.
Get by with a little help from your friends

Socialization is extremely important for a healthy brain, and we've found it goes hand in hand with mental activity. Social interaction forces you to use your brain's memory circuits—you have to remember people's names and follow along in conversation. And if you're doing something like playing bridge, you have to remember the rules. There has been some research on how social activity maintains brain vitality and reduces your risk of developing Alzheimer's or dementia, but there are many other good reasons to stay socially engaged as well, so join a club, travel with friends or sign up for volunteer work.

—Maria Carrillo, Ph.D.,
senior director of Medical and Scientific Relations for the Alzheimer's Association

2.
P.S., I love you!

I used to have a bionic memory. I could remember everyone's name and everything in their chart, no problem. I still know everything in the charts, but I don't necessarily remember names. When I need to know who everybody is—say, before a big event—I take phosphatidyl serine (PS). PS is the major phospholipid found within the membranes in the nerve cells in our brains. The results of 10 double-blind human studies in the United States and Europe demonstrate pretty conclusively that PS can help maintain concentration and memory. When I recommend it to my patients, they report a sense of well-being, better concentration and improved memory. Take 50 to 100 milligrams, once or twice a day, up to 200 milligrams a day.

—Janet Zand, O.M.D., L.Ac.,
coauthor of Smart Medicine for Healthier Living

3.
Nosh on foods that are good for your noggin

Eating a plant-based diet is essential for brain health. The complex carbohydrates found in plants are brain fuel; carbohydrates also aid in the production of serotonin, a chemical that affects mood.

Another crucial diet move: Be careful about the kind of fat you eat. Everyone knows that solid fats, such as butter and lard, are correlated with heart disease, but they also increase the risk of brain diseases like Alzheimer's. All the fat we eat ends up in our cell walls; solid fats make cell walls stiff so that it's difficult to get messages through from one cell to another. On the other hand, liquid fats (such as olive oil) make cell walls more liquid and flexible, so that they can communicate with each other more easily.

—Katherine Tallmadge, R.D.,
spokeswoman for the American Dietetic Association

4.
Pay attention to your scalp

In ayurveda, many memory and concentration problems are due to an imbalance of the vata dosha, which is sensitive to stress and governs circulation, thinking and movement. To balance vata quickly, give yourself a daily head massage. Put an ounce of sesame oil or brahmi oil in your hand and begin to rub your scalp in a clockwise motion, starting small and getting bigger and bigger. Once you reach your hairline, stop making circles and give yourself an all-over head massage with your fingertips. Put a towel on your pillow and sleep with the oil on your head for an even more calming effect on the brain.

—James Bailey. L.Ac., Dipl OM., Dipl. Ayu, *founder of Sevanti Wellness in Santa Monica, Calif.*

5.
Steer clear of toxins

Skip caffeine, which constricts blood vessels, prevents the sleep you need to think clearly and dehydrates you—a big problem, considering that the brain is 80% water. It's also wise to limit your alcohol intake. People are walking around thinking it's good to drink red wine every day, but alcohol is bad for the cerebellum, which controls our processing speed and coordination. Be careful with prescription painkillers and anti-anxiety medications, such as Xanax, Ativan and Valium. These kinds of drugs can diminish overall brain performance when used improperly.

—Daniel G. Amen, M.D., *founder of the Amen Clinics and author of* Change Your Brain, Change Your Life *and* Making a Good Brain Great

6.
Wake up your brain

One of my favorite mind boosters is acetyl-L-carnitine. It's a powerful antioxidant that has been found in animal studies to regenerate brain tissue. Acetyl-L-carnitine is the thing to take if you're having trouble focusing on work, you just can't get motivated or you're not able to get through the day without feeling mentally tired. I recommend taking it in capsule form, anywhere between 200 and 500 milligrams on an empty stomach in the morning—you'll need to experiment with the dose to find what works for you (start with the smallest dose first). It's great to take on an as-needed basis because most people feel the effects within a day, and possibly even within an hour.

—Ray Sahelian, M.D., *integrative physician and author of* Mind Boosters

7.
Drink your vegetables

A recent study published in the *American Journal of Medicine* found that drinking fresh vegetable juice may help delay the onset of Alzheimer's disease. It can also help you with day-to-day brain performance. To make your own brain booster, juice some broccoli, celery, carrot and peeled cucumber (cucumber, especially, has some well-balanced minerals that are beneficial for brain health). If you'd like, add an apple for sweetness. Drink it, and you'll feel like someone turned the lights on in your head. It's like an IV infusion of the vitamins and minerals your brain needs to function well.

—**Dharma Singh Khalsa, M.D.,**
author of Brain Longevity *and president of the Alzheimer's Research and Prevention Foundation*

8.
Press ahead

We do acupressure naturally when we have mental stress by instinctively rubbing our temples. When we gently hold our foreheads to clear our minds, we're holding acupressure points that can help us with concentration. To stimulate memory quickly and clear the mind, find the "gallbladder 14" points, which are located on your forehead, over each eye, about one finger-width above your eyebrows and in line with your pupils; you'll feel a slight indentation there. With your right hand, use your thumb to lightly press the point above your right eye and your middle finger to lightly press the point above your left eye.

With your other hand, reach around and stimulate the "gallbladder 20" points, which are also known as "the gates of consciousness." They are just below the base of the skull on either side of the top of your neck, about two inches apart (you'll feel a little hollow there). Use firm pressure on these points, pressing your thumb into the left side and your pointer or middle finger on the right side. When you stimulate the "gallbladder 14" and "gallbladder 20" points together, it creates a powerful environment for rejuvenating the mind.

—**Michael Reed Gach,**
Ph.D., founder of the Acupressure Institute (acupressure.com) and author of Acupressure's Potent Points

9.
Do it (yoga, that is) doggie style

Downward-Facing Dog pose is a great way to freshen up your thinking. It puts your head lower than your heart, which helps bring oxygenated blood to your brain. I think of it as the great neutralizing pose—if you're tired and foggy, it will pick you up; if you are overwrought and scattered, it will calm you and help you focus.

To do the pose, start on your hands and knees, with knees just below your hips and hands out in front of your shoulders. Inhale deeply. As you exhale, lift your knees away from the floor and push your thighs back so that you form an inverted V shape. Keep your ears between your upper arms and spread your palms and soles widely on the floor. Hold the pose for a few minutes to get the full effect. When you're done, bend your knees back down to the floor as you exhale, then rest for a few breaths.

—**Richard Rosen,**
founder of the Piedmont Yoga Studio in Oakland, Calif., and author of The Yoga of Breath, *and* Pranayama: Beyond the Fundamentals *and* Yoga for 50+

10.
Handle your hormonal side

If you're a woman who is walking around feeling foggy-headed, depressed, irritable or indecisive, you may very well be suffering from a hormonal imbalance—especially if you're in your 40s. Take action to regain your balance: The North American Menopause Society recently issued a position statement saying that the earlier you start with hormone replacement therapy, the more likely you'll experience brain-boosting benefits, including mood improvement, enhanced intelligence and protection against Alzheimer's. Stick to bioidentical hormones for best results, and opt for creams or patches over pills. Bioidentical progesterone cream is available over the counter and can really help if you're starting to feel like you just can't juggle things the way you used to. Start with a dose of 50 milligrams every day, starting on day 15 of your menstrual cycle; increase by 50 milligrams on day 15 of every cycle until you start to see improvements in your mood and focus, and/or reductions in premenstrual symptoms. Typically, it takes three cycles for best results.

Hormones can also help if you're postmenopausal, but it's best to talk to your doctor about what bioidenticals to use.

—**Erika Schwartz, M.D.,**
founding director of the Bioidentical Hormone Initiative, Natural Health *adviser and author of* The Hormone Solution

11.
Get playful

Games and puzzles can help keep your brain sharp. But if you're already really good at crossword puzzles, more crosswords probably won't help you. You need to challenge new circuits in your brain to reap the most benefits (for example, crossword lovers should try sudoku). One of my favorite activities for boosting concentration and building coordination? Ping-pong.

—Daniel G. Amen, M.D.

12.
Choose rosemary for remembrance

The old adage "Rosemary is for memory" dates back to medieval times, and there's a lot of truth to it. In fact, science has proved it: In 2003, a study published in the *International Journal of Neuroscience* found that rosemary not only improves memory, but it also boosts alertness and overall cognitive performance thanks to its ability to increase circulation to the surface of the brain.

To reap those benefits, put one or two drops of rosemary essential oil on the top of each foot; deoxygenated blood must return quickly to the lungs from there, because it's the end of the circulatory line. Choose a high-quality, organic essential oil, such as those made by Simplers, Oshadhi, Original Swiss Aromatics or Acqua-Vita. You can use rosemary several times a day as needed, but don't use it anywhere near bedtime or you'll be lying in bed wide awake, thinking clearly.

—Suzanne Catty,
Toronto-based master aromatherapist and author of Hydrosols: The Next Aromatherapy

13.
Listen carefully

Hearing is incredibly important to brain function—it is the way we receive and process information. If you do activities that require you to be a careful listener, you can gradually improve the accuracy of your speech-perception abilities and speed up your brain in general. To improve your hearing skills, turn the volume on the television down from your normal setting. Concentrate as you watch, and see if you can begin to hear just as clearly as you did before. This will help you focus on conversations so you can catch every word.

—Michael Merzenich, Ph.D.,
Frances A. Sooy professor of otolaryngology at the W.M. Keck Foundation Center for Integrative Neuroscience at the University of California, San Francisco

Yoga

The question here is less "How can yoga help me?" than "Who *isn't* yoga helping already?" LeBron James claims his performance on the basketball court is grounded by the practice; Maroon 5 singer and "Sexiest Man Alive" Adam Levine attributes his stamina and sanity on tour to yoga; and supermodel yogi Christy Turlington Burns founded women's health foundation Every Woman Counts as a result of her passion. There's a sitcom about yoga. The Disney Store sells yoga pants. Even McDonald's uses yoga in a commercial, as hot young yogis drool over cherry pies. (*Ommmm...* cheeseburger?)

Its celebrity advocates are many, but glitz aside, yoga is about more than being seen in class, or attaining a perfectly rounded derriere (though this is one of its happy side effects). The health benefits are undeniable: A Mayo Clinic report published in 2012 unequivocally promotes yoga's power in reducing stress and boosting vitality, strength and flexibility. Yoga has been found to very significantly reduce risk factors associated with chronic diseases such as high blood pressure and heart disease, and is being used to alleviate other chronic conditions such as depression, anxiety, insomnia and pain. According to *Yoga Journal*, thousands of studies have shown that the practice of yoga can help you control certain bodily functions and improve your health, which is the reason an estimated 16 million people in the U.S. now practice regularly. If you have chronic pain of any kind, but especially back pain, you should try yoga and massage (see page 254) before even thinking about surgery. In fact, if you have any problem, physical or mental, try yoga. It just makes you feel good.

Old school

Yoga also has longevity on its side: It is *the* oldest-known health system in the world. It has been practiced for thousands of years in India as a complete method of physical, mental and spiritual training—and an integral part of ayurvedic medicine. First introduced to the West in the 1800s, yoga has been growing steadily in the United States since the 1960s, when it was popularized by BKS Iyengar (founder of the Iyengar method) and Sri K. Pattabi Jois (think of him as the godfather of ashtanga yoga).

Now, there are nearly as many different types of yoga on offer, from classic hatha yoga through to laughter yoga and Yoga Booty Ballet (we're not making this up). There really is something for everyone, even the most endorphin- and adrenalin-seeking exerciser; and many doctors, including cardiologist Dean Ornish, M.D. (author of *Reversing Heart Disease*), prescribe yoga as part of a health care and disease risk-reduction program.

Essential Concepts

Yoga in Sanskrit means "union." Yoga originated more than 4,000 years ago in India, where it was practiced by Hindu yogis as a path to spiritual enlightenment—realizing the oneness (union) of all things. In its purest form, yoga is practiced in all aspects of your life, from making healthy eating decisions and practicing good personal hygiene to being socially conscious and compassionate. Sounds like common sense, right? The aim of yoga is to quiet the fluctuations of the mind. That endless chatter you hear when you sit still and quiet for a few minutes? That's called *vrittis* in Sanskrit, and a solid yoga practice will begin to calm down the mind's whirring. Progress is made along the path with the practice of physical postures called *asanas*, breathing techniques (*pranayama*) and meditation; the eventual goal for serious yogis is a supreme level of consciousness, or nirvana. For the rest of us, attaining peace of mind and a healthy body into old age may be bliss enough.

The most widely practiced version of yoga is *asana*, or hatha ("balance") yoga. This is the kind of yoga you do on your mat, based on a series of physical postures and movements and usually paired with breathing techniques. Its health benefits are impressive: Hatha yoga's therapeutic *asanas* have been proven to lower blood pressure, regulate heart rate, reduce stress, improve respiratory function, slow the aging process and even reduce insulin dependence for diabetics. Twisting moves can ease back pain and improve the digestive and lymphatic systems, while going upside-down (in headstands, for example) allows blood to flow freely, stimulates overall good circulation and is

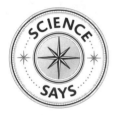

You'd think that feeling good and getting stronger and more flexible would be plenty, but yoga actually has tons of research to prove its benefits. One very famous study back in the 1990s showed that it worked better than anything else for chronic low back pain (96% of participants reported significant improvement), and conclusions from a NCCAM 2011 study of chronic or recurring low back pain suggested that 12 weekly yoga classes resulted in better function than usual medical care, so the research is holding up. Studies are ongoing: The NIH's NCCASM, the American Cancer Society, the Mayo Clinic, even Harvard have conducted, published and endorsed research that promotes yoga for eating disorders, cancer treatment side effects, migraines, stress, inflammation and insomnia. Nearly every condition that can benefit from stress reduction has been shown to improve with a regular yoga practice, and even one session can relieve pain and muscle tension.

Are medical doctors recommending yoga to their patients? Well, yes and no; certainly Dr. Oz is a big fan, and integrative physicians such as Frank Lipman, M.D., who runs Eleven Eleven Wellness Center in New York City, do without hesitation. Lipman marvels at the adaptabilty of yoga, saying on his website that "When you are tired there are poses to restore you, when stressed out, poses to relax you, when depressed, poses to elevate your mood, or when you can't sleep, poses to help the insomnia." It's far-fetched to imagine that other, more conventional docs are doing the same, or that new health care plans will cover it, so you might be on your own.

believed to promote longevity. Forward bending moves stretch leg and back muscles and improve circulation to the brain. Back bends energize and can reboot your day.

The combination of breathing exercises, physical movements and mental prompts (in some classes, teachers recite poetry or play music, even hip-hop) can transport you to an altered state. You can practice yoga on your own or as part of a class, but regularity is key to improving strength and boosting cardiovascular function.

If you're suspicious of anything New Age-y, the idea of chakras may seem a little hokey, but yogic scriptures teach that chakras are the centers of life energy, the seat of human emotions, intellect and senses. They're a big deal, in other words. Seven chakras are situated in ascending order of spiritual refinement, from the root chakra at the base of the spine, which is associated with our sense of stability, via the fourth, or heart chakra, linked to our immune systems and compassion, to the seventh, or crown chakra, which is the most purely spiritual and intellectual. In yoga, your asana and meditation practice aim to channel your prana, or life force, into the body's midline, making a clear path through the chakras. When you orgasm, it's thought that all seven chakras open up completely—and then contract and close immediately afterwards. Adam Levine, give us a call.

* BEST FOR: Studies repeatedly have found that yoga is one of the best, possibly the most effective, therapy for back pain when practiced appropriately. It also works to reduce stress, fatigue, depression and headache pain, including migraine. Improvement has been shown for digestive and circulatory disorders, asthma, arthritis, menstrual and menopausal issues; and flexibility and mobility are often restored through regular practice. Yoga is particularly useful in the prevention and management of stress-related chronic health problems.

Precautions

During menstruation, a restorative practice is recommended and inversions should be avoided.

Seek advice when practicing yoga during pregnancy. A yoga practice can be tremendously beneficial but certain postures are strongly contraindicated (twists across the body, belly-down poses, back bends, and inversions at certain points in the pregnancy).

Make sure to tell your instructor if you are pregnant or have any injuries.

Headstands and shoulder stands are not advised if you have a back or neck injury, high blood pressure, heart disease or circulatory problems, or injuries to the eyes, ears or brain.

Wait two hours after eating to practice, so that your body can digest properly and you won't be farting during class. No one wants to be that guy.

Take care to not push your body too far or ignore pain or injuries.

Find It

Yoga classes can be found in studios, health clubs, churches and community centers nationwide. For information on Iyengar Yoga, check out iyila.org. *Yoga Journal* magazine regularly publishes a list of yoga teachers nationwide. To find a yoga therapist, go to the International Association of Yoga Therapists website (iayt.org).

Try It Out
What type of yoga is right for you?

Understanding the distinctions among the five biggest styles will help you get the most out of every breath and pose.

"To say there is a variety of methods and interpretations of yoga is an understatement," says Judith Hanson Lasater, Ph.D., a physical therapist and yoga instructor and author of *30 Essential Yoga Poses*. Truth be told, even experienced practitioners may not always have a clear grasp of the nuances and varied benefits of each type of yoga, which can affect results (if you're sweating profusely when you're seeking calm, for instance)—or possibly even lead to injury. That's why we put together this guide to five of the most popular practices. While each style includes a series of asanas, or poses—which may include vinyasas, or breath-synchronized movements—the way in which they are done can be quite different, from vigorous and athletic to slow and meditative. The execution varies, but the underlying goal is the same, says yoga therapist Carol Krucoff, author of *Healing Yoga for Neck and Shoulder Pain:* to connect our minds and bodies through conscious movements and breathing, to bring our attention inward, recognize where we habitually hold tension and learn how to release it.

Of course, a lot also depends on the instructor—so even after you've decided which type (or types) appeal to you most, you may need to look around for the perfect fit. Ultimately, it will be well worth the effort. "By finding the styles and teachers that meet both your physical and mental needs, you develop a physical practice that also brings a sense of purpose and passion into your life, and one you'll stick with," says Kim Shand, a certified yoga instructor based in New Jersey, and founder of Rethink Yoga. So prepare to be enlightened, and to get more out of your yoga practice; we even have included some basic yoga moves for you.

Ashtanga Vinyasa

Often promoted as a modern-day form of classical Indian yoga, ashtanga vinyasa—also known simply as ashtanga—is a vigorous practice comprising a series of sequential postures, developed by one of modern yoga's true pioneers, Sri K. Pattabhi Jois. It begins with Sun Salutations (*Surya namaskara*), followed by one of six main series of poses: primary moves for beginners, followed by intermediate poses, then four variations of advanced moves. To give you an indication of how challenging ashtanga can be, few practitioners get beyond the first or second series!

Ashtanga also incorporates a breathing style called *ujjayi*, which is characterized by an ocean sound that resonates from the throat—an audible sighing out of the breath in sync with specific movements. While ashtanga can be fairly fast-moving, this focus on the breath means it can have a wonderfully meditative quality. Often called "flow yoga," ashtanga focuses on continuous movements, leaving less time for instruction, says Lasater; but a well-trained teacher will take the time to adjust you properly. Most sport and "power" yoga classes are also derived from ashtanga.

* **BEST FOR:** Skilled exercise enthusiasts seeking a calorie-blasting, body-sculpting workout, or an intense experience of yoga.

✻ **SKIP IT IF:** You have physical limitations, or prefer to stretch and move gently.

Iyengar

This is a great place to begin your yoga practice, wherever you're at with your body, due to its careful attention to physical alignment. Iyengar yoga is also the least overtly "mystical" yoga practice, so it attracts a lot of sporty types, especially those working with injuries. Developed over a period of 50 years by B.K.S. Iyengar, this practice emphasizes stability and good health. In Iyengar, poses are generally held longer than in other types of yoga, with more attention paid to both muscular and skeletal alignment. It's a slow-going practice, with regular stops to position blocks and blankets and to check on postures. "Iyengar yoga focuses heavily on proper execution," says Lasater. The idea is that precision will help build strength, stamina, balance and flexibility. Practitioners often use props, such as belts, chairs, blocks, blankets or the wall, which help them to perform poses correctly and minimize the risk of injury. Iyengar is one of the most therapeutic types of yoga, with many programs targeted to ease specific ailments such as backaches, high blood pressure, insomnia or symptoms of menopause.

* **BEST FOR:** Patient seekers of calm, steady strength and healing.

✻ **SKIP IT IF:** You like to keep moving swiftly or your mind wanders easily.

Vinyasa

Vinyasa yoga is the most popularly practiced form of yoga in the U.S., and it's easy to see why it's become so big. The term vinyasa is a Sanskrit term, *nyasa* meaning "to place" and *vi* meaning "with intention." Taught well, the practice combines the flowing movement of ashtanga yoga with the precision of Iyengar yoga, and a good deal of imagination on your teacher's part. Vinyasa teachers will design sequences according to the needs they perceive in their students on any given day, whether that's in response to students' injuries or aptitude, or finding a sequence that works in harmony with the season or even the time of day. Vinyasa classes often open with a brief instructional talk which relates to the practice, and will likely feature *pranayama* (seated breathing practices), chanting, mantras and meditation to influence the mind as well as the body.

   ✱ **BEST FOR:** Those seeking emotional release and spiritual development as well as physical strength.

   ✖ **SKIP IT IF:** You have trouble with physical coordination; its flowing sequences may be challenging for you.

Hip Hybrids

If you're looking for something beyond the traditional yoga offerings, there's no shortage of programs that pair *asanas* with heart-pumping aerobic exercise. Just note that these hybrids often focus on sweat factor more than proper form, so make sure you've mastered your yoga poses (and your teacher has, too!) before trying a dual discipline.

CORE FUSION YOGA (exhalespa.com) melds three concentrations: yoga sequences for breath awareness and stretching; Pilates exercises to strengthen your core and abdominal muscles; and slow, deliberate qigong postures for balance.

KOGA (kogaworkout.com) pairs yoga's meditation, stretching and breathing techniques with kickboxing's fat-burning intensity.

YAS (go2yas.com) is a self-described "no om zone" designed for athletes, and mixes popular yoga postures such as Sun Salutations with indoor cycling.

YOGA BOOTY BALLET (beachbody.com) combines short yoga sequences with stretching, dance moves and ballet conditioning to target the abs and—you guessed it—butt.

Bikram

Bikram classes (bikramyoga.com) usually run for 90 minutes and include the same, slow series of 26 poses and two breathing exercises. "All Bikram studios are designed to meet strict guidelines so they all look essentially the same, and each teacher is trained to the same basic script," Shand says. With upwards of 1,600 studios around the world, Bikram is the most popular form of hot yoga (others include TriBalance yoga, which is performed in even hotter but less humid conditions). It is practiced in a room heated to 105 degrees Fahrenheit with a humidity of 40% in order to mimic the climate of India, yoga's birthplace.

Its creator, Bikram Choudhury—who brought Bikram to the United States in the 1970s—says that performing poses in such high heat helps to loosen and stretch the muscles and open the joints without injury, as well as to aid in body detoxification through excessive sweating (bring a towel!). The heavy perspiration also may reduce stress and tension, and help with weight management. Just keep in mind that you might become dehydrated, dizzy or nauseous from the heat, so check with your doctor to make sure the soaring temps will be safe for you, and listen to your body: If you need to take a water break, lie down or leave the class, do so.

✱ BEST FOR: Those who like some predictability—and serious sweat—in their practice.

✖ SKIP IT IF: You can't stand the heat or want more variation or a little philosophy sprinkled in with your asanas.

Kundalini

Most of us know someone who is suspicious of yoga, and if this is the case, they may well be thinking of kundalini yoga, whose dedicated follows often wear white when they practice and look, we'll admit it, a little bit like cult members. But kundalini yoga is far from a cult and has its own beautiful benefits.

Often called "the yoga of awareness," kundalini (kundaliniyoga.org) is regarded as an advanced form of yoga and meditation focused on developing a higher consciousness and spiritual strength. It was introduced in the U.S. in 1968, when Yogi Bhajan, an Indian kundalini master, visited Los Angeles and decided that he must stay and teach the '60s generation, whose destiny it was to usher in a new era. According to yogic philosophy, *kundalini* is a spiritual energy located at the base of the spine, often depicted as a coiled or sleeping serpent. kundalini yoga is a way to prepare the body for and aid in the awakening of that energy, and to work it through the seven chakras of the body. The movements and breathing are very rhythmic, and some teachers use visualizations—of energy, thoughts, light—to help students clear their minds and sink deeper into each pose. "The physical postures and sequencing may be rigorous," says Shand, "but most classes focus more on the spiritual components." Classes often start with chanting or the repetition of mantras (for example, *sat nam,* or "I am truth"), and end with a meditation. There is often a strong emphasis on breathing techniques. Intense breathing and the intake of extra oxygen often helps practitioners to reach an "altered" meditative state. It's a radically different style of practicing, compared to the other four types of yoga listed here, which focus on *asana*.

✱ **BEST FOR:** Those seeking emotional release and spiritual development as well as physical strength.

✖ **SKIP IT IF:** You're not into spirituality, chanting or deep breathing.

YOGA FOR BEGINNERS

Classic poses for stretching, strengthening and de-stressing

Yoga's rather exotic history stretches back 5,000 years to India, where its earliest practitioners entered deep states of meditation in order to attain enlightenment. The dedicated few who have traveled down this path have been known to develop extraordinary abilities, like being able to spontaneously move into strange contortions or hold the breath for extended periods of time. But even in that magical-sounding time, yoga's sense of abiding calm prevailed. In Patanjali's Yoga Sutras (think of these as ancient yogic instructions), the sage wrote in Sanskrit, *"Sthira sukham asanam"*—which means that our physical practice should be steady and sweet, an equal balance of effort and ease.

If you're able to find this balance in class and really listen to what's going on with your breath and in your body, then yoga's benefits will start to really blossom. Besides helping you manage your weight, gain muscle tone, and increase strength and flexibility, yoga will recharge your nervous system, and studies show that yoga can help to mitigate a wide range of ailments, from back pain to heart disease.

The lessons you'll learn in class extend far beyond the mat. If you topple over in a balancing pose, you may realize there's another area in your life where you feel unstable. Or perhaps you ignore your body's messages and hurt yourself by moving too ambitiously, thus prompting you to ponder whether perhaps you push too hard in your relationships or career as well. If you feel shame when you can't get into a challenging pose, that may shine light on your need to accept yourself and your limitations. "Yoga provokes you to honor yourself, to compassionately observe yourself in order to understand your motivations and aspirations in all your interactions, and to recognize the expansive and downright beautiful qualities of your own heart," says Elena Brower, founder and co-owner of Virayoga in New York City.

That's why we're bringing you this series of *asanas*—so that you can practice yoga the way it was originally intended, keeping your focus on the movement of your breath, the sensations in your body and the thoughts in your mind. In between each pose and series, bring your hands to the gesture of *namaste* (palms together in prayer at your heart center) to feel a sense of beginning or completion—and see if you can turn the corners of your mouth upwards. You got it. A smile. Giving thanks for your health and the well-being of others can get you through the trickiest of poses.

What to Do

Begin your practice with a round of Sun Salutations, a flowing series of poses on the next page. This warms up your muscles, helps to lubricate your joints, and creates energy in your body, as well as helping to focus your mind and prepare you for the grounding poses. Then do the seven postures (aka asanas) in the order shown three to four days a week as part of your regular practice. Breathe through the nose if possible, and try to keep your inhales and exhales long and smooth. Use your breath as a guide to where you are with the poses: If the breath becomes shallow, rapid or strained in any way, you know it's time to back off!

Hold each posture for three to five breaths, or longer to increase your stamina and stability.

End each session by relaxing and rebalancing your muscles in the *savasana*, Corpse pose: Lie on your back, letting your feet fall open. Keep your arms relaxed at your sides, palms up. Breathe deeply, inhaling and exhaling down into your belly, expanding and closing your rib cage with each breath. Use this time to de-stress; visualize your breath moving into tight areas and releasing. After breathing deeply, let the breath become natural as you relax even more. Stay here for at least 10 minutes.

SUN SALUTATION

1.

Start in Mountain pose, with feet together and legs straight. Inhale and sweep your arms up overhead keeping them slightly apart and parallel.

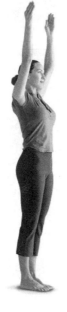

2.

Exhale, hinging forward at the hips to a forward bend.

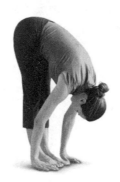

3.

Release the arms and head toward the floor. Keep your legs straight or slightly bent if the hamstrings are tight, with fingertips touching the floor. Inhale and look forward, elongating your spine so it's straight.

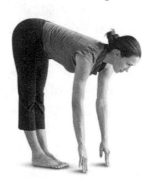

7.

Exhale, lowering your torso to the floor. Inhale, turning the toes under, then exhale, lifting your hips up to form an inverted "V" to Downward Facing Dog.

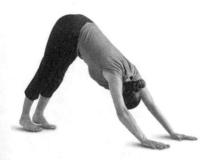

8.

Inhale, and bring your right leg forward between your hands, then the left leg, so the feet are together in Forward Bend.

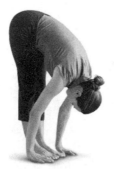

9.

Inhale and lengthen your spine.

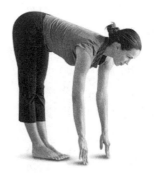

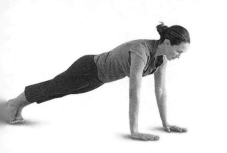

4.

Exhale and step back with your right foot, then your left, so feet and legs are together. Lower your hips so your body forms a straight line in Plank pose.

5.

Put your knees on the floor if you need to. Inhale, then exhale and lower your torso to the floor, keeping your elbows close to your sides.

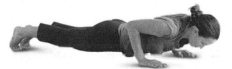

6.

Inhale, straightening the elbows and pushing your upper torso off the floor to Upward Facing Dog.

10.

Then exhale deeper into the bend, releasing your head down. Inhale, and sweep your arms back up and straight overhead to Mountain pose.

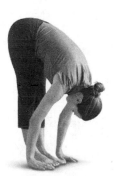

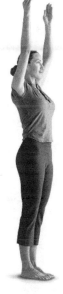

11.

Exhale and release the arms to your sides. Repeat four to six times.

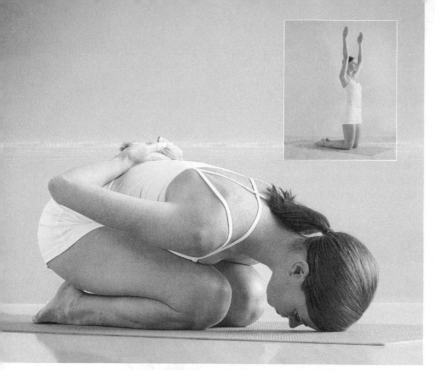

1. BALI SEAL

Kneel and sit back on your heels, keeping the tops of your feet flat on the mat, ankles and knees together. Hinge forward from your hips, placing your belly and chest on your thighs, and let your forehead touch the floor (top left). Keep your neck long, hands at the base of your spine, palms up. Inhale, lifting your arms out and up toward the ceiling as you rise onto your knees (inset). Exhale, bend your knees and lower yourself to start position. Repeat four to six times as a flow series.

As you hold the grounding postures, breathe steadily to maintain your stillness and your inner reflection on how you feel.

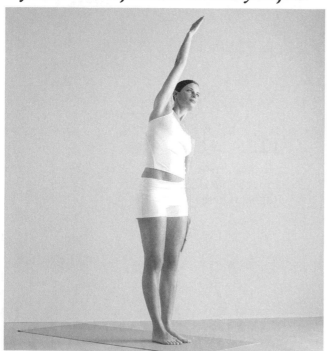

3. BLOWN PALM

Standing in Mountain pose, inhale, then exhale and slowly lean to your left, drawing your left arm down to your side. Keep your right arm aligned with your ear, extending up and out through the fingertips (bottom left). Root your feet firmly to the ground, engage your thighs and buttocks, and allow your entire being to be supported. Hold for three to five breaths, then inhale, lifting the left arm up, and return to start position. Repeat on the opposite side.

2. CHAIR

Stand in Mountain pose with feet together and legs straight. Pressing your thighs, knees and ankles together, bend the knees as if you were to sit. Inhale and extend your arms up and overhead, forearms parallel to each other (right). Draw the shoulder blades down and back, keeping your breastbone lifted, your spine long and your abs firm to maintain a strong, erect torso. Hold for three to five breaths, sitting a little deeper and extending your arms a little higher.

To deepen your practice, move in and out of each posture with intention, thought and care. If your mind wanders during a pose, come back to your breath and find a soft gazing point, or drishti.

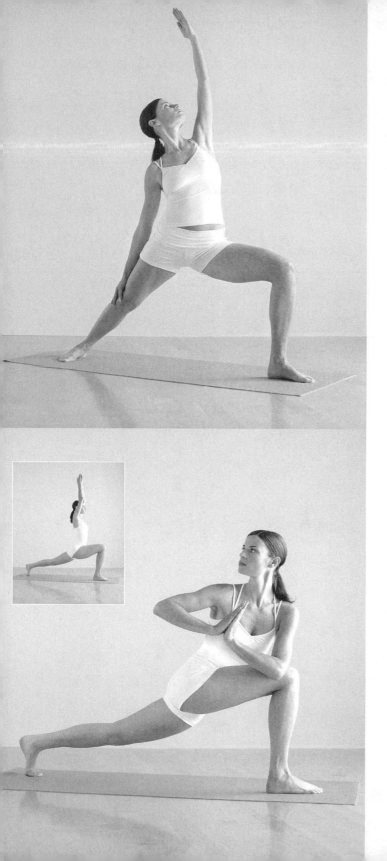

4. REVERSE WARRIOR

Standing in Mountain pose, put your hands on your hips and take a step backward about three to four feet with your right foot, turning the foot out 45 to 60 degrees and lining up the arch to the left heel. Keeping the right leg straight, hips squared and torso centered, bend the left knee to align over the left ankle. Place your right hand on your right thigh. Inhale, lifting your left arm up and overhead as you lengthen your spine into a mild back bend (top left). Exhale and stay here for three to five breaths. Inhale, bringing your torso to a centered position, then place your hands on your hips and step forward to start position.
Repeat with the opposite leg.

5. LUNGE IN PRAYER

Standing in Mountain pose, place palms together at your breastbone and take a step back with your left foot. Keep the left heel lifted and bend the right knee to align over the right ankle. Inhale, lifting both arms overhead (inset). Stabilize in the pose, rooting your feet and grounding through the strength of your legs. Keeping your palms together, exhale and lower your arms to place the left elbow on the outside of your right thigh. Inhale, then exhale and rotate into a twist, looking over your right shoulder (bottom left). Stay here for three to five breaths, then inhale and untwist so the torso is centered, bringing the palms to the breastbone. Step back to start position and repeat with the opposite leg.

6. WIDE-ANGLE FORWARD BEND

From Mountain pose, separate your feet slightly more than hip-width. Lift your breastbone, drawing the shoulder blades down your spine as you interlace your fingers behind your back (top right). Inhale into a slight back bend, then exhale, folding forward from your hips, bringing your torso toward the floor. Keep your breastbone lengthening away from your hips, reaching the arms up and overhead. Hold for three to five breaths, lower your hands to the small of your back, bend your knees and roll up slowly.

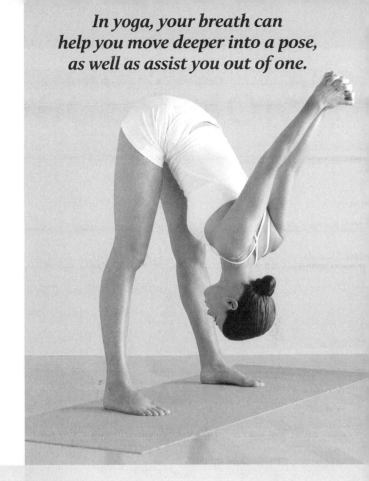

In yoga, your breath can help you move deeper into a pose, as well as assist you out of one.

7. BOUND BRIDGE

Lying face-up on the floor, bend your knees, keeping them aligned over the ankles. Place the feet flat, hip-width apart. Relax your arms by your sides (below left). Inhale and lift the tailbone off the floor, drawing the torso up until your body forms a straight line from shoulder to knees. Interlace your fingers underneath you, forefingers pointing forward along the floor (below right). Continue to draw your shoulder blades down and back as you press your hands toward your feet. Hold for three to five breaths, then slowly lower your torso.

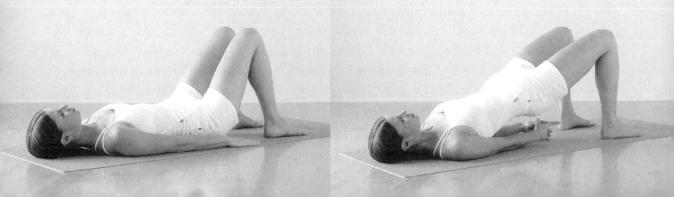

Biofeedback

THERE'S A SCENE IN **The Matrix** when Neo bends a spoon with his mind. It's sci-fi, but not that far off from the way you control your body. For example, as you read this sentence, you direct your eyes to scroll from left to right—just as you can tell your gut to keep quiet because it's not time for lunch, or your legs to move faster because you want to beat your record mile.

But that's child's play, everyday stuff—think bigger.

Could you tell your heart, for instance, to beat slower? Could you direct blood to the bottom of your toes? Could you heal a wound through sheer will?

Biofeedback proponents believe, yes, we can. Using a series of machines, their systems give you information about your body so you can then manipulate it, using your mind to heal. Imagine controlling "involuntary" processes such as blood pressure and skin temperature, or even tightening the muscles in your vagina. That's worth at least one Keanu-sized "Whoa."

Essential Concepts

Biofeedback looks like a 1960s science experiment (and was in fact invented then): You are attached by electrodes on your head and/or body to electronic sensors—the feedback devices—that monitor your physical responses to stimuli and mental exercises. The devices give you signals—beeps, flashes, needles on a dial—and you use this feedback to learn how to regulate your body's function.

Try It Out

Say you had a problem with anxiety—a biofeedback therapist may recommend galvanic skin response training, in which sensors measure how much you're sweating, alerting you to when the feeling's kicking in biologically. That may then lead to you being able to anticipate the next attack.

Sometimes there's a physical component, as well. An emerging field of gynecological physical therapy helps women with pelvic floor issues, including uterine prolapse—when the uterus slips down, due to weakened muscles—and incontinence. The therapist inserts a tampon-shaped device into the woman's vagina, and she then does Kegels or similar pelvic-floor exercises. The monitor tells her how much pressure she is exerting, and—just like doing bicep curls—she learns how to strengthen her pelvic floor muscles.

✱ **BEST FOR:** Biofeedback is most often used as a relaxation and stress-relieving technique; it has proven useful for stress-related conditions such as high blood pressure, migraines and other headaches,

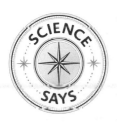

Here's a shocker: Western medical doctors actually *believe* in biofeedback. Numerous studies support its efficacy, especially for muscle tension and weakness, and pain. Research suggests that thermal biofeedback may ease symptoms of Raynaud's disease (a condition that causes reduced blood flow to fingers, toes, nose or ears) while EMG biofeedback has been shown to reduce pain, morning stiffness, and the number of tender points in people with fibromyalgia. And a new review of scientific clinical studies found that biofeedback may help people with insomnia fall asleep.

A landmark study by the Agency for Health Care Policy and Research that has since been put into nursing home protocol found that patients could learn to control incontinence using biofeedback. The Women's Health Physical Therapy department at Northwestern Memorial Physicians Group in Chicago—along with other cutting-edge PT departments—has been studying biofeedback for years, and uses it with great success to treat pelvic-floor disorders such as uterine prolapse.

insomnia, asthma and IBS. Muscle-related conditions such as weakness after surgery and incontinence and other pelvic-floor disorders (especially ones that materialize during pregnancy and after childbirth), have improved with biofeedback.

Precautions

Biofeedback is virtually risk-free, but let your medical doctor know if you are trying it.

FIND A PRACTITIONER

The best way to find a biofeedback therapist is by a referral from your doctor.

Specialists who provide biofeedback training range from psychiatrists and psychologists to nurses, dentists and physicians. Of course, the usual caveats apply, including:

- Check the credentials and education of the therapist.
- Since there's not a lot of personal interaction, a pre-appointment interview is not really necessary, but do make sure you feel comfortable with your therapist. Especially if, you know, you're going to have a tampon-shaped device inserted into your vagina.
- Typically, 10-week sessions are prescribed; make sure to check if your insurance covers it.
- The Association for Applied Psychology and Biofeedback (aapb.org) is a good resource for finding qualified biofeedback practitioners in your area.

Homeopathy

Homeopathy is much more popular in Europe than here at home. It's reportedly favored by Paul McCartney, Orlando Bloom and other famous Brits, including the Royal Family. (The U.K. health care system even hosts homeopathic hospitals.) But the 200-year-old holistic healing system—which actually can be traced back to the writings of Hippocrates dating back to the fifth century—is inexpensive, completely natural and rarely has side effects. It could be the next big British Invasion.

Essential Concepts

Two laws govern most homeopathic remedies: The law of similars, or "like cures like," means that a patient's symptoms are seen as a clue to the appropriate remedy; remedies are derived from substances that induce symptoms similar to those of the illness. For example, a remedy made from highly diluted coffee may cure your insomnia; barely perceptible traces of onion can ease allergic, watery eyes.

A 2010 piece in *Alternative Medicine Review,* for instance, suggests using conventional allergy testing to determine a patient's most significant allergen, and then administering a 30C dose of this substance (available at homeopathic pharmacies). The law of potentization calls for a dilution of a remedy so that its side effects are limited. (See "Science Says" on page 368.)

"Giving a person a remedy that matches her symptoms slightly magnifies the existing disease process and encourages the body to react to this stimulus by activating its own power to heal," explains Kathy Thorpe, M.A., a certified homeopath in Boulder, Colo.

Quite a few studies back her up, including one published in 2010 that might put to rest Western medicine's biggest criticism of homeopathy: How can it work when the remedies appear to have nothing of substance in them? Using an EEG to measure electrical activity in the brain, researchers in Germany showed that the brain responds strongly to homeopathic treatments. Ironically, the more diluted, the higher the impact. In a landmark double-blind study published in the journal *Rheumatology,* homeopathic remedies for fibromyalgia outperformed a placebo, and a 2010 review published in *The Rheumatologist* concludes that because the efficacy of conventional analgesic drugs for chronic pain is modest at best, "We should be particularly aggressive about using more non-pharmacological therapies in treating patients with chronic pain."

✱ BEST FOR: Homeopathy has been shown to work best for allergies, colds and flu, anxiety, nervous tension and shock, long-term and relapsing chronic conditions, skin conditions, fatigue, insomnia, headaches, nausea, menopause and PMS.

Try It Out

Choose a remedy that addresses your most intense symptom(s) as well as your emotional state, advises one of the best-known homeopaths in this country, Dana Ullman, M.P.H., *Natural Health* advisory board member and coauthor of *Everybody's Guide to Homeopathic Medicine.* If it doesn't work within the prescribed time, simply try a different one. The idea, he says, "is to give as few doses of the remedy as possible, but as many as necessary." You don't need to continue using a remedy once you feel better, unless the benefits wear off. Some people like single-ingredient, under-the-tongue dissolvable pills; others prefer combination remedies. Here are several options for six common conditions, based on your primary symptoms and/or emotional state.

Allergies

Santa Barbara, Calif., homeopath Mary Aspinwall, author of *A Basic Guide to Homeopathy* and founder of Homeopathy World, suggests taking a dose of one of these remedies and repeating it if the same symptoms return.

ARSENICUM ALBUM: Violent sneezing; watery, burning eyes and nose; you're anxious about not being able to breathe.

NUX VOMICA: Violent sneezing; nose may run during the day but be stuffed up at night; you may feel irritable, headachy, chilled and sensitive to noises.

SABADILLA: Sneezing; red, watery eyes; itchy eyes, nose, ears, throat and roof of mouth; ears are sometimes blocked.

Combination solutions: Hyland's Seasonal Allergy Relief ($7; amazon.com); Similasan allergy relief formulas ($11; similasanusa.com)

Anxiety

Self-prescribed remedies work well for in-the-moment anxiety, but more serious distress requires the attention of a professional homeopath. Ullman and Margo Marrone, a London-based pharmacist and homeopath and founder of The Organic Pharmacy, suggest taking one of these remedies up to four times a day during an anxiety attack.

ACONITE: For sudden-onset anxiety and intense fear following a traumatic event.

ARGENTUM NITRICUM: For performance anxiety, fear of heights or claustrophobia, generally accompanied by stomach cramps and loose stools.

IGNATIA: For acute anxiety and depression, especially after the breakup of a relationship or a death in the family.

Combination solution: Bach Flower Essence's Rescue Remedy ($13 for 10 milliliters; bachflower.com)

Colds

Thorpe suggests taking one of the following every hour for three doses, then once every three hours.

ACONITE: For the first 24 hours of a cold that appears suddenly after exposure to cold or wind; you feel hot and dry, anxious and may be very thirsty.

ALLIUM CEPA: For the early stages of a cold when there is a lot of sneezing; clear, watery nasal discharge; and profuse tearing; you feel worse in warm rooms and better in the open air.

PULSATILLA: For the later stages of a cold when there is thick, yellow-green mucus, a lack of thirst and changeable symptoms.

Combination solution: Dr. Hauschka's Agropyron Cold Relief ($14; drhauschka.com)

OSCILLOCOCCINUM: It's one of the most popular homeopathic remedies and is marketed to relieve flu-like symptoms (Boiron Oscillo-coccinum $23; vitaminshoppe.com)

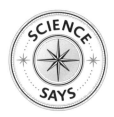

According to the most recent numbers from the NIH National Health Interview Survey, which includes a survey of the use of complementary practices used in the U.S., approximately 3.9 million adults and 910,000 children use homeopathy. While it has been studied much more extensively in Europe, still more research needs to be done on the practice; a recent report by the British Homeopathic Association reported that 43% of the randomized controlled trials carried out have been positive, 6% negative and 49% inconclusive. A 2012 review of eight studies published in *Cochrane Summaries* showed that homeopathic remedies outperformed placebos in treating the adverse effects of cancer treatment. Studies on homeopathy are constantly being called for because anecdotal evidence of its efficacy is so strong.

But its use is controversial, in large part because it is not possible in scientific terms to explain how a remedy containing little or no active ingredients can have any positive effect. And since treatments are highly individualized and there are hundreds of different homeopathic compounds, prescription is challenging. The NCCAM is currently funding research on homeopathy, including its effect on symptoms of fibromyalgia.

Fatigue

Occasional bouts of fatigue respond well to these remedies, Aspinwall says. Take one dose and repeat if fatigue returns.

ARNICA: Best following extreme physical exertion like giving birth or running a marathon; also helps with jet lag.

CHINA: For exhaustion and weakness brought on by dehydration; helpful after diarrhea, vomiting or sweaty fevers.

PHOSPHORIC ACID: For nervous exhaustion and brain fog brought on by intense mental activity; you may feel heaviness and a burning sensation in your spine and limbs.

Headaches

Ullman suggests taking three doses one-half hour apart, then one dose three times a day.

BELLADONNA: For throbbing pain aggravated by noise, light, touch, motion or lying down; pain is relieved by applying cold compresses or firm pressure.

NUX VOMICA: For headaches resulting from drinking too much coffee or alcohol or working too hard; often accompanied by constipation and extreme irritability. Pain is relieved by applying warm compresses, sitting quietly or lying down.

PULSATILLA: For headaches aggravated by heat, stuffy rooms or overeating; may be relieved by being in the open air or applying cold compresses.

Insomnia

The naturopathic docs at Arizona Natural Health Center in Tempe suggest these remedies. Take two to three pellets under the tongue once or twice a day.

ARSENICUM ALBUM: If you're anxious, especially about your health, and have trouble staying in bed at night due to extreme restlessness; you feel better with company, worse when alone.

COFFEA CRUDA: If you feel wide awake from too much excitement and an overly active mind.

IGNATIA: If you can't stop thinking about your troubles; you avoid sharing problems with others and feel best when busy and distracted.

Precautions

Do not use homeopathy as a replacement for proven conventional care or vaccines; do not postpone seeing a health care provider about a medical problem.

Tell your regular doctor about any complementary treatments you use or plan to use.

If you are considering using a homeopathic treatment, bring it with you when you see your medical doctor, who can determine if it might pose a problem.

Pregnant or nursing women—or those considering using homeopathy on a child—should consult with their medical providers.

Take extra care when using homeopathic treatments that are not diluted and/or that contain heavy metal, such as mercury or silver.

FIND A PRACTITIONER

You can find homeopathic remedies (single pills, combination remedies and kits) at most natural food stores like Whole Foods Market and on a variety of websites, including vitaminshoppe.com, amazon.com, heelusa.com, drhauschka.com and homeopathyworld.com.

Homeopaths are licensed in some states; some conventional medical doctors also practice homeopathy. To find a homeopath, the best place to start is with a referral from friends or family. You also can walk into a homeopathic pharmacy and therapists will help you choose a course of treatment based on your symptoms. Because a homeopath treats every patient and every disease as unique, a practitioner will ask not only about your physical symptoms, but also about your physical condition, emotional state, personality traits, fears and phobias. She might ask about your home environment and family situation, so be prepared to be brutally honest. Also:

Check credentials and education. For homeopaths, these include the American Board of Homeotherapeutics, the Society of Homeopaths , the North American Society of Homeopaths and the Council for Homeopathic Certification.

When you're looking for a practitioner for an office visit, call ahead for a five- to 10-minute interview. Be wary of one who won't talk to you.

An initial examination involves lots of questions. Use your intuition to judge whether you're comfortable and it's working for you or not.

Inquire up front about costs; most health care plans in this country do not cover homeopathy.

Be wary of any practitioner who makes excessive claims and guarantees a cure. Also be wary of one who wants to sign you up immediately for a specified number of treatments.

The above-mentioned certifying organizations maintain databases of their members.

You also can find a directory at nationalcenterforhomeopathy.org.

Hypnotherapy

Your eyes are getting heavy, your breath is growing deeper, you can feel your shoulders relax, the tension melt away into your chair... deeper... deeper... As kitschy as this scenario sounds—"It'd never work for me," you're thinking—hypnosis has gotten very hip, especially the self-hypnosis used to break bad habits, boost self-confidence and even reduce the pain of childbirth. Nowadays, hypnotherapy is even recommended by the NIH for chronic pain; a 2009 review in the *Journal of Behavioral Medicine* supports the NIH recommendation, and clinical studies show that using hypnosis may reduce your need for medication, improve your mental and physical condition before an operation and reduce the time it takes to recover.

It also has been found particularly effective for treating anxiety, depression and addiction. A 2008 smoking cessation study conducted by San Francisco V.A. Medical Center and the University of California, San Francisco found hypnotherapy to be effective as standard behavioral counseling when combined with nicotine patches. You are getting very... very... convinced.

Essential Concepts

Hypnotherapy is a form of psychotherapy in which the conscious, rational part of the mind is bypassed, making the subconscious extremely susceptible to suggestion. It's mainly used to change behaviors, attitudes and responses. (A hypnotherapist will not make you do tricks or strip in front of a Vegas audience. That's a hypnotist.)

The word hypnosis comes from *hypnos*, the Greek word for sleep, but practitioners do not induce sleep—hypnosis is a type of trance during which breathing, heart rate and metabolism slow and suggestions that can help you change unwanted thoughts and behaviors are made by the therapist.

Changing behavior and thoughts takes practice; when something happens to us, we have a response, and if that response is repeated over and over, it becomes tough to break the pattern. A hypnotherapist teaches you what led to those reactions and how you can replace them with different, healthier reactions.

They believe that during the deep meditative state induced by hypnosis, the brain produces intense alpha waves, and that during this quiet state, the body and mind are highly receptive to suggestions. Practitioners may implant a suggestion or response that has a trigger, aimed at overcoming problems such as smoking, overeating or a lack of confidence.

Try It Out

A hypnotherapist will induce a hypnotic trance, usually by speaking in a slow, soothing voice. Some also use a ticking clock to enhance the rhythmic breathing and suggest to you that you are starting to feel heavy and deeply relaxed. Indeed, after a few sessions, it might take just the word "relax" to make you feel relaxed.

The goal is for you to remain alert, hear every word and also respond to questions and suggestions. During your deeply relaxed state, the therapist will give you posthypnotic suggestions, meaning instructions to do or not do something, such as "stop smoking" now; the therapist may frame it as an indirect suggestion, too, like "I wonder how it would feel for you to not use heroin?" Your unconscious mind will absorb the suggestion, and that should make it easier to stick to your goals and learn healthier behaviors.

Clinical hypnotherapist Jon Rhodes says it's better to start with a hypnotherapist and learn self-hypnosis techniques, but you can teach yourself, too: Start by thinking about what you want to change, and state your goal in a single sentence. Sit or lie down comfortably (if you can find a ticking clock, even better), close your eyes and, slowly counting from 10 to one, breathe in through your nose and out through your mouth. As you exhale, say the word "relax." Then, imagine you are walking down 10 steps, and there is a door at the bottom. When you get there, open the door and discover your favorite place ever. A beach, a garden, anyplace you really want to be. When you are deeply relaxed, you can state your goal, imagine the behavior you want to adopt, the responses you'd like to change, then let go and count back up from one to 10.

✷ **BEST FOR:** Stress and anxiety, fears and phobias, weight management and eating disorders, addictions, depression, allergies and asthma, pain relief and digestive disorders. Recently, self-hypnosis has been taught for use during childbirth.

Precautions

Always let your medical doctor know about any alternative therapy you are considering.

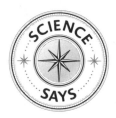

The medical community has come to accept that hypnosis works, but they don't know how. Research published in the *American Journal of Clinical Hypnosis* in 2009 showed hypnosis to be effective in treating irritable bowel syndrome, and recent studies in Australia and the U.S. found that it could control anxiety and be used for relaxation during dental surgery. A 2012 Stanford University School of Medicine study published in the *Archives of General Psychiatry* found that the ability to slip into the mental state known as hypnosis varies among people, and that 10% of us are highly hypnotizable, one-third are not at all, and the rest fall in between. Study author David Seigel of Stanford's Center for Integrative Medicine suggests that people who were highly imaginative as children are more easily hypnotized. In a 2008 study, also at Stanford, researchers used hypnosis to properly diagnose children who appeared to be epileptic. Doctors seem to place more confidence in self-hypnosis than hypnotherapy.

Do not attempt hypnotherapy or self-hypnosis if you are psychotic; practice extreme caution if you are deeply depressed.

Find a trustworthy, qualified practitioner.

FIND A PRACTITIONER

The best way to find a hypnotherapist is by referral from a friend, family member or even another health provider, possibly a psychotherapist. Also:

Look for a therapist with the proper credentials and education. Most hypnotherapists are licensed family counselors, social workers, medical doctors or registered nurses who have received additional training in hypnotherapy. Members of the American Society of Clinical Hypnosis (ASCH) must hold a doctorate in medicine, dentistry, podiatry or psychology, or a master's-level degree in nursing, social work, psychology or marital/family therapy with at least 20 hours of ASCH-approved training in hypnotherapy. The American Psychotherapy and Medical Hypnosis Association provides certificates for licensed medical and mental health professionals who complete a six- to eight-week course.

Call for a five- to 15-minute interview before booking an appointment, and be wary of a therapist who will not talk to you on the phone. The voice is very important, and you need to feel you can be honest and trusting with this person.

Don't feel you have to book a number of appointments in advance; in fact, beware of a therapist who insists on this.

The National Board for Certified Clinical Hypnotherapists (NBCCH) certifies therapists and maintains a website that can be used as a resource (natboard.com).

Naturopathy

Naturopathy is probably the most natural-sounding of the complementary and alternative modalities in this book—and it's also the one many experts feel will be integrated into our future health care systems. It's a multidisciplinary approach to healing that uses natural resources, such as herbs, fresh air, sunshine, nutrition and exercise to encourage the body to heal itself—often with disdain for modern science.

Essential Concepts:

Naturopaths believe that the body will strive on its own toward balance, the vital force called "homeostasis," which can be thrown off by unhealthy lifestyle, stress, lack of exercise and sleep, poor diet, pollution and even negative mental attitudes. Poor lifestyle habits, they feel, allow toxins and waste products to build, which weakens the immune system, making the body susceptible to viruses, bacteria and allergens, and preventing it from maintaining good health. Emphasizing prevention, a naturopath uses a variety of diagnostic and therapeutic methods—including acupuncture, homeopathy, soft-tissue manipulation and therapeutic counseling—to encourage a patient's natural self-healing process. Other therapies a naturopath uses include:

YOGA, which promotes deep relaxation and breathing, as well as strength and flexibility

HERBAL REMEDIES, prescribed to support the body's own healing powers

A WHOLE-FOODS DIET, rich in antioxidants and anti-inflammatory
foods, organic fruits and vegetables and unprocessed whole grains

DETOXING CLEANSES, commonly prescribed, along with fasting
and juicing

MASSAGE, to promote circulation and relax muscles

OSTEOPATHY, crucial to a healthy body structure and well-being

HYDROTHERAPY, is one of the most ancient therapies, using water
in all forms—ice, steam, baths, colonic irrigation—to maintain
health and treat disease

A naturopath is a teacher who strives to educate and motivate
patients to accept personal responsibility for their health by adopting
a healthy lifestyle. They also recommend many self-help treatments,
such as juicing and fasting, herbs and supplements, self-massage and
breath work.

So does it work, or what? More and more research is being conducted. *The Journal of Alternative and Complementary Medicine* (JACM) has
been publishing pilot studies that look at naturopathy for multiple sclerosis, diabetes, menopause and other tricky, chronic and lifestyle-effect-
ed conditions. The NIH has been funding studies that include looking at
a naturopathic approach to diet for type 2 diabetes. Naturopathy seems

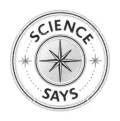

Many of the naturopathic
principles—such as
the benefits of exercise
and relaxation; a diet
based on whole, organic
foods; sleep and stress
reduction—are well-
researched. A study by the American Association of Naturopathic
Physicians found that naturopathy
was an effective alternative to
antibiotics or surgery for ear infections in children. A study at Bastyr
University in Seattle followed
16 HIV-positive patients who
received naturopathic treatments
for a year and found that 12 experienced improved well-being and
none developed AIDS. There's
absolutely no dispute that conventional preventative medicine owes
much to naturopathic theory,
but well-designed research needs
to continue.

to work best treating the "whole" person; a 2013 study of overweight and obese adults with osteoarthritis published in the *Natural Medicine Journal* found that an intensive 18-month course of naturopathic diet and exercise resulted in more weight loss, less knee pain and better function than diet or exercise alone.

So far, pretty much across the board, research is finding that naturopathic medicine is at least as effective as conventional approaches. Many states are starting to license N.D.s as primary-care providers, which allows them to prescribe drugs (such as antibiotics) and perform minor office procedures. And when conventional approaches don't work, many are turning to naturopathy with success.

But while specific treatments have been studied, there's not a lot of scientific research on naturopathy as a whole. Currently, the track record goes from support to allegations of quackery (controversial health buff John Kellogg, of Corn Flakes fame, was an early adopter), but it's also considered one of the fastest-growing and most exciting alternative methods of health and healing; many believe it to be the health care system of the future. An estimated 729,000 American adults and 237,000 children used a naturopathic treatment last year.

Try It Out

Start by making sure your contact is a state-licensed naturopathic doctor (N.D.); N.D.s attend a four-year accredited naturopathic medical school and are trained to be primary-care physicians who emphasize gentle, noninvasive, natural therapies that facilitate the body's inherent ability to restore and maintain good health. They are different from integrative M.D.s in that they are trained to identify the root cause of an illness and treat it with natural interventions; conventional therapies are generally used as a last resort. N.D.s also are trained to perform minor surgery and prescribe medications; however, their scope of practice in these two areas varies from state to state. Currently, according to the American Association of Naturopathic Physicians (AANP), 17 U.S. states, the District of Columbia, Puerto Rico and the U.S. Virgin Islands have licensing or regulation laws for naturopathic doctors.

How to Eat Naturopathically

Naturopaths are all trained to help clients make nutritional changes to their diets to boost their health. In fact, several studies have included or focused on a naturopathic 30-day diet. The diet looks a bit like the Mediterranean Diet of the '90s, and a bit like an anti-inflammatory or detox diet.

Here's a sample of one, designed by San Diego-based clinical naturopath David Getoff, who has extensive experience with nutrition. He gently reminds us that we are not going on a diet, just eating in a way that is healthier for 30 days. His diet calls for you to avoid all processed foods, including meats, grains, snack foods and dairy foods. Here are his guidelines:

NO Hot dogs, luncheon meats, or fish high in mercury such as shark, swordfish or orange roughy.

OK Fresh turkey, chicken, beef, lamb and fish are OK. Eggs should be whole and fresh.

NO Dairy, except for raw milk (stop this if you have a reaction). No cheese, yogurt, ice cream or cream

NO Grains, potatoes, beans or bread (unless it's made from almond flour, the only flour allowed).

NO Frozen, canned or starchy vegetables, including corn, squash, potatoes.

OK Only raw, fresh fruit—no frozen, canned or dried fruit.

OK Butter, olive oil, coconut oil, all are OK. Fats that come with the food, such as skin, are OK. All other oils are not.

NO Sugar of any kind, including honey and artificial sweeteners.

NO Caffeine or alcohol; drink two quarts of water a day.

OK Only single spices, no spice combos.

OK Go for organic and hormone-free whenever possible, and be careful about eating in restaurants, Getoff says. Make sure you are eating two to three portions of protein daily, and do not go hungry. (There's the challenge!)

✱ BEST FOR: Long-term degenerative conditions such as arthritis and asthma, fatigue, colds and flu, sinus infection, gastrointestinal issues, depression and PMS. Research is promising also for type 2 diabetes and multiple sclerosis. Naturopathic physicians are trained in natural childbirth and many work in conjunction with midwives.

Precautions

Make sure your medical doctor knows you are working with a naturopath, especially if you are pregnant or being treated for an illness.

Seek a reputable, licensed, qualified practitioner.

FIND A PRACTITIONER

It's always best to get referrals from friends, family or health care providers for a good naturopathic doctor, but you also should do some research. A great place to start is by inquiring at one of the accredited U.S. schools: Bastyr University in Seattle, Wash.; National College of Natural Medicine in Portland, Ore.; National University of Health Sciences in Lombard, Ill., and Southwest College of Naturopathic Medicine (SCNM) in Tempe, Ariz. Naturopaths are quoted throughout this book as well, and that can be a good starting source. Also:

Always check credentials and education. Licensing for N.D.s is slowly happening; currently 17 states offer it, but in a state that doesn't check for certificates from the above schools.

When you're looking for a practitioner, always call ahead for a five- to 10-minute interview. You'll be spending lots of time with this doctor, and you need to have a sense that you can be comfortable with and trust him/her. Be wary of one who won't talk to you.

An initial examination is a lot like a conventional medical visit, but lasts longer, about 1½ hours. You'll be asked to bring any test results you have, and also will be asked lots of questions; the doctor will discuss treatment plans that may include diet and exercise plans, herbs, supplements and/or homeopathy. Use your intuition to judge whether it's working for you or not.

Be wary of any practitioner who makes excessive claims and guarantees a cure. Also be wary of one who wants to sign you up immediately for a specified number of treatments.

Inquire up front about costs and find out what your insurance will cover; some health care plans will cover treatments by an M.D., but not a yoga or massage therapist.

The American Association of Naturopathic Physicians in Washington, D.C. (aanmc.org) maintains a database of local practitioners along with their credentials and education.

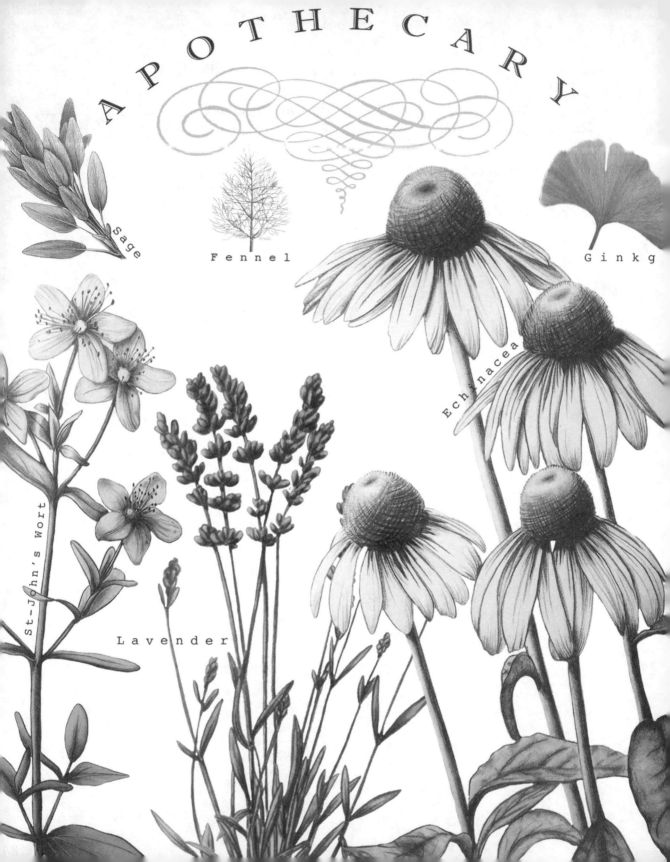

APOTHECARY

Sage

Fennel

Ginkg

St-John's Wort

Lavender

Echinacea

Botanical Medicine

Live longer, naturally, with no side effects. That's been the irresistible sales pitch for herbal remedies since plants first grew on the Earth. So why are you hearing so much about them now, in this advanced new millennium? Because they'll also save you cash—an insane amount of cash, especially on drugs.

Americans spend more per capita on medicines than any other developed country, and buy more generics, too—and even the generics can cost $80 and up, since prices rose 5.3% in 2012. As a result, the natural foods aisle is suddenly flooded with people trying to tell their cramp root from their dong quai. Vulnerable, hurting for money, we want to believe these cheaper remedies work. And do they?

This chapter tells you, definitively, which ones do—and which ones don't. We've combed through the most up-to-date research on botanical medicines, studying the latest breakthroughs and debunking the false claims. And we're proud to report that relief is here for cancer, diabetes, even jet lag (also, NSFW: Our "boost-your-sex-drive" section is a must-read, even if you have no issues down below).

The idea behind herbal remedies is wonderfully simple: Herbalists believe whole plants are more effective than the isolated elements and synthetic ingredients used in drugs—with the added bonus of fewer unintentional effects. Its medicines should be seriously considered for ailments like colds and flu, insomnia, autoimmune diseases—the worries that typically cause conventional docs to throw up their hands. Yet herbs are also proven to help ease the symptoms of more serious ailments, like heart disease and cancer.

(Chinese, Egyptian, Indian and indigenous American civilizations might say, "Welcome to the club, America, what took you so long?")

If trends here continue, it won't be long before this "boom" becomes common practice. While still not fully accepted by Western medicine or every M.D., herbal medicine is now taught more in medical and pharmacy schools. Extensive studies are ongoing not just overseas, but now in the United States. And because some medical doctors realize that plants are the source of many synthetic drugs, an increasing number accept that herbs have benefit.

Just how much benefit? In the following chapter, we recommend products that fared well in evidence-based or double-blind studies—giving an honest look at what to buy and what to avoid. You'll find an A-Z Guide to Herbs, the 12 best herbs for women, and sections on plants that can boost your mood, your energy and your sex drive. As a sales pitch, it's irresistible; as medicine, it's sound.

✳ BEST FOR: Herbs are used to treat many conditions, including persistent conditions such as asthma, migraines and arthritis; autoimmune conditions; respiratory, digestive and circulatory problems; skin conditions; depression; insomnia; PMS and menopausal symptoms; and cancer.

What to Know Before You Buy

So, how safe are these products? And do they do what they promise? Well... it's tricky. Manufacturers do not need FDA approval to put their product on the market, and are allowed to put claims on the label, as long as they also note that the FDA hasn't approved the claim.

Once a product is on the market, the FDA does monitor its quality and safety, and if it's if deemed unsafe, it can issue a warning or require the maker or distributor to remove the product from the marketplace. (In Europe and Australia, herbal products must provide scientific proof before any medicinal claims can be printed on labels.)

These guidelines do not, however, guarantee that an herb is safe for anyone to take—there may be dangerous interactions with other herbs or drugs, so always tell your medical doctor, and the herbal dispensary, about any drugs or herbal supplements you're on. Also:

Do your own research. We've done a lot for you and provide current warnings and precautions, but it's always a good idea to do some of your own and find out what support groups, studies and experts say about a particular herb.

Be especially careful if you are taking warfarin, aspirin or any other blood-thinner; some herbs may increase their anticoagulant effect and increase the risk of bleeding. Some of these herbs are very innocent-sounding, like chamomile and ginger. Also be careful if you are taking any immunosuppressant drugs—drugs that are used to suppress the immune system after a transplant or to control symptoms of autoimmune disease such as lupus and type 1 diabetes—such as corticosteroids (prednisone). Herbs that boost immunity, such as licorice, astragalus and ginseng may counteract these drugs.

Look for reputable brands. Many good companies are represented in these pages; try to buy from companies that have been in business for a long time and have an established reputation.

Learn how to read labels. A reputable brand will not just tell you its product will cure your headache—it should tell you how, and you should be able to find ingredient descriptions and actions on the product website. Then, you can cross reference with unbiased, evidence-based research.

Follow label instructions. Duh. Don't think that if a little works well, a lot will work better. Just don't do it. And don't mix one herb with another herb, unless a professional tells you to.

Be smart. If you're pregnant or nursing, have severe allergies or ailments, then don't take herbs without talking to your doctor. Don't give to children without talking to your doctor.

Tell your medical doctor what you're up to. Unfortunately, a *New England Journal of Medicine* study found that 70% of people (mostly well educated and with a high income) do not tell their doctors that they are using complementary or alternative treatments.

FIND A PRACTITIONER

Herbalists, naturopathic physicians, Traditional Chinese Medicine practitioners, acupuncturists, chiropractors and medical doctors all may use herbs to treat illness. So the guidelines that apply to those therapies (see those chapters) apply to anyone dispensing or recommending herbs. But if you go to an herbalist:

Check education and credentials. Find out where he was trained, and look for credentials and membership in respected organizations such as the American Herbalists Guild. The AHG requires that its members follow a code of ethics and are open to constant peer review. Also, many herbalists are also licensed acupuncturists (L.Ac.).

Be wary of anyone who guarantees a cure, makes outrageous claims, or wants you to sign up for a course of treatment right away, especially if it's before you have even started treatments.

For more information and to find a qualified herbalist, contact the American Herbalists Guild (americanherbalistguild.com). And for more information on herbal and botanical medicine, contact the American Botanical Council (herbalgram.org).

Healing Herbs A–Z

This is it: The List. The 25 herbs that have been proven to work—with a few bliss boosters and serenity savers as a bonus. Stick to the dosages specified here, in the studies or on the label—and make sure to tell your doctor about any herbs you plan to take, especially if you are pregnant or nursing, have a chronic condition or take medication regularly; remember that even though herbs are natural, they can still be contraindicated.

1. ALOE VERA (*Aloe barbadensis*)

BEST FOR: Burns

Aloe vera is *the* herb for minor (second-degree) burns, confirmed by a 2009 *Surgery Today* study, among others that have shown aloe vera gel has a dramatic effect on burns, wounds and other skin conditions. The gel provides a protective layer for the affected area, and speeds healing due to aloecin B., which stimulates the immune system. The gel also can be used orally for ulcers and irritable bowel and as a laxative; it creates an internal protective coating and also stimulates the digestion.

DOSAGE: Apply 100% pure gel to burns several times a day—or, better yet, keep a potted plant on your windowsill and snip off a thick leaf, slit it open and apply the gel to the burn. For ulcers, drink 50 milliliters a day.

PRECAUTIONS: Do not use the yellow gel at the base on skin. Do not take internally while pregnant or nursing, or if suffering from kidney disease or hemorrhoids.

2. BOSWELLIA (*Boswellia serrata*)
BEST FOR: Arthritis and joint injuries

Also known as Indian frankincense, this gummy resin has been clinically proven to have strong anti-inflammatory effects. Boswellia is known to reduce congestion and heat (kapha and pitta elements in ayurveda) in the joints, and is also used to promote appetite and digestion. In a 2008 study published in *Arthritis Research and Therapy*, researchers gave people with osteoarthritis of the knee an extract of boswellia (5-Loxin). After three months, the herb group showed significantly greater relief than a group given a placebo.

DOSAGE: Take one 300-milligram capsule three times a day, with food.

3. ECHINACEA (*Echinacea angustifolia*)
BEST FOR: Common cold

Studies on the effectiveness of echinacea for treating the common cold have been mixed. The largest so far was in 2012 at Cardiff University Common Cold Centre in the U.K.; found that three doses daily, taken for four months reduced the number of colds, and reduced the duration by 26%. The study was peer-reviewed and published in the journal *Evidence-Based Complementary and Alternative Medicine*. The study was funded by the Swiss manufacturers of Echinaforce. But our experts advise ignoring the naysayers, and looking to traditional usage. "Native Americans used *Echinacea angustifolia*—not *Echinacea purpurea*—and they used only the root," explains Sheila Kingsbury, N.D., chair of the Botanical Medicine Department at Bastyr University. "Clinically speaking, accessing the root is the best place to start. It can shorten the length of a cold significantly."

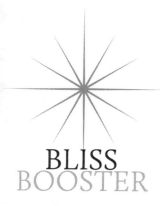

BLISS BOOSTER

CHOCOLATE

Yes, chocolate is an herb, says "medicine hunter" Chris Kilham, ethnobotanist at the University of Massachusetts at Amherst. "Cocoa is one of the great herbal mood enhancers," he says. Chocolate contains a substance called anandamide—aka the bliss molecule—which is known to bind to human cannabinoid receptors (the same ones that interact with marijuana) to create a sense of well-being. "It's a bliss-enhancer—*ananda* means bliss in Sanskrit," Kilham says. "We know that chocolate boosts natural levels of serotonin, the feel-good neurotransmitter. You can happily self-medicate with chocolate and greatly improve your brain chemistry."

Dosage: One teaspoon of echinacea root glycerite liquid every two hours beginning at onset of symptoms; decrease the dose to once every three to four hours after symptoms ease.

4. EVENING PRIMROSE OIL (*Oenothera*)
BEST FOR: Eczema

Evening primrose seeds contain an oil with a high concentration of compounds rarely found in plants: the essential fatty acid gamma-linolenic acid. There are more than 30 human studies reporting its benefits; in one, 1,207 patients found that the oil helped relieve the itching, swelling, crusting and redness of eczema, which a 2013 University of Maryland Medical Center review confirms. Also has been found to lower blood pressure and reduce PMS and some multiple sclerosis symptoms when taken internally.

Dosage: Apply topically for skin conditions; follow label instructions for internal use.

5. FENNEL (*Foeniculum vulgare*)
BEST FOR: Intestinal gas

Fennel seeds contain phytonutrients that are thought to reduce spasms in small muscle fibers like those found in the intestines, helping to reduce gassiness. The aromatic quality of the seeds will also help freshen your breath. And a 2011 review published in *Pediatrics*, for instance, found that fennel tea can be useful for treating a baby's gas-caused colic.

Dosage: Chew a pinch (¼ to ½ teaspoon) of whole fennel seeds after a meal. Your body will let you know—with one last burst of gas—when to stop.

6. FLAXSEED (*Linum usitatissimum*)
BEST FOR: Heart health

Nearly twice as many American women die of heart disease and stroke as from all forms of cancer, including breast cancer, according to the American Heart Association (AHA). One reason: high cholesterol. In fact, women tend to have higher cholesterol levels than men from age 45 on, according to the AHA. Flaxseed, which is rich in the omega-3 fat alpha-linoleic acid, may help lower it.

An Italian study of 40 male and female patients with cholesterol levels greater than 240 mg/dL found that consuming ground flaxseed (20 grams, or about 0.7 ounces, daily) could significantly lower levels of total and LDL cholesterol (the artery-clogging kind), while also improving the ratio of total cholesterol to HDL. (Low levels of HDL may be a greater risk factor for women, according to the AHA.) In a Harvard study of 76,763 women participating in the Nurses' Health Study, researchers also noted that women consuming a diet rich in alpha-linoleic acid seem to have a lower risk of dying from heart disease and stroke, compared to women whose diets were lacking this fat.

Flaxseed also provides fiber; two tablespoons of ground flaxseed have 4 grams of fiber—almost 20% of the 25 grams recommended by the U.S. Department of Agriculture. Lignans, which are a particular type of fiber found in flaxseed, may also be beneficial for preventing breast and prostate cancer, according to preliminary studies. (Lignans are not present in flaxseed oil, however, notes integrative physician and herbalist Tieraona Low Dog, M.D.)

DOSAGE: Low Dog recommends adding 1 to 5 tablespoons of ground flaxseed to your diet several days a week; sprinkle it on cereal or yogurt, or stir it into protein shakes. Flaxseed oil—which must be kept refrigerated to prevent rancidity—should be added to salads and not used for cooking.

PRECAUTIONS: Flaxseed and its oil are safe if consumed in normal amounts, although they can produce a laxative effect. "If you eat huge amounts of flaxseed meal, you could develop cyanide toxicity, but this hasn't, to my knowledge, ever occurred in humans," says Low Dog.

7. GARLIC (*Allium sativum L.*)

BEST FOR: Ear infections and cancer prevention

Garlic's antibiotic compound, alliin, has no medicinal value until the herb is chewed, chopped or crushed. Then an enzyme transforms alliin into a powerful antibiotic called allicin. Raw garlic has the most antibiotic potency, but garlic still has benefits when cooked. Garlic is antimicrobial and anti-inflammatory, so it will treat any infection, but when combined with mullein oil (*Verbascum densiflorum*), it's especially effective for ear infections, says a 2010 report in *Natural News*; the mullein oil is soothing, and helps draw out fluid to relieve pain and decrease pressure. According to the National Cancer Institute, preliminary studies in 2008 suggest that garlic consumption may also reduce the risk of developing several types of cancer, especially those of the gastrointestinal tract.

DOSAGE: Put three drops of oil in each affected ear, two to three times a day as needed. (The oils are sold in a premixed formula.) For internal use, fresh garlic or capsules may be used; follow label directions.

PRECAUTIONS: Don't put drops—or anything else—into your ear if you think the eardrum may be perforated.

8. GINGER (*Zingiber officinale*)

BEST FOR: Nausea and vomiting

A Danish study showed that new sailors prone to motion sickness had less vomiting than a placebo group. Research published in *Obstetrics and Gynecology* found that 88% of nausea-plagued pregnant women got relief when they took 1 gram a day of ginger powder for no longer than four days. And a 2008 study by the *Journal of Alternative and Complementary Medicine* found that powered ginger paired with high-protein meals eased chemotherapy-induced nausea .

DOSAGE: For motion sickness, take a 1 gram capsule of powdered ginger root about an hour before you embark, and another every two hours or as needed. For morning sickness, take 250 milligrams, four times a day. Cooking with the herb may also be helpful.

PRECAUTIONS: Few side effects are linked to normal ginger consumption, but powdered ginger may produce bloating or indigestion. Ginger may also exacerbate heartburn in pregnant women.

SERENITY SAVER

MOTHERWORT (*Leonurus cardiaca*)

When you're feeling anxious and want to run away, hide in that bag of Mint Milanos, try motherwort, a member of the mint family. "The Latin name means 'heart of the lion,'" says Susun Weed, master herbalist and author of the *Wise Woman Herbal* book series. "That's exactly what motherwort does. It gives you the courage of the great cat. It's like sitting in your mother's lap."

9. GINKGO (*Ginkgo biloba*)

BEST FOR: Alzheimer's and antidepressant-induced sex problems

In a landmark study published in the *Journal of the American Medical Association*, researchers gave 202 people with Alzheimer's either a placebo or 120 milligrams a day of ginkgo extract. A year later, the ginkgo group retained more mental function. According to new research in rats (2013), supplementation with an extract from *Ginkgo biloba* may help to battle memory loss and cognitive impairments associated with dementia by encouraging the growth and development of neural stem cells. From upstairs to downstairs: In a University of California, San Francisco study, investigators gave 209 milligrams of ginkgo a day to 63 people suffering from antidepressant-induced sex problems, including erection impairment, vaginal dryness and inability to reach orgasm; the herb helped 91% of the women and 76% of the men to return to normal sexual function.

DOSAGE: Traditional usage is 80 to 240 milligrams of a 50:1 standardized leaf extract daily or 30 to 40 milligrams of extract in a tea bag, prepared as a tea, for at least four to six weeks.

10. GINSENG

BEST FOR: Immune enhancement and diabetes

Many studies show that ginseng has "adaptogenic" powers, which means it helps the body adapt to stress and revs up the immune system. Most studies have used *Panax ginseng* (Asian ginseng); a 2013 University of Maryland review found that Asian ginseng may help boost the immune system, reduce risk of cancer and improve mental performance and well-

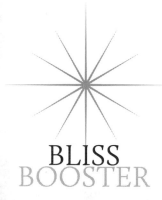

BLISS BOOSTER

KAVA KAVA (*Piper methysticum*)

Native to Polynesia and Melanesia, kava kava was traditionally used as an intoxicating herb for ceremonies and celebrations. "It's my favorite herb for coping with anxiety because it relaxes the musculature while it clears the mind," says herbalist Rosemary Gladstar, author of *Herbal Healing for Women*. "It makes you feel very present in the body—relaxed, but very much in charge." Kava was withdrawn from European markets because of concern that it could be toxic to the liver, but a 2010 study out of Melbourne finds its efficacy so impressive that the Kava Anxiety-Lowering Medication (KALM) project was established to lobby for its re-introduction.

being. And that subjects who took daily doses of ginseng got fewer colds and less severe symptoms than a placebo group. Ginseng also reduces blood-sugar levels. A study in Toronto, Canada, found that Korean red ginseng improved glucose and insulin regulation in well-controlled type 2 diabetes. (Of course, diabetes requires professional treatment, so consult your physician about using ginseng.) Studies also have found ginseng supports liver function and one preliminary study suggests that American ginseng (*Panax quinquefolius*), in combination with ginkgo (*Ginkgo biloba*), may help treat ADHD.

DOSAGE: 500 milligrams daily, best for short-term, stressful events

PRECAUTIONS: Should not be taken for more than six weeks. Avoid caffeine when taking ginseng, and do not take if pregnant.

11. GOLDENROD (*Solidago virgaurea*)

BEST FOR: Nasal congestion

Goldenrod is particularly effective for treating congestion caused by allergies. Surprised? That's because goldenrod gets a bad rap. "People blame goldenrod for their allergies because they look across the field and see the beautiful yellow flowers," says herbalist Margi Flint, author of *The Practicing Herbalist*. "But it's the blooming ragweed they can't see that causes all the trouble. In nature, the remedy often grows right next to the cause." Also used for urinary infections and cystitis, and to flush out kidney and bladder stones.

DOSAGE: Place three drops of the extract under the tongue; repeat as necessary until nasal passages are clear.

12. GOLDENSEAL (*Hydrastis canadensis*)

BEST FOR: Digestive-tract infections

Goldenseal, an herbal antibiotic, is often marketed in combination with echinacea as a treatment for infections, but it is effective only in the digestive tract, not for colds or flu. A 2012 University of Maryland study reported in *Clinical Advisor* found that goldenseal is an effective antibacterial agent and an aid to digestion. For gastrointestinal infections (e.g., ulcers, food poisoning, infectious diarrhea), ask your doctor about using goldenseal in addition to medical therapies. Also can be used topically for wounds and infections.

DOSAGE: For internal use, take a 300-milligram capsule three times a day; apply a dilution as needed for external use.

PRECAUTIONS: Can be toxic if taken to excess. May interact with antidepressants and codeine. Do not use if pregnant, nursing or suffering from high blood pressure.

13. LAVENDER (*Lavandula angustifolia*)
BEST FOR: Headaches

"The scent of lavender triggers a calming response, releasing tension in the scalp muscles a bit, which eases the pain," explains Kingsbury Herbalist Rosemary Gladstar, author of *Rosemary Gladstar's Herbal Recipes for Vibrant Health.* She recommends using lavender oil in a pain-relieving foot soak: Add a few drops to a hot footbath, and then put a cold lavender-infused pack on the forehead. "This draws heat away from the head, and is guaranteed to make you feel better," she says.

DOSAGE: Dab a few drops of essential oil on each temple and rub some around the hairline. Breathe deeply and relax; repeat as needed.

PRECAUTIONS: Do not take the essential oil internally unless under the care of a professional.

14. LEMON BALM (*Melissa officinalis*)
BEST FOR: Anxiety and herpes

Science has shown that lemon balm is tranquilizing. Several double-blind studies have found that a 600-milligram dose promoted calm and reduced anxiety. The herb and its oil have been used in Alzheimer's care units to calm those who are agitated. To decompress after a tough day, try a cup of lemon balm tea; for extra benefit, mix with chamomile. Lemon balm also has antiviral properties and has been shown to reduce the healing time of both oral and genital herpes. German researchers gave people in the early stages of herpes simplex virus outbreaks lemon balm cream or a placebo. The herb group had milder outbreaks that healed faster.

DOSAGE: Available in capsule form, tincture and essential oil; follow label instructions.

PRECAUTIONS: Do not take the essential oil internally unless under the care of a professional.

15. MEADOWSWEET (*Filipendula ulmaria*)

BEST FOR: Heartburn

The Native American herb, high in salicylic acid, calms inflammation in the stomach, often working within a day or two, says Kingsbury. "For people on protein pump inhibitors who are desperate to get their heartburn under control without medication, I have them drink one cup of meadowsweet tea a day, and that's all they need," she says. "They're always shocked that it's so easy."

DOSAGE: Pour two teaspoons of the dried herb in one cup of hot water; steep 20 minutes and drink once a day (the slightly sweet tea has a mild almond flavor).

PRECAUTIONS: Do not take meadowsweet if you're allergic to aspirin.

16. MILK THISTLE (*Silybum marianum*)

BEST FOR: Liver health

Silymarin in milk thistle seeds has a remarkable ability to protect the liver. This herb has been shown to help treat hepatitis and alcoholic cirrhosis. "In our analysis," says Mark Blumenthal, executive director of the American Botanical Council, "a clear majority of studies support milk thistle seed extract for liver conditions." A 2010 NIH-NCCAM study on the effects of silymarin on hepatitis C hepatology showed multiple positive effects demonstrating its antiviral and anti-inflammatory properties. Because most drugs are metabolized through the liver, many herbalists recommend silymarin for anyone who takes liver-taxing medication. Can ease symptoms of a hangover. Also used to increase breast-milk production and to treat depression.

DOSAGE: 500 milligrams daily for liver health; also can be steeped in a tea.

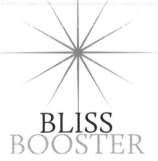

BLISS
BOOSTER

STINGING NETTLE (*Urtica dioica*)

Stinging nettle made its rep as an anti-allergy herb. But it's also a terrific energizer for women, says Weed.

"If you touch the wild stinging nettle plant, you will feel a shock—and that electricity and energy is available to us when we drink nettle infusion," says Weed. The benefits, she explains, are nearly endless: Nettle restores and rebuilds the adrenal glands, tonifies the kidneys, rebuilds the pancreas and stabilizes blood sugar.

17. PSYLLIUM (*Plantago spp.*)

BEST FOR: Digestive problems

Psyllium is a tiny seed that contains mucilage, a soluble fiber that swells on exposure to water. For diarrhea, psyllium can absorb excess fluid in the gut. For constipation, psyllium adds bulk to stool, which presses on the colon wall and triggers the nerves that produce the urge to go. Also helps relieve hemorrhoids and helps remove toxins. May be used topically to draw out infections such as boils.

DOSAGE: Follow label directions; also available in capsule form.

PRECAUTIONS: When using psyllium, drink plenty of water; do not exceed recommended dose.

18. ST. JOHN'S WORT (*Hypericum perforatum*)

BEST FOR: Depression and pain

"Long before it was ever used for depression or anxiety, St. John's wort was used as a pain reliever and an anti-inflammatory for muscle pains, burns and bruises," explains Gladstar, adding that blending the oil with the alcohol-based tincture helps draw the active constituents into the skin for faster healing. For mild depression, St. John's wort often works as well as some antidepressants, but with fewer side effects. "We recently concluded a comprehensive review of the scientific literature on St. John's wort, and 21 of 23 studies support it for mild to moderate depression," says Blumenthal. It's not clear if St. John's wort is as effective as selective serotonin reuptake inhibitors (SSRIs) such as Prozac or Zoloft, but a 2013 Mayo Clinic overview states that scientific evidence supports its use for mild to moderate depression; for severe depression, the evidence remains unclear.

DOSAGE: For depression, studies showing benefits have used 600

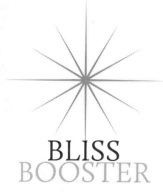

BLISS BOOSTER

GOTU KOLA (*Centella asiatica*)

It's hard to be happy when you can't think straight. According to Sheila Kingsbury, N.D., R.H., chairwoman of the Botanical Medicine Department at Bastyr University in Seattle, the solution for the inner muddle is gotu kola. "It's terrific for mood because it improves the flow of oxygen to the brain, making you feel awake and stimulated without feeling wired." (And this without a Diet Coke.)

to 1,800 milligrams a day; most have used 900 milligrams a day. For pain, make a liniment by mixing equal parts St. John's wort tincture and St. John's wort oil. (Most concoctions come in 2-ounce bottles.) Mix vigorously before using, apply topically to affected area (avoiding the eyes), and massage into skin as needed.

PRECAUTIONS: Stomach upset is possible, and St. John's wort interacts with many drugs, including possibly reducing the effectiveness of birth control pills; so seek professional advice if you are taking a prescription medication. Depression requires professional care; ask your physician about St. John's wort. May cause sensitivity to light.

19. TEA (*Camellia sinensis*)
BEST FOR: Heart health

Tea, particularly green tea, has rocketed to prominence as an herbal medicine. It's high in antioxidants, which help prevent heart disease. In a study published in the *Journal of the American Medical Association,* researchers tracked the consumption of green tea by 40,530 adults over an 11-year period. Women who drank five or more cups a day reduced their risk of dying from cardiovascular disease by 31% and from stroke by 42%, compared to those who drank less than one cup per day. And scientists at the University of Western Australia discovered in 2011 that drinking three cups of tea a day lowers systolic and diastolic blood pressure.

DOSAGE: One to five cups of tea per day; choose according to taste and conditions.

PRECAUTIONS: Read labels and avoid certain herbs and plants if you are pregnant or nursing.

20. TEA TREE OIL (*Melaleuca alternifolia*)
BEST FOR: Athlete's foot and other skin conditions

Tea tree is an Australian plant with an antifungal, antiseptic oil. In a double-blind trial, 158 people with athlete's foot were treated with placebo, a 25% tea tree oil solution or a 50% tea tree oil solution for four weeks. Results showed that the tea tree oil solutions were more effective than placebo. (In the 50% tea tree oil group, 64% were cured; in the 25% tea tree oil group, 55% were cured; in the placebo group, 31% were cured.)

Also helpful for a range of vaginal yeast infections.

DOSAGE: Apply essential oil mixed with a base cream or carrier oil to skin; for vaginal infections, use suppositories.

PRECAUTIONS: Do not take the essential oil internally unless advised by a professional.

21. TRIPHALA (*Emblica officinalis, Terminalia chebula* and *Terminalia belerica*)

BEST FOR: Constipation and digestive problems

Triphala ("three fruits" in Sanskrit), a bowel-regulating formula in ayurvedic medicine, is a combination of the powdered fruits of amalaki, bibhitaki, and haritaki, all of which are rich sources of antioxidants with anti-inflammatory, adaptogenic, antistress, antibacterial, analgesic, anticancer and immune-enhancing properties. A 2012 review published in the *Chinese Journal of Integrative Traditional and Western Medicine* (we're guessing that in China "traditional" means Eastern) confirms the extensive healing properties of this amazing herbal compound. "Triphala treats the entire digestive system, helping with constipation, hemorrhoids, diarrhea, indigestion, bloating and liver detoxification," explains ayurvedic herbalist Will Foster, L.Ac., who trained with traditional ayurvedic healers in India. Because it operates as a bowel tonic (helping to maintain proper function) rather than a laxative, triphala is safe to take every day.

DOSAGE: Take two to four 500-milligram tablets just before bedtime.

PRECAUTIONS: Do not take during pregnancy or if underweight; can cause weight loss.

22. TURMERIC (*Curcuma longa*)

BEST FOR: Arthritis and cancer prevention

Curcumin, the active compound that gives the spice turmeric its bright-gold color, has long been known as an anti-inflammatory and antioxidant. In combination with boswellia, ashwagandha and ginger, it may treat osteoarthritis, according to a study published in the *Journal of Clinical Rheumatology.* Turmeric may cause indigestion; try using it or yellow curries in cooking. And a recent study published in the journal

Phytotherapy Research found curcumin to be "comparable" in efficacy to diclofenac sodium, a prescription anti-inflammatory, for treating rheumatoid arthritis.

The American Cancer Society has reported that large studies are being conducted to see how curcumin might prevent and treat cancer; one of the challenges is that it doesn't absorb well from the intestines, but that could be an advantage for targeting cancer precursors in the colon and rectum. For women with recurrent breast cancer, curcumin might prove especially useful; animal models have shown that curcumin may help prevent metastasis, even after failed treatment with the drug tamoxifen. In women with HER-2 receptor-positive cancer, curcuminoids also seemed to behave much like the highly successful chemotherapy drug Herceptin, although research is highly preliminary.

Dosage: It's best to get your curcumin by using turmeric in curries and other foods. If you aren't a fan of Indian food, take one 500-milligram capsule of curcumin—standardized to 95% curcuminoids—each day.

Precautions: Side effects are rare but include flatulence, diarrhea and heartburn. Do not take turmeric if you're on blood thinners.

23. UMCKALOABO (*Pelargonium sidoides*)
BEST FOR: Cough and cold

A really fun herb to pronounce, "umckaloabo" means "heavy cough" in Zulu. The South African herb is a powerhouse with antiviral and antibacterial properties, says herbalist Mark Blumenthal. "There are good

SERENITY SAVER

MILKY OAT SEED (*Avena sativa*)

Been burning the candle at both ends for so long your gut's on fire? This herb's for you, says David Winston, R.H., coauthor of the resource guide *Winston and Kuhn's Herbal Therapy & Supplements.* Milky oat seed is—as the name implies—the extract of the whole milky oat produced by the oat plant in seed form only; you can't get similar benefits from, say, upping your morning oatmeal intake. "It creates a stronger and more balanced emotional foundation so that you're not as reactive to every little thing," Winston says. "It's an especially good choice for those people who make themselves sick with stress."

clinical studies on the use of umckaloabo for treating bronchitis as well as tonsillitis," he says, adding that taking umckaloabo at the onset of symptoms will bring relief within a day or two. Recent German studies of the preparation found that it significantly reduced symptoms and duration of colds and cough.

DOSAGE: Take as drops, syrup, chewable tablets or spray. Follow package instructions.

24. VALERIAN (*Valeriana officinalis*)
BEST FOR: Insomnia

Many studies have affirmed the safety and efficacy of valerian for treating garden-variety insomnia. "It works in the same way Valium or Xanax does, but the effect is much milder; there is no hangover afterward nor any risk of addiction," says Kingsbury. There's just one catch: "It's a reliable sedative for most people, but a small percentage will get jazzed up instead," she cautions. In a study published in the *European Journal of Medical Research,* investigators gave 202 insomniacs valerian or a Valium-like tranquilizer. After six weeks, both treatments were equally effective.

DOSAGE: Take two 500-milligram capsules one hour before bedtime as needed.

PRECAUTIONS: Don't take valerian if you're taking prescription sleep aids; and it can interact with drugs such as antidepressants and antianxiety medications. Be sure to let your doctor know if you are considering it.

SERENITY SAVER

MARIJUANA (*Cannabis sativa*)

OK, we know: It's illegal in the United States, legal for medicinal purposes in only 19 states and for recreational use in just two. But that doesn't mean it's not a powerful herbal medicine with long traditional usage as an anxiolytic (antianxiety agent). "Of all the relaxers in nature's pharmacy, cannabis is one of the most immediate. It produces near instant calming effect, and goes to work more quickly than a cup of coffee would," Kilham says. The substance—taboo though it may be in some circles—is well-known to reduce tension, headaches and pain associated with conditions ranging from multiple sclerosis to cancer.

Condition Reference

ALZHEIMER'S
Ginkgo

ANXIETY
Lemon balm

ARTHRITIS/ JOINT PAIN
Boswellia
Turmeric
Willow bark

ATHLETE'S FOOT
Tea tree oil

BACTERIAL INFECTION
Garlic
Goldenseal

BURNS
Aloe vera

CANCER
Garlic
Turmeric

COLDS
Echinacea
Umckaloabo

COLIC
Fennel

COUGH
Umckaloabo

CONSTIPATION
Triphala

DEPRESSION
St. John's wort

DIABETES
Ginseng

DIGESTIVE PROBLEMS
Goldenseal
Psyllium
Triphala

EAR INFECTIONS
Garlic

ECZEMA
Evening primrose oil

HEADACHES
Lavender
Feverfew
Willow bark

HEARTBURN
Meadowsweet

HEART HEALTH
Flaxseed
Tea

HERPES
Lemon balm

HIGH CHOLESTEROL
Evening primrose oil

IMMUNE HEALTH
Ginseng
Goldenseal

INFECTION
Garlic

INTESTINAL GAS
Fennel

INSOMNIA
Valerian

LIVER HEALTH
Milk thistle

MENOPAUSE/ HOT FLASHES
Black cohosh
Willow bark

MIGRAINES
Feverfew

NASAL CONGESTION
Goldenrod

NAUSEA/ VOMITING
Ginger

PAIN
Red pepper
St. John's wort
White willow bark

PMS
Chaste tree

SEXUAL DYSFUNCTION
Ginkgo
Ginseng

YEAST INFECTIONS
Tea tree oil

URINARY TRACT INFECTIONS
Cranberry

25. WHITE WILLOW BARK (*Salix alba*)

Best for: Pain relief

White willow bark contains salicin, a close chemical relative of aspirin. A study in *Phytomedicine* followed people with severe back pain for 18 months. In the group taking white willow bark, 40% were pain-free after just four weeks; the same was true of only 18% of the second group, who were allowed to take whatever prescription drugs they wanted. In another well-designed study of nearly 200 people with low back pain, those who received willow bark experienced a significant improvement in pain compared to those who received placebo. People who received higher doses of willow bark (240 milligrams salicin) had more significant pain relief than those who received low doses (120 milligrams salicin).

It has also been shown to relieve arthritis, inflammation, headaches and fever and hot flashes.

DOSAGE: Follow label directions; the bark can be made into a tea.

PRECAUTIONS: Like aspirin, willow bark can cause stomach distress, and shouldn't be given to children or used if pregnant or breast-feeding. Avoid if you are allergic to aspirin.

Know Your Source

Recently there has been concern in the herb industry about the adulteration of herbs. "Whether accidental or deliberate, some companies are mixing or cutting their high-quality herbs with cheaper powders," says Mark Blumenthal of the American Botanical Council. "To be safe, always know your supplier and use the same products that have been used in the research whenever possible."

The 11 Best Herbs for Women

Managing the monthly cycle of hormonal ups and downs—mood swings, headaches, menstrual cramps, assorted energy drains—drives many of us to reach routinely for ibuprofen, antidepressants, sleeping pills and other drugs. And we're just talking about the husbands. (Hey-o!)

But for generations, herb-savvy women have been turning to the plant world for nontoxic, natural remedies for these common complaints. It's time we revisited those simple cures, urges Rosemary Gladstar, founder of Sage Mountain Herb Center in Barre, Vt., and author of the classic *Herbal Healing for Women.* Given the high price of health care and the stresses of daily life, herbs are more relevant than ever, she says. "Treating yourself with home remedies is the easiest, least invasive and oftentimes most effective treatment." You just need to know your cramp bark from your feverfew.

1. BLACK COHOSH (*Cimicifuga racemosa*)

BEST FOR: Hot flashes and night sweats.

"This herb is one of the best-studied—and perhaps most popular—treatments for hot flashes," says Tieraona Low Dog, M.D., author of a review of botanical supplements for menopause published in the *American Journal of Medicine.* A 2013 Mayo Clinic overview confirms the findings. In fact, most studies have found it to be effective in reducing the hot flashes and night sweats associated with menopause, according to the National Center for Complementary and Alternative Medicine (NCCAM), a division of the National Institutes of Health (NIH). Despite all the research, however, no one is quite sure how it works. One long-held theory asserted that black cohosh exerted a positive estrogenic effect. (Declining estrogen levels are principally responsible for menopausal symptoms.) But newer data suggest that it may actually decrease levels of other hormones (including luteinizing hormone) that cause hot flashes, according to a research review published in the journal *American Family Physician.* Black cohosh isn't effective at relieving other menopausal issues, such as vaginal dryness, however.

DOSAGE: The recommended dosage is 20 milligrams twice daily. It's available as a fresh or dried root or in pill form; Lane P. Johnson, M.D., M.P.H., author of *The Pocket Guide to Herbal Remedies,* recommends the brand Remifemin, a standardized extract that has been used in more than 90 studies.

PRECAUTIONS: "Anyone with any kind of liver disorder or on any type of hepatotoxic medication" should put the kibosh on black cohosh, cautions Johnson. It should not be taken during pregnancy or while breast-feeding.

2. CHASTE TREE BERRY (*Vitex agnus-castus*)

BEST FOR: Premenstrual syndrome

"There's very good data to suggest chaste tree berry as a general remedy for PMS," says Ellen Hughes, M.D., clinical professor of medicine at the University of California, San Francisco. A study of 170 women published in the *British Medical Journal* showed that 52% found relief from PMS-related irritability, mood changes and headaches by taking this herb.

DOSAGE: Hughes recommends one or two capsules of dried herb standardized to 0.6% acubin (the active ingredient). "Capsule is preferable," she says, "because you'd have to drink about 24 ounces of tea a day—and it's difficult to find a standardized tea preparation." Alternately, you can take chaste tree berry as a tincture of 40 to 80 drops daily.

PRECAUTIONS: Rarely, the herb can cause skin rash, and it should not be taken during pregnancy or while breast-feeding. Chaste tree berry may also interfere with drugs that inhibit the effect of dopamine in the brain, such as certain antidepressants.

3. CRAMP BARK (*Viburnum opulus*)

BEST FOR: Menstrual cramps

This Native American herb is a safe and effective alternative to ibuprofen. Cramp bark is a uterine sedative that reduces inflammation, relaxes spasms and calms an overactive uterus so effectively it's often used by midwives to halt premature labor. Research, including a 2008 study on herbal remedies for dysmenorrhea, has shown that cramp bark has an antispasmodic effect on smooth muscle fibers like those found in the uterus and large intestine, so it's also useful as a muscle relaxant.

DOSAGE: Take one to two droppers of tincture in water every two hours as needed.

4. CRANBERRY (*Vaccinium macrocarpon*)

BEST FOR: Prevention of UTIs

For reasons that aren't well understood, women are more likely than men to develop a urinary tract infection (UTI). In fact, one in five women will get one in her lifetime, according to 2012 National Institute of Diabetes and Digestive and Kidney Diseases statistics. Some women are more prone to UTIs than others—diaphragm users, for instance, are at a high risk—and almost 20% of women who develop one will eventually develop another. Most infections arise from an overgrowth of E. coli bacteria in the urethra (urethritis) and/or bladder (cystitis). Cranberry prevents bacteria from adhering to the walls of either organ, making it difficult for infection to take hold. It will not, however, kill the bacteria once they're established; in that case, only prescription antibiotics can provide relief.

DOSAGE: Johnson recommends drinking at least one eight-ounce glass of cranberry juice a day. Choose a high-quality juice with a large concentration of cranberry; Northland brand, for instance, contains up to 27% cranberry. Pure unsweetened cranberry juice is available in health food and vitamin stores, but it's so tart that it's hard to drink. The recommended dosage is 15 to 30 milliliters per day; you can dilute it in water to improve the flavor. "You can also take cranberry capsules," says Johnson. "But studies show the effects aren't as strong."

PRECAUTIONS: There are no known medical precautions to consider when drinking cranberry juice, but if you suffer from gastroesophageal reflux disease or a peptic ulcer, the acidity may aggravate your symptoms.

5. DONG QUAI (Angelica sinensis)
BEST FOR: General female wellness

Also known as angelica root or dong quai, this Chinese herb is often called the "female ginseng" because of its usefulness in treating irregular periods, fatigue, and premenstrual irritability and anxiety, says Dana Price, D.O.M., L.Ac., Dipl.OM. Scientists aren't clear on how it works; dong quai may have a weak estrogenic effect, but this remains unconfirmed. In Traditional Chinese Medicine (TCM), dong quai is used in combination with other herbs to strengthen the blood of people with excess yin energy; females are generally more yin than yang, according to the ancient practice.

DOSAGE: TCM is highly individualized, so it's best to consult an accredited specialist for a correct herbal prescription, explains Price.

PRECAUTIONS: Avoid dong quai if you're pregnant—it can stimulate uterine contractions, warns Price. "It may also cause diarrhea and/or abdominal distension," she says. If you're on a blood thinner such as warfarin, you shouldn't use this herb. Dong quai can increase your sensitivity to sunlight, so be sure to wear sunscreen.

6. FEVERFEW (Tanacetum parthenium)
BEST FOR: Migraines

Nearly three times as many women as men experience migraines, according to the National Headache Foundation, but men who were diagnosed with headache were most often diagnosed with migraine headaches (36%). An estimated 7.5 million men in the United States suffer from migraines. Feverfew may help relieve the nausea and vomiting associated with these debilitating headaches and/or reduce the need for traditional prophylactic pharmaceuticals, according to Mark Blumenthal, executive director of the American Botanical Council in Austin, Texas.

DOSAGE: Blumenthal recommends 100 to 150 milligrams of dried leaves or 2½ fresh leaves daily (with food or after eating).

PRECAUTIONS: Blumenthal recommends that pregnant women and anyone taking a blood thinner steer clear of feverfew. If you're allergic to ragweed (a member of the feverfew family), marigolds or chrysanthemums, it's also wise to stay away. (In the German study, some subjects reported mouth ulcerations as a side effect.) Feverfew may also increase the risk of sun sensitivity caused by prescription medications like Retin-A.

7. GINGER (*Zingiber officinale*)
BEST FOR: Nausea

Whether your queasy stomach is caused by PMS, pregnancy-related morning sickness or an upcoming visit from the in-laws, ginger can most likely help. A review of six double-blind randomized controlled clinical trials published in the journal *Obstetrics & Gynecology* concluded that ginger was an effective treatment for nausea and vomiting during pregnancy. Studies from 2009 to 2012 showed great success combating the nausea from chemotherapy.

DOSAGE: Low Dog recommends taking dried ginger for the best effects. "Stick with 250 milligrams, four times a day." Cooking with the herb may also be helpful.

PRECAUTIONS: Few side effects are linked to normal ginger consumption, but powdered ginger may produce bloating or indigestion. Ginger may also exacerbate heartburn in pregnant women.

8. GREEN TEA (*Camellia sinensis*)
BEST FOR: Cancer prevention

A growing body of research suggests drinking this Asian staple may help ward off cancer. According to an American Cancer Society 2012 overview, many lab studies in cell cultures and animals have shown that green tea has chemopreventive properties. Two meta-analyses, one published in the journal *Carcinogenesis* and the other published in *Integrated Cancer Therapies*, found that green tea consumption may prevent the growth of lung cancer and breast cancer tumors, especially in the early stages. Do not replace any therapy that's working, with green tea.

DOSAGE: Drink 6 to 10 cups of organic green tea a day, suggests Christine Horner, M.D., author of *Waking the Warrior Goddess: Dr. Christine Horner's Program to Protect Against and Fight Breast Cancer.* Also, choose caffeinated, unless you are pregnant or must otherwise limit your intake of caffeine. (A cup of green tea contains 20 milligrams, about a quarter of the amount in coffee.) "Some research has found that removing the caffeine reduces the chemoprotective potential," says Horner.

9. NETTLE (*Urtica dioica*)
BEST FOR: Anemia

Nettle tea is a rich plant-based source of iron, chlorophyll and folic acid; a 2013 study found its analgesic properties can benefit anemia as well as seasonal allergies and UTIs (also enlarged prostate—just covering our bases). It also contains vitamin K, which helps blood clot, so it's great if you tend to get a little anemic because of heavy periods. Also a detoxifying herb that increases urine production, and may be useful for skin conditions.

DOSAGE: Make a tea of one tablespoon dried nettle herb steeped in a cup of hot water for at least 30 minutes (or overnight); drink warm, three cups a day.

10. SAGE (*Salvia officinalis*)
BEST FOR: Hot flashes

"Sage has been passed down from generation to generation in Western herbal tradition as the sure-fire cure for hot flashes," explains Sheila Kingsbury, N.D., chair of the Botanical Medicine Department at Bastyr University. It's such an effective astringent that it's been approved in Germany as a treatment for excessive sweating for both men and women. "Sage was also used in Native American cultures to clear negative energy so it may help ease some of the irrational fears that can cycle through your head during menopause," says herbalist Margi Flint, author of *The Practicing Herbalist.*

DOSAGE: Make a tea of one tablespoon dried sage steeped in one-cup hot water for 15 minutes or more; strain and cool. Drink up to three cups a day. If you don't like the taste, put the tea in a spray bottle (after it has cooled completely) and spritz it on your neck.

PRECAUTIONS: Avoid therapeutic doses of sage during pregnancy, or if epileptic.

11. YARROW (*Achillea millefolium*)

BEST FOR: Heavy periods

Yarrow is the go-to herb for heavy menstrual bleeding, says Gladstar. "It slows excessive bleeding, relieves pelvic congestion, reduces cramping and flushes out the liver so estrogen and progesterone are processed more efficiently," she says. A 2013 University of Maryland Medical Center report says it may work by relaxing the smooth muscle in the uterus; also eases menstrual cramps.

DOSAGE: Take two droppers of tincture every half hour until bleeding slows.

PRECAUTIONS: Do not use during pregnancy. Rarely, may cause allergic reaction. Use essential oil internally only under professional supervision.

Herbs from the East

Herbs are extremely "2014" in the United States—very trendy, very in. But we're way behind Asian countries like China and India. There, the plants have been at the core of Traditional Chinese Medicine (TCM) and ayurvedic medicine for thousands of years.

Catch up now. The recommendations below are *known*—for what they can do and can't do, and also for any cautions you should be aware of before taking them.

ASAFOETIDA (*Ferula vesceritensis*)

This ayurvedic herb's name comes from the Farsi *aza* (resin) and the Latin *foetidus* (smelly), and its fetid odor was thought to repel illness. Known primarily as a spice, asafoetida is used in ayurvedic medicine to promote gastrointestinal function. It's a digestive stimulant that relieves intestinal cramping from gas; it also promotes laxative action and can eliminate intestinal parasites. A 2012 review published in *Organic and Medicinal Chemistry Letters* attested to the microbial powers of the essential oils of this herb.

DOSAGE: Use asafoetida under supervision of an ayurvedic physician.

PRECAUTIONS: There are no reports of side effects in adults, but it should not be given to infants or used by pregnant or nursing women.

GOTU KOLA (*Centella asiatica*)

Because the leaves of this herb are enjoyed by elephants, gotu kola (no relation to the kola nut) is traditionally considered a longevity promoter. Indian animal studies showed it improved learning and memory. It also boosts blood flow, especially through the smallest blood vessels, which is useful for diabetics prone to blood vessel problems. Topical gotu kola cream speeds wound healing. In a study of 100 pregnant women, a cream containing the herb along with vitamin E helped prevent stretch marks, and a 2013 University of Maryland review showed that the triterpenoids in the herb healed wounds in lab and animal studies.

DOSAGE: In tea, 600 milligrams dried leaves three times a day; or 60 to 120 milligrams of extract per day.

PRECAUTIONS: Gotu kola is safe in advised doses, but in excess may cause liver damage.

ASHWAGANDHA (*Withania somnifera*)

This superstar herb, revered in ayurvedic medicine, is known as the "Indian ginseng" because it's an overall restorative. It strengthens the body, and treats fatigue, weakness, debility and problems of old age. Animal studies have found ashwagandha's adaptogenic activity boosts antibody and red-blood-cell levels and spurs white blood cells to devour germs. A 2011 review in the *African Journal of Traditional, Complementary and Alternative Medicines* found it protects against stress and has anti-tumor effects. It was also found useful in the treatment of Parkinson's and Alzheimer's. Diabetics and people with high cholesterol who took ashwagandha daily lowered their cholesterol and blood sugar levels significantly after one month.

DOSAGE: 1 to 6 grams per day in capsules or tea; in tincture or liquid extract, 2 to 4 milliliters, three times a day.

PRECAUTIONS: Ashwagandha does not cause significant side effects in recommended amounts. But large doses may cause gastrointestinal distress. Pregnant women should not use it.

CINNAMON

Beyond its traditional use as a spice, cinnamon has a long history in ayurvedic medicine. It's warming, so it's good for colds, congestion, and high cholesterol. Cinnamon is a traditional remedy for digestive problems like nausea and diarrhea. Recent research has confirmed cinnamon's antibacterial and antifungal qualities; and it has been shown to kill salmonella, a type of bacteria that causes food poisoning.

A 2012 Mayo Clinic review concluded that the use of cinnamon had a potentially beneficial effect on glycemic control. One study published in 2009 found that a 500-milligram capsule of cinnamon taken twice a day for 90 days improved hemoglobin A1C levels.

DOSAGE: 0.5 to 1 gram of powdered bark in tea three times a day; in liquid extract, 0.5 mL three times daily. This tasty spice is easily added to many foods, not just toast, oatmeal and cookies.

PRECAUTIONS: There are no significant side effects, but remember that diabetics should be under the care of a specialist, and cinnamon should be used only to complement other treatments.

BOSWELLIA (*Boswellia serrata*)

A close relative of frankincense, this tree's transparent gold resin has been traditionally used as an astringent and anti-inflammatory. Recent studies in India and Germany [2012] found boswellia has a positive effect on pain and stiffness resulting from rheumatoid arthritis, leading to speculation that the plant could aid sufferers of other chronic inflammatory diseases like ulcerative colitis and psoriasis; the herb significantly reduces pain and swelling.

DOSAGE: 350 to 400 milligrams per day.

PRECAUTIONS: There are no known side effects.

DONG QUAI (*Angelica sinensis*)

Dong quai is a major herb in TCM, and is typically used to relieve pain and strengthen blood flow. Researchers at China's Fourth Military Medical University found dong quai inhibits blood clots that trigger heart attack, while a study at Wuhan University determined it helps restore blood flow through the brain after a stroke. In the West, it's often prescribed for menstrual complaints such as cramps and PMS. Look for products whose labels specify *Angelica* (or *A.*) *sinensis*.

DOSAGE: 4 to 6 grams of the powdered root with meals; or 20 to 40 drops of liquid extract with meals.

PRECAUTIONS: Dong quai causes no significant side effects, but pregnant women should avoid it and you should avoid if you are on blood thinners.

LICORICE (*Glycyrrhiza glabra*)

Licorice is the most widely used Chinese herb. Dubbed "the great harmonizer," it moderates the effects of harsh herbs and sweetens the taste of bitter ones. It's known as a safe, gentle and effective remedy for inflammation like sore throats, allergies, food poisoning, stings and muscle-spasm pain. Licorice also helps treat ulcers and, according to a study at the University of Texas, stimulates the immune system.

DOSAGE: 1 to 4 grams powdered root three times a day; 1 teaspoon chopped licorice root added to hot water to soothe a sore throat.

PRECAUTIONS: Look for DGL or deglycyrrhizinated licorice.

At high doses, licorice may cause laxative effects, fluid retention, and hypertension. Those with heart disease or hormone-sensitive cancers shouldn't take licorice as an herbal treatment. Eating it is fine.

REISHI (*Ganoderma lucidum*)

Called "the mushroom of immortality," this fungus treats fatigue, respiratory and liver complaints, cancer and heart disease. Reishi's immune effect was confirmed at the Free University of Berlin and at Peking University Health Science Center. Korean studies noted antibacterial and antiviral activity. A potent antioxidant, reishi may help prevent cancer-causing cell damage. Lab and animal studies in Japan and at Methodist Research Institute in Indianapolis found reishi suppressed growth of colon, prostate and breast cancers.

DOSAGE: Use reishi in consultation with a TCM practitioner.

PRECAUTIONS: Reishi may lead to dizziness, skin irritation and GI upset; avoid it if you're pregnant.

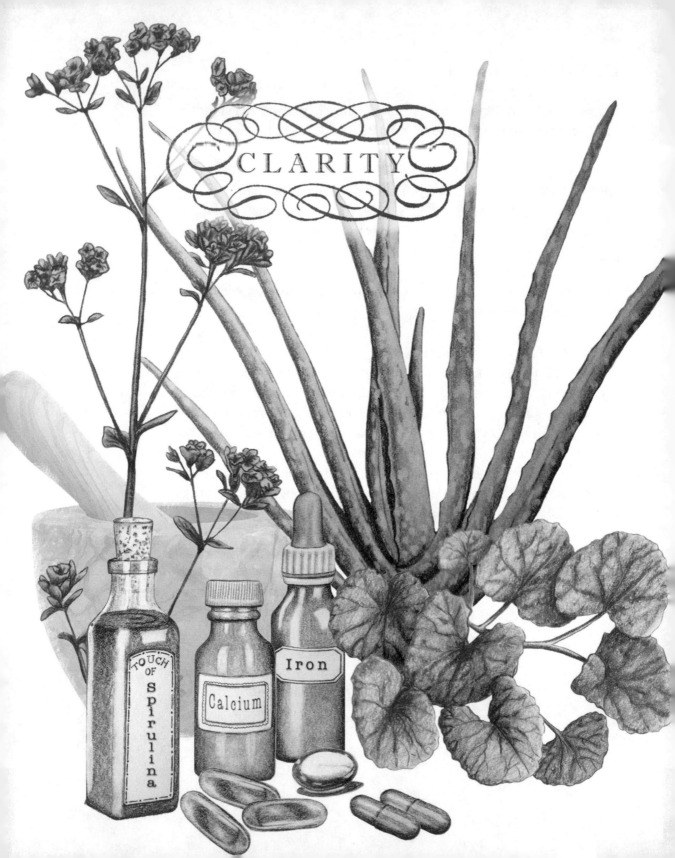

CLARITY

TOUCH OF Spirulina

Calcium

Iron

PART

IV

Supplements

In 2014, we have become, as a nation, both more open to trying supplements and more—much more—confused about what works when. Who wouldn't be? Lock down the one surety —that the human body needs vitamins, minerals, amino acids and omega oils to function—and then the questions begin. Do we get enough from the food we eat, or do we need extra supplements? Can they cure diseases? Ease chronic pain? Help us concentrate? Will they make me run faster, sleep better, live forever? Universities, doctors, patients, insurance companies, pharmaceutical makers, entrepreneurs and hucksters shout over one another to claim, once and for all, that they have the answer—with differing agendas and differing answers.

In this chapter, *Natural Health* gives you the definitive answers. And we get there by going way deep under the hood, combing through every important study—the landmark cases, and the brand-new, up-to-the-minute 2013 research—to tell you whether a supplement is worth taking for a specific ailment, or whether you're rolling the dice. The results are sometimes inspiring (when the evidence is strong), and often frustrating (when "more studies need to be done"), but always the straight truth.

The chapter is organized alphabetically, so it's easier to use in the supplement aisle, or when you're searching for one supplement in particular. You'll find a running theme, as supplements fall into a few different types:

AMINO ACIDS: Amino acids are the building blocks of protein. Twenty amino acids are found in protein; the human body can produce 10 of them, the other 10—called "essential" amino acids—come from the food we eat. Unlike fat and sugar, we can't store amino acids, so they must be replenished daily. And failure to get just one of the amino acids results in a breakdown of proteins to supply the one that is missing.

ANTIOXIDANTS: An antioxidant is a molecule that protects cells from oxidation or cell damage. They are especially of interest in the prevention of chronic diseases such as heart disease, cancer and those caused by chronic inflammation. Vitamins C and E, selenium, and carotenoids such as beta-carotene, lycopene, lutein and zeaxanthin all are antioxidants. Vegetables and fruit are rich sources of antioxidants, and research continues to find benefits for using supplements to fill in nutritional gaps.

COMPOUNDS: Dietary supplements are sometimes formulated to contain several vitamins, minerals or other chemical compounds; usually these formulations are created because the elements benefit each other, such as calcium and vitamin D, for instance.

MINERALS: Minerals are the inorganic chemical elements all living organisms need for growth and function; the seven most important minerals for humans are calcium, phosphorous, potassium, sulfur, sodium, chlorine and magnesium; "trace" or minor minerals, necessary for mammalian life, include cobalt, copper, iron, iodine, molybdenum, selenium and zinc.

OMEGA OILS: Omega-3s are essential fatty acids, meaning that we do not produce them and so must get them from food or supplements. Most omega-3s come from fish and fish oil, but they are also available from plants such as flax and algae (which is what the fish eat). Researchers are busy finding ways to support claims that omega-3 supplements can prevent heart disease, cancer, chronic diseases associated with inflammation and aging in general.

VITAMINS: Vitamins are organic compounds that we need for growth and for health, and that cannot be synthesized in sufficient amounts by our bodies, and so must be ingested. Pretty much anything that's not a mineral, an essential fatty acid or essential amino acid is probably a vitamin. Thirteen vitamins are universally recognized: A, B_1, B_2, B_3, B_5, B_6, B_7, B_9, B_{12}, C, D, E and K.

There you go: from A to Z, with no BS in between.

The Big 30 Supplements

OUR METHODOLOGY

Forgive us for getting technical for a second, but we want you to understand how deeply we researched these supplements—and what our terms mean.

GOOD EVIDENCE FOR: Hooray! This means we found that multiple randomized clinical studies and/or meta-analysis (i.e., methods that focus on comparing multiple studies) have supported the use of this supplement for a specific condition.

SOME EVIDENCE FOR: Hmm... some reliable clinical studies have supported the use of this supplement for a specific condition. But more research is needed.

LIMITED EVIDENCE FOR: You can guess this one. This means there is some research connecting a compound to a specific condition, but the evidence is limited by the quality or quantity of studies. Or in some cases, dietary research points to health benefits, but research on supplements is limited.

NO EVIDENCE FOR/POSSIBLY DANGEROUS: Red alert! Red alert! Research has found no benefit or has found that a particular supplement actually causes harm.

1. ARGININE (L-ARGININE)

This amino acid can be found in red meat, poultry, fish, eggs and dairy. In the body, it is converted to nitric oxide, which is a vasodilator—meaning it widens the blood vessels. So if you've had a heart issue, perhaps you've heard of it.

GOOD EVIDENCE FOR:

Heart Disease: Along with decreasing fluid buildup after congestive heart failure, arginine may help decrease inflammation and increase vasodilation (that aforementioned blood vessel widening), which might help people suffering from coronary artery disease, angina or atherosclerosis.

Healing Wounds: Supplemental arginine can improve wound healing by increasing new blood vessel growth around the wound, according to some studies, which brings vital oxygen and nitrogen to healing tissue.

LIMITED EVIDENCE FOR:

Erectile Dysfunction: The studies that have shown that arginine helps with erectile dysfunction have used a combination of arginine and other herbal ingredients; there isn't enough evidence to suggest that arginine works by itself.

Exercise Endurance: Some studies suggest it might improve exercise endurance in untrained athletes.

NO EVIDENCE FOR/POSSIBLY DANGEROUS:

High Blood Pressure: Since arginine causes the blood vessels to widen, it's often marketed as a treatment for high blood pressure, but the studies do not back up this claim.

PRECAUTIONS: There is evidence that arginine might actually be harmful for those who have suffered a heart attack. Do not take if you've had one. Arginine may cause abdominal pain or gastrointestinal problems. In some people it can cause an allergic reaction or worsen existing allergies. It can also lower blood pressure and increase the risk of bleeding. Do not take if you are about to undergo surgery.

BUT WAIT, THERE'S MORE!

For a steamy Viagra-like L-arginine lotion, see the "Sexual Dysfunction" section on page 208.

2. ALPHA-LINOLENIC (ALA)

You can find alpha-linolenic acid in vegetable oils like flaxseed, canola and walnut oils—it's an essential omega-3 fatty acid.

LIMITED EVIDENCE FOR:

Heart Disease: Studies suggest that increasing dietary ALA can reduce the risk of fatal heart attack, decrease the amount of plaque in the coronary arteries and improve heart disease risk factors like high blood pressure, but there is no clinical evidence that supplemental ALA does the same.

PRECAUTIONS: Some studies have linked ALA with an increased risk of prostate cancer. Diets rich in ALA may increase the risk of macular degeneration.

3. BETA-CAROTENE

We've all heard of the plant carotenoid that gives some vegetables, fruits, nuts and grains a red, orange or yellow pigment. In supplement form, it comes from palm oil, algae or fungi. You may also see it called pro-vitamin A. So does it work?

SOME EVIDENCE FOR:

Photosensitivity: Some studies have shown that beta-carotene can provide some protection from sun sensitivity by increasing the pigmentation of the skin (carotenemia). A review of studies using beta-carotene published in *Cellular and Molecular Biology* found mixed results.

Age-related Macular Degeneration (AMD): A large-scale study by the National Eye Institute called the *Age-Related Eye Disease Study* (AREDS) found that beta-carotene, along with vitamin C, vitamin E and

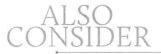

ALSO CONSIDER

CHROMIUM

What It Is:
Chromium is a mineral, considered an essential "trace" element, because very little is required for optimal human health.

What It's Commonly Used For:
Chromium picolinate is thought to regulate blood sugar and help insulin work better for people with type 2 diabetes, and research is being done to see if it also can help those with type 1 diabetes. There's some evidence that it might help lower cholesterol when taken in higher doses.

Any Proof It Works?
Studies have confirmed that a chromium deficiency can result in subnormal glucose utilization and even insulin resistance. Research into improved performance benefits is as yet inconclusive.

zinc, reduced the risk of vision loss associated with AMD by 25% in those with advanced stages of the disease.

LIMITED EVIDENCE FOR:

Breast Cancer: Dietary beta-carotene intake is associated with a decreased risk of breast cancer. A 2009 study in *The American Journal of Clinical Nutrition* found that a diet high in it reduced risk of breast cancer in post-menopausal women. It's unclear whether supplementation with beta-carotene provides the same benefit.

NO EVIDENCE FOR/POSSIBLY DANGEROUS:

Cataracts: No dice. Studies have not confirmed the use of beta-carotene supplements for cataracts. The AREDS study mentioned earlier found no protection against cataracts with beta-carotene supplementation. And a study in the *Archives of Ophthalmology* also found no correlation between beta-carotene and cataracts.

Cancer: Numerous studies have confirmed no correlation between cancer incidence and beta-carotene supplementation. Breast cancer and ovarian cancer studies have shown some protective effect for diets high in beta-carotene.

PRECAUTIONS: Numerous, unfortunately. Multiple studies have found an increased risk of lung cancer in people who smoke and take supplemental beta-carotene. While some studies have found a protective effect for men against prostate cancer, other studies have not replicated this effect, and one study in the *Journal of the National Cancer Institute* found that men who take high-dose multivitamins along with a beta carotene supplement *increase* their risk of developing advanced aggressive prostate cancer by 32%.

4. BIOTIN

Also known as vitamin H, biotin is a water-soluble B vitamin that helps our bodies turn food into fuel.

SOME EVIDENCE FOR:

Brittle Nail: A few small, older studies have found supplemental biotin to be an effective treatment for brittle nail syndrome. One study in the journal *Cutis* found a 25% increase in nail thickness after six moths of supplementation. This study only looked at 44 people. And a German study from 1989 found that of the 45 people they treated with biotin, 41

BUT WAIT, THERE'S MORE!

Low levels of beta-carotene may be linked to eczema. See page 106 for more.

had stronger nails after treatment. Why mention these moldy oldies now? Because a review of studies done by Columbia University researchers concluded that biotin is, indeed, an effective treatment for brittle nail.

LIMITED EVIDENCE FOR:

Diabetes: Preliminary studies have found that a combination of biotin and chromium might improve fasting blood glucose levels in those with type 2 diabetes, but studies on biotin alone have not found any of the same protective effect.

NO EVIDENCE FOR/POSSIBLY DANGEROUS:

Cradle Cap: While studies have shown that children who suffer from seborrhoeic dermatitis (aka cradle cap) might have a disruption in the way they process biotin, no studies have linked biotin supplementation to reduced symptoms of it.

PRECAUTIONS: Antibiotics may decrease biotin levels in the body. Raw egg whites contain protein called avidin, which binds biotin, blocking it from being absorbed in the body.

5. CALCIUM

The most abundant mineral found in the body, 99% of our calcium is stored in our bones and our teeth. The rest is used throughout the body—in the blood, muscles, and other fluids—where it assists with muscle contraction, nerve transmission, vasodilation, and acts as a messenger for hormones and enzymes. To absorb calcium you also need vitamin D. Got milk?

GOOD EVIDENCE FOR:

Osteoporosis: Many studies have found that supplementing with calcium increases bone density and decreases the risk of osteoporosis, especially for women over the age of 30. A recent longitudinal study in

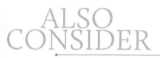

ALSO CONSIDER

COLLOIDAL SILVER

What It Is: Colloidal silver is, obviously, a mineral, but not an essential mineral and has no known benefits to the body. It's available in oral supplements and also in cream form.

What It's Commonly Used For: Health claims made by manufacturers include that colloidal silver can boost immunity, kill bacteria and viruses, prevent cancer and cure HIV/AIDS, herpes and many chronic diseases.

Any Proof It Works? In a word, no. And it could be dangerous.

the *British Medical Journal* of 61,000 women found that moderate intake of calcium (around 1,000 milligrams) taken with vitamin D can help prevent the bone fractures associated with osteoporosis in women. Note: The study also found that both high levels of supplementation (2,000 milligrams) and low levels of supplementation (<300 milligrams) were associated with increased fracture risk.

SOME EVIDENCE FOR:

PMS: There is some evidence that supplementing with calcium can ease the discomforts of premenstrual syndrome. One oft-cited study from the *American Journal of Obstetrics and Gynecology* found that supplementing with calcium carbonate (1,200 milligrams a day) decreases the water retention, food cravings and pain of PMS by 18% compared to placebo.

LIMITED EVIDENCE FOR:

Weight Loss: You wish. Multiple studies have linked dietary calcium intake with weight loss and reduced body fat. But the research on supplements is mixed: A large study on postmenopausal women found that supplementing with 1,200 milligrams of calcium might decrease the risk of weight gain. But others, like a study in the *American Journal of Clinical Nutrition,* using data from the Health Professionals Follow-up Study, found no link between dietary or supplemental calcium intake and weight gain or body fat levels.

NO EVIDENCE FOR/POSSIBLY DANGEROUS:

Heart Disease: A recent study in *JAMA Internal Medicine* found an increased risk of death from cardiovascular disease in men over the age of 50 who supplemented with high doses (1,000 milligrams of calcium a day). This effect was not seen in women. Dietary calcium did not carry a similar risk. However, another recent study in the *British Medical Journal* found that women who take more than 1,400 milligrams of calcium a day doubled their risk of death from heart disease.

Precautions: Supplemental calcium may cause gastro problems like constipation or nausea. People with kidney problems or a history of kidney stones should not take calcium. High amounts of calcium (>2,000 milligrams) have been linked to increases in prostate cancer; and doses greater than 1,200 milligrams have been linked to heart attack.

BUT WAIT, THERE'S MORE!

To see how calcium could be the key to curing osteoporosis, turn to page 193.

The Calcium-Rich Diet

Women are often warned to monitor their calcium intake, lest their bones crumble like some Ray Harryhausen skeleton. So how much is enough? Official recommendations encourage women between the ages of 19 and 50 to get 1,000 milligrams of calcium a day, and women older than 50 to get 1,200 milligrams. Amy J. Lanou, Ph.D., senior nutrition scientist for the nonprofit Physicians Committee for Responsible Medicine and coauthor of *Building Bone Vitality* suggests lowering that to 500 to 800 milligrams, preferably from dairy-free food sources. Lanou explains that a higher calcium intake is unnecessary and, if it comes from supplemental sources, may cause constipation and negatively impact the absorption, production or metabolism of other nutrients.

Dairy foods—cheese and ice cream in particular—are highly acidic, but the body prefers a slightly alkaline pH; to neutralize the acidity from dairy, your body pulls calcium from the bones. Hip fracture rates are highest where calcium intake from dairy foods is highest, including in the U.S. and Northern European countries.

Almond Milk

Almond milk—ground almonds with water, and sometimes sweeteners—has 300 milligrams of calcium per 8 oz., and can be used in recipes and smoothies in lieu of cow's milk.

Arugula

Classified as a cruciferous vegetable, this brother of broccoli has a leg up on lettuce. Arugula contains about eight times the calcium, five times the vitamin A, vitamin C and vitamin K, and four times the iron as the same amount of iceberg lettuce—not to mention more fiber, folate, protein, potassium and magnesium. Add it up and arugula can help defend against heart disease, osteoporosis, sun damage and certain cancers. Arugula has a peppery, slightly bitter taste and can be used in salads or even to make pesto. Two cups = 60 milligrams of calcium.

Broccoli

Broccoli is among nature's richest sources of sulforophane, a compound that's thought to strongly inhibit cancers. Research suggests that sulforophanes stimulate the body's own cancer-fighting enzymes, slowing the rate of breast and prostate cancer cell growth. Two cups = 80 milligrams of calcium.

Kale

Arguably the king of the leafy greens, kale scored No. 1 in a ranking of 84 veggies by the Center for Science in the Public Interest in Washington, D.C. Crammed with nutrients, notably vitamins K, A and C and calcium, kale is also a cancer-fighting superpower. Kale's 45 flavonoids combine antioxidant and anti-inflammatory benefits to help fend off bladder, breast, colon, ovarian and prostate cancer. Noggin-nourishing antioxidants in kale also keep the brain sharp as you age. Use three cups to make kale crisps and you'll be snacking on 270 milligrams of calcium.

Sesame Seeds

Just one tablespoon of sesame seeds has 90 milligrams of calcium and only 52 calories. Sprinkle over salads or sautéed greens.

Turnip Greens

Dark, leafy greens are the rock stars of the produce department: Nutrition powerhouses like turnip greens have been shown to prevent everything from cancer to heart disease while keeping your body and brain in top shape. Sauté turnip greens like spinach. Two cups = 210 milligrams of calcium.

Oranges

One medium orange contains about 70 milligrams of calcium and 60 milligrams of the antioxidant vitamin C. Oranges also supply flavonoids—among them hesperetin, which regenerates vitamin C, helps fight cancer, protects the heart and prevents viral infection. In addition, because of the potassium they contain, oranges lower the risk of developing hypertension. Eat oranges whole and fresh; the fruit's rind and membranes protect the juice from oxygen, which destroys fragile vitamin C. In addition, the flavonoids are found in the membranes surrounding each orange segment, as well as in the pith and in the fuzzy stem-like structure running through the center of the fruit.

Mustard Greens

This peppery plant is jam-packed with vitamins K, A and C, a triple threat of antioxidants that battle the effects of aging and disease. Heart-healthy nutrients like folate, fiber, potassium and beta-carotene also protect the heart and lungs, while calcium builds stronger teeth and bones.

"By providing us with a diverse array of antioxidants, mustard greens help protect our bodies from damaging free radicals," says Christine Avanti, C.N., holistic nutritionist in Los Angeles and author of *Skinny Chicks Don't Eat Salads*. Raw or cooked, the pungent green works as a side or combined with a casserole or stir-fry. Two cups = 120 milligrams of calcium.

Figs and Prunes

Dried fruits such as figs and prunes are concentrated versions of all the fiber and vitamins in regular fruit. They also have high concentrations of sugar, so it's best to eat them in small portions, and with nuts or whole grains so you're getting additional fiber and protein to help maintain steady blood sugar. A study published in the *British Journal of Nutrition* found that women who ate about eight to 10 prunes a day had significantly higher bone mineral density in their forearms and spines compared with those who ate dried apples. Prunes provide boron and potassium, two elements that help suppress the breakdown of bone. Two dried figs have 60 milligrams of calcium and two prunes have 40 milligrams of calcium.

Almonds

Nutrient-dense almonds are packed with potassium, vitamin E, iron, magnesium, calcium and protein. Loaded with monounsaturated fat and fiber, cholesterol-free almonds are also good for your heart. Almonds contribute to longer satiety, preventing those peaks and valleys of blood sugar levels that keep so many of us snacking throughout the day. ¼ cup (28g) = 70 milligrams of calcium.

6. CARNITINE

Call it the workhorse. Derived from the amino acid lysine, it is essential for turning fatty acids into energy. It is produced by the body and is stored in tissues that use fat for fuel, like the heart, skeletal muscles, brain and sperm, where it helps shuttle fatty acids into the mitochondria to be burned for energy. It's found in red meat, poultry, fish and dairy. Confusingly, carnitine is a general term used to describe L-carnitine, acetyl-L-carnitine, and propionyl-L-carnitine and other acyl-carnitine esters.

SOME EVIDENCE FOR:

Angina: A few older studies have found L-carnitine to be effective for treated exercise-induced chest pain (angina) by improving the heart muscle metabolism and increasing exercise tolerance.

Male Sexual Function and Infertility: Things are looking up, gentlemen: One study in the journal *Fertility and Sterility* found that supplementing with a combination of L-carnitine and acetyl-L-carnitine increased sperm quality and motility.

Age-related Fatigue: A placebo-controlled, randomized, double-blind study in the *American Journal of Clinical Nutrition* found that supplementation with carnitine can increase muscle mass, decrease fat and improve cognitive functions in elderly adults.

LIMITED EVIDENCE FOR:

Heart Attack: A few studies have found evidence that carnitine supplementation, in addition to standard medical care, helps the heart heal after a heart attack; but results have been mixed, with one study finding that it can preserve the heart tissue and shape after an attack and other studies finding no protection.

Athletic Performance: Slow down, ballers: Studies have been mixed and experts disagree on the role of supplemental carnitine in improving athletic performance. Since carnitine can improve blood flow and maximum oxygen uptake, it seems logical that it would improve your playing time. And while there are some studies showing that carnitine content in muscles does increase with supplementation—and the onset of exercise-induced fatigue is prolonged—there is no evidence that it'll make you stronger or jump higher.

Depression: While some older studies found a correlation between

BUT WAIT, THERE'S MORE!

Integrative physician Ray Sahelian, M.D., calls acetyl-L-carnitine one of his favorite "mind boosters." See page 338.

depression and carnitine supplementation, a recent placebo-controlled trial found no evidence that carnitine has any antidepressant effects.

NO EVIDENCE FOR/POSSIBLY DANGEROUS:

Alzheimer's Disease: Many studies have tried to find a benefit for carnitine supplementation in treating Alzheimer's; but recent large, double-blind, placebo-controlled studies have found zero benefit.

PRECAUTIONS: Carnitine can cause nausea, vomiting, abdominal cramping, diarrhea and a fishy body odor. Carnitine supplementation might interfere with thyroid hormone medications, and might exacerbate hypothyroidism.

7. CLA (CONJUGATED LINOLEIC ACID)

A fatty acid found in meat and dairy. Supplemental CLA is often processed from vegetable oils high in linoleic acid, like safflower or poppy seed.

SOME EVIDENCE FOR:

Obesity: Could this be the cure America needs? A recent randomized, double-blind, placebo-controlled trial published in *Nutrition* found that supplementing with 1.7 grams of CLA twice a day for 12 weeks decreased total fat mass, fat percentage, subcutaneous fat mass and waist-to-hip ratio in study participants. Researchers believe that CLA might actually reduce body fat by increasing fat cell metabolism. However, a recent meta-analysis of randomized studies concluded that while research points to small decreases in body fat and body weight with CLA supplementation, more research is needed. Other research has found that CLA can reduce hunger and improve satiety.

LIMITED EVIDENCE FOR:

Immunity: Supplementing with CLA increases the levels of immune-boosting antibodies in the blood, according to animal studies and a few human studies. One small study in the *European Journal of Clinical Nutrition* found that CLA decreased the levels of two pro-inflammatory cytokines—a "cytokine" regulates your body's response to pain—and increased the levels of anti-inflammatory cytokines in healthy young study subjects. However a similar study in the journal *Lipids* found zero benefit to the immune system with CLA supplementation in healthy young women.

Cancer: Many dietary studies have linked CLA with a decrease in cancer. A study in Nutrition and Cancer found a link between dietary CLA from cheese and a reduction in breast cancer. Another study in the *American Journal of Clinical Nutrition* found that dietary CLA might reduce the risk of colon cancer. Yet another study found that CLA might be associated with a decreased risk of certain types of breast cancer tumors, but not others. There's no research indicating that supplemental CLA has any effect on cancer risk.

PRECAUTIONS: CLA supplementation is associated with a risk of constipation, diarrhea and soft stools. Supplemental CLA has been associated with increased insulin resistance and metabolic syndrome. It has also been shown to reduce the fat content in breast milk.

8. COENZYME Q10 (COQ10)

A fat-soluble antioxidant found in every cell of the body. It helps the mitochondria in our cells to use carbohydrates and fats to create ATP (adenosine triphosphate), the kind of energy used by cells, while working as an antioxidant, protecting mitochondrial from free radical damage. All that's a long way of saying, this could be quite powerful if you have one of the symptoms below.

GOOD EVIDENCE FOR:

Congestive Heart Failure: Wow: A recent study found that supplementation with CoQ10 decreased all-cause mortality in heart failure patients by half, cut the occurrence of a second major adverse cardiac event

GLUTAMINE

What It Is:
Glutamine is an amino acid (a building block of protein), stored primarily in the muscles. Dietary sources include meat, dairy, cabbage, beets and fish.

What It's Commonly Used For:
Glutamine is favored by bodybuilders because it's believed to be a powerful tool in maintaining muscle mass (it wants to pump—[clap]—you up!). While our bodies are able to produce enough for typical needs, under extreme stress—such as hitting the bench press hard—they need much more (although a caveat: critics say higher levels of glutamine were used in studies than would normally be found in supplements).

Any Proof It Works?
Studies suggest that glutamine can help the body recover from surgery, infections, burns and other injuries and that it can improve symptoms of inflammatory bowel disease and Crohn's disease, although more research is needed.

in half, decreased hospitalizations and adverse events after heart failure. This study comes after years of research pointing to beneficial effects of CoQ10, used in conjunction with standard treatment, for heart failure patients. There have been a few large studies that found no benefit with CoQ10 supplementation.

Migraine: Numerous studies have found CoQ10 supplementation to be successful at decreasing the number of migraine headaches, the nausea associated with migraine, and the duration of pain in both adults and children.

SOME EVIDENCE FOR:

Heart Attack: One study published in *Molecular and Cellular Biochemistry* found that people who've recently had a heart attack reduce their risk of a second heart attack and other heart-related problems. More research is needed.

Diabetes: There are some studies showing that CoQ10 supplementation can decrease insulin resistance. A study in the *European Journal of Clinical Nutrition* found that 200 milligrams of CoQ10 might long-term improve blood sugar control in subjects with type 2 diabetes. And a recent open label study of CoQ10 found that it improves glycemic control by improving insulin secretion without any adverse effects. However, numerous other studies have found no benefit for insulin resistance and glycemic control.

LIMITED EVIDENCE FOR:

Parkinson's Disease: While some placebo-controlled studies found that high doses of CoQ10 (1,200 milligrams) slowed the progression of early Parkinson's disease, new, larger studies have not repeated these results in early or later stages of the disease. A recent clinical trial by the National Institute of Neurological Disorders and Stroke (NINDS) on CoQ10 for Parkinson's was terminated because it was clear that no benefit was seen.

Cancer: Some preliminary studies have shown benefit for a few cancers, most notably breast cancer, but more conclusive evidence is needed.

NO EVIDENCE FOR/POSSIBLY DANGEROUS:

Aging: Since aging is associated with decreased mitochondrial function due to the oxidative damage caused by free radicals, and since tissue levels of CoQ10 decrease with age, it's been theorized that supplementing with

BUT WAIT, THERE'S MORE!

For more on Coenzyme Q10 and how it zaps migraines, see our doctor's advice on page 182.

CoQ10 would slow the aging process. But research has found no such link.

PRECAUTIONS: May cause gastro issues like nausea and upset stomach. Might interfere with blood pressure medications, chemotherapy treatments, blood thinning medications and warfarin.

9. CREATINE

This one's familiar to anyone who's ever been to the gun show [kisses biceps]. Creatine is an amino acid stored in the muscles that is converted to phosphocreatine and then ATP (adenosine triphosphate), the energy source for our cells. It is made in the body, but we also get it by eating meats and fish.

GOOD EVIDENCE FOR:

Exercise Performance: There have been numerous, double-blind studies showing that creatine supplementation increases athletic performance during high intensity exercise. Studies have found increases in muscle mass, bone mass and strength with creatine. However, studies in older men and in women have found no benefit. The results are mostly seen with intense short bouts of exercise (like swimming and weightlifting) and not necessarily seen for endurance and aerobic exercise (like running and cycling). Most of these studies, however, have included small groups of people and more research is needed.

LIMITED EVIDENCE FOR:

Heart Disease: One study found slight reductions in triglyceride levels with creatine supplementation. A few others have found that creatine can increase exercise capacity in those who've suffered a heart attack. But further research is needed.

Parkinson's Disease: Preliminary research points to creatine as a treatment for slowing the progression of Parkinson's disease. A study in *Neurology*, for example, found creatine supplementation successful in easing the symptoms of early Parkinson's.

PRECAUTIONS: Weight gain, dizziness, muscle cramping, high blood pressure, kidney and liver damage have all been reported. Because of the positive evidence with creatine and muscle mass, many people are taking excessive amounts, and this can lead to sudden kidney failure. Because creatine draws water from the rest of your body, be sure to hydrate well when taking it.

10. FIBER

There's nothing more aggravating than feeling bloated, unclean, unfinished or plugged up. (According to one theory, if everyone in the world had regular bowel movements daily, there'd be world peace.) If only we all ate more fiber. Found in fruits and vegetables, grains, legumes, nuts and seeds, it keeps your digestive tract moving along in a healthy manner (preventing constipation). It also has been shown to reduce the risk of many diseases, including heart disease, obesity and diabetes. Most processed foods are lacking in fiber so best to choose fresh, whole foods whenever possible. The world's counting on you.

GOOD EVIDENCE FOR:

Bowel Health: Dietary fiber bulks up in your bowels, which makes the food and toxins easier to pass, and prevents constipation and diarrhea. A diet high in fiber also can reduce your risk of developing diverticulitis (small pouches in your colon) and hemorrhoids. A 2013 study published in the *Journal of Nutrition* showed improved laxation and minimal intolerance with a soluble fiber supplement.

Heart Disease: Studies have shown that soluble fiber—found in oats and bran—lowers LDL (bad) cholesterol, and also may reduce blood pressure and chronic inflammation.

Diabetes: Very strong studies have shown that dietary fiber—both soluble and insoluble (found in fresh vegetables, nuts and beans)—can slow the absorption of sugar and lead to better blood sugar control; a diet

Fiber can make you smell better—really. See page 71 for how.

PHOSPHOROUS

What It Is: Phosphorous is the second-most abundant mineral in the body, next to calcium and, like calcium, is used to build bones and teeth. Phosphorous is also crucial for energy transport and storage and essential for transporting waste materials from the kidneys and muscles.

What It's Commonly Used For: Athletes often supplement after training, because phosphorous is important for rebuilding tissue and has been found to reduce muscle pain after a hard workout. Most of us get enough phosphorous from our diets, since it's found in grains, milk and any protein-rich food.

Any Proof It Works? The key to phosphorous is balance: Having too much can actually be worse than too little. Excessive phosphorous levels have been shown to cause brittle bones as well as gum and teeth issues, and getting too much is more common in the West, because of our consumption of meat, poultry and carbonated beverages. Most people don't need supplements.

high in insoluble fiber has been found to reduce the risk of type 2 diabetes.

Weight Control: Fiber is dense, so it takes longer to chew, which gives your body time to register satiety; it also expands in your belly, so you feel full faster, and longer.

LIMITED EVIDENCE FOR:

Calcium Absorption: It's all about the probiotics: Some studies have found that fiber supplements may increase specific strains of beneficial bacteria in the gut, and therefore facilitate calcium absorption, but more evidence is needed.

NO EVIDENCE FOR/POSSIBLY DANGEROUS:

Apart from excessive gas while your gut gets used to the rough stuff, there have been no serious dangers associated with consuming the recommended amounts of fiber. Pro tip: sit near a dog and blame him.

PRECAUTIONS: Getting too much (more than 50 grams a day) might interfere with the absorption of the minerals and other nutrients in the foods you eat, as well as some medications you take, because the fiber could make the food fly through your intestines too fast. Best to gradually increase the amount you get through supplements and food, and be sure to drink lots of water.

11. FISH OIL (OMEGA-3 FATTY ACIDS), DHA/EPA

Until the probiotics craze hit the supplement scene, omega-3s were the headliners. Found in, yes, fatty fish such as salmon, trout, herring,

POTASSIUM

What It Is: Potassium is a mineral that's vital for the function of organs, cells and tissues, and also is an electrolyte, a substance that acts as a conductor of electricity in the body. It plays an important role in muscle contraction, and so is key to proper digestion and muscle function, and also to heart function. Potassium is readily available in meat and fish, fruits and vegetables and legumes. Dairy also is a good source.

What It's Commonly Used For: Potassium supplementation is not generally recommended; it's often used to treat symptoms of hypokalemia, or low levels of potassium, which include muscle weakness and abnormal heart function. Athletes down electrolyte drinks during training and competition; diets rich in potassium.

Any Proof It Works? Diets rich in potassium have been shown to lower risk of stroke and osteoporosis and to reduce high blood pressure. Certain conditions such as Crohn's and IBD may need supplementation, but most experts suggest supplementing only under medical supervision. Instead, stick to the bananas and sports drinks.

sardines and anchovies, the two omega-3 fatty acids (EPA/DHA) without a doubt reduce the risk factors of chronic diseases—heart disease, high blood pressure, high cholesterol, arthritis, maybe even cancer—by reducing inflammation. Vegetarian sources include flaxseed oil and algae.

GOOD EVIDENCE FOR:

Heart Disease and Hypertension: Numerous studies have proven that taking fish oil supplements can lower triglyceride levels and reduce the growth rate of arterial plaque; sudden death in study participants dropped by 45% compared to patients not taking the capsules.

Joint Health: Most studies looking at fish oil and arthritis have been done on rheumatoid arthritis, and shown great success. Most done on osteoarthritis have been anecdotal or inconclusive. However, a 2011 animal study (it was done on guinea pigs, which are prone to arthritis, OK?) showed a 50% reduction in the stiffness and pain of the disease in the poor things. (Recent research done in New Zealand on humans supports these findings.)

Osteoporosis: According to the University of Maryland, recent studies have shown that women getting sufficient omega-3 essential fatty acids—through diet or supplementation—can slow the rate of bone loss.

SOME EVIDENCE FOR:

Cancer: Although not all experts agree, people who get plenty of fish oil, through foods or supplements, tend to have lower rates of certain types of cancer. Eskimos, for instance, have a low rate of colorectal cancer, and animal and human studies have found that omega-3 fatty acids can stop or slow the progression of colon cancer. Studies show that a lifelong diet rich in omega-3s may prevent breast cancer.

LIMITED EVIDENCE FOR:

Depression: The debate still rages: Does supplementation of omega-3s help with mental health disorders, primarily depression (though research is also being done on bipolar disorder, ADHD and schizophrenia)? It does appear that fish oil can help medications work more effectively; more evidence is needed, but a diet high in omega-3s is good for anyone.

NO EVIDENCE/POSSIBLY DANGEROUS:

Prostate Cancer: While fish and fish oil may prevent prostate cancer, some studies show that alpha-linolenic acid (ALA), which the body converts to EPA and DHA (the more readily available form), may be associated with increased risk.

PRECAUTIONS: Always buy from a reputable source, since fish may contain contaminants such as pesticides and heavy metals.

12. FOLATE

Folate is the naturally occurring form of the man-made folic acid, which every woman of childbearing age knows about, or should: It came to fame when a very important study found that taking folic acid reduces birth defects, most notably spina bifida. You'll find it in dairy, leafy green vegetables, fruits, whole grains, poultry, nuts and fish. (Folic acid is taken in supplements and added to foods.) Folate helps grow tissues, red blood cells and DNA, and helps cells work.

GOOD EVIDENCE FOR:

Prevention of Birth Defects: A landmark study in 1997 showed that taking folic acid before and during pregnancy significantly reduces the risk of birth defects including spina bifida, anencephaly and some heart defects. Now, prenatal folic acid is a given, and experts recommend taking it before you get pregnant and for at least three months after. And because many women don't know they're pregnant till weeks in, anyone who is trying to or could become pregnant should take some, too.

BUT WAIT, THERE'S MORE!

Mark Hyman, M.D., recommends a folate formula to aid depression. It's on page 97.

Heart Health: Harvard Medical School reports that folate is a key nutrient in heart health because of its effect on blood levels of homocysteine. The ongoing Nurses' Health Study has found that folic acid supplements can lower levels of homocysteine (an amino acid found in the majority of people with cardiovascular disease) and even reverse cardiovascular damage.

Cancer: Folate is crucial to normal cell division and growth. The Nurses' Health Study found lower levels of breast cancer and colon cancer in participants who took daily folic acid supplements; supplementation has been found beneficial for patients with Crohn's disease and ulcerative colitis.

Diseases of Aging: Studies show that low levels of blood folate are associated with Alzheimer's disease and hearing loss; a British study found that Alzheimer's was 3.3 times more likely in subjects with the lowest levels of folate.

PRECAUTIONS: Too much folic acid could mask a type of anemia associated with a B_{12} deficiency which could lead to permanent nerve damage; so some experts suggest limiting folic acid from supplementation. Alcohol lowers folate levels (although the Nurses' Health Study found that women who took 600 milligrams of folic acid did not increase their risk of breast cancer).

13. GLUCOSAMINE/CHONDROITIN

You can thank your dog for this one: Well before it was accepted for human use, glucosamine was given by vets to aging canines to help repair cartilage and ease joint pain. Glucosamine is a naturally occurring compound found in healthy cartilage; glucosamine sulfate is believed to strengthen cartilage and aid in the production of glycosaminoglycan, a molecule used to make cartilage.

GOOD EVIDENCE FOR:

Osteoarthritis: Strong evidence from many randomized studies shows that glucosamine/chondroitin sulfate is highly effective in treating arthritis, especially in the knee.

LIMITED EVIDENCE FOR:

Rheumatoid Arthritis: The theory is that supplemental glucosamine could ease the pain of RA, but more research is needed.

IBD: Some studies have suggested glucosamine might benefit children with inflammatory bowel disease, Crohn's disease and ulcerative colitis, but the studies were small, and lacked a control group.

PRECAUTIONS: Glucosamine has been found to be well tolerated, but in some cases may cause drowsiness, headache, insomnia and digestive issues. There is some evidence that use of glucosamine may worsen blood sugar control, so diabetics should work with their doctors. Rarely, the combination of glucosamine and chondroitin has caused an elevation in blood pressure and heart rate. Glucosamine is most effective when taken for two to four months.

14. IRON

This isn't a contest, but if we had to choose the most essential vitamin or nutrient in this chapter, iron may be it: It is crucial for life, most particularly the production of red blood cells, which carry oxygen to the body and contribute to cell growth. Iron also is involved in producing

ATP, which transports energy within cells—you know, cells, the things you're made up of. Without iron, there's no you.

"Heme" iron, which is easiest to absorb, comes from animal products such as meat, poultry and fish; "non-heme" comes from plant sources, including leafy greens (spinach and kale), tofu, legumes and fortified cereals. You can boost your absorption by pairing these with high vitamin C foods like sweet potatoes, broccoli, red peppers and blueberries.

BUT WAIT, THERE'S MORE!

It's Iron vs. Anemia: Help yourself win on page 44.

Sounds plentiful. If only: Iron deficiency, or anemia, is the most common nutrient deficiency worldwide, affecting 1.62 billion people; the World Health Organization estimates that as much as 80% of the global population may be iron deficient, and a quarter of the world's population has iron-deficiency anemia, a shortage of red blood cells or blood cells that are too small due to a lack of iron.

GOOD EVIDENCE FOR:

Anemia: Anemia, usually characterized by extreme fatigue, can be caused by poor nutrition, menstrual blood loss, pregnancy, bleeding ulcers, surgery and other conditions; treatment should be guided by your doctor, but iron supplements have been found to be very effective.

SOME EVIDENCE FOR:

Athletic Performance: Some studies have suggested that even a low level of iron deficiency may cause low energy, and found that iron supplementation improved performance for those who already were deficient.

LIMITED EVIDENCE FOR:

ADHD: Some preliminary studies have found that iron supplements might help children who are deficient, but iron can be toxic to children with normal levels; so never give them to your child (or any infant or child younger than 18) without your doctor's recommendation.

PRECAUTIONS: Too much iron may lead to hemochromatosis, which is usually an inherited disease but can occur in people who take large amounts of iron supplements. Side effects of taking supplements include digestive problems such as constipation, diarrhea and heartburn, and many people's poop turns black. Pregnant women may be especially plagued; look for an easy-to-digest form such as Floradix. Never give iron supplements to a child under 18 without a doctor's supervision.

15. LUTEIN/ZEAXANTHIN

Lutein and its coexistent isomer (or sidekick), zeaxanthin, are carotenoids—the yellow, red and orange pigments synthesized by plants—that are present in the body because of foods or supplements that you consume. And you care why? Because they also are the only carotenoids found in the lens and the retina of the eye, where light enters. Studies have found that they provide protection against damaging rays for the eyes and for skin, where lutein and zeaxanthin are found as well. Dietary sources include egg yolks, green vegetables (especially spinach and collard greens, kiwi, grapes, orange juice, zucchini, squash and corn).

GOOD EVIDENCE FOR:

Eye Health: Lutein and zeaxanthin have been studied extensively for use in treating cataracts and preventing macular and retinal degeneration with some success due to their abilities to trap short-wavelength light and their antioxidant capabilities. Four large studies found that men and women who had diets rich in lutein and zeaxanthin, particularly spinach, were less likely to require cataract surgery. And 2013 data published in the *Journal of the American Medical Association* (*JAMA*) showed significant reduction in the progression of macular degeneration with supplement use. However, experts call for more research.

Cardiovascular Disease and Cancer: The role of carotenoids in the prevention of heart disease and cancer has been established since the 1990s, and while their antioxidant effects (which can reduce inflammation and may prevent and reduce atherosclerosis),

RED YEAST RICE

What It Is: This traditional Chinese remedy looks like you think it would: It's fermented rice with a deep reddish hue caused by mold (when cultivated correctly) or by food dye (when tampered with). It works like statin drugs, inhibiting the body's cholesterol-making enzyme.

What It's Commonly Used For:

Lowering cholesterol.

Any Proof It Works? Results are encouraging. In a double-blind placebo-controlled randomized trial, 52 doctors and their wives were tested, and red yeast rice was proven "very effective," as reported in the journal *BMC Complementary and Alternative Medicine*, July 2013. So we're getting closer to a definitive answer. Because of its power, red yeast rice is best taken under the guidance of a naturopath or physician. If you have hepatic or renal disease, check with a doctor before taking.

more research is called for. A Finnish study suggests that dietary lutein and zeaxanthin may reduce lung cancer risk.

16. LYCOPENE

Why are tomatoes red? It's because of lycopene, which is also a powerful antioxidant that may help protect cells from damage. Another carotenoid (like lutein) common in North American diets, lycopene is also responsible for the color of pink grapefruit, guava and watermelon, though most of the lycopene in the U.S. diet comes from tomatoes and tomato products. (It can only come from diet and supplements.)

GOOD EVIDENCE FOR:

Cardiovascular Disease: Cardiovascular disease is the leading cause of death in Western societies, and accounts for a third of deaths worldwide. And compared to the United States and Northern Europe, the CVD rates in the Mediterranean areas of Europe are very low. This is attributed at least in part to the diet of those regions, which is high in many antioxidants, but especially lycopene from tomatoes. (Maybe Tony Soprano didn't die in the finale after all.) And a 2011 analysis in *Current Medical Chemistry* confirms that supplementation of lycopene is an effective preventive measure for reducing many risk factors of CVD.

Prostate Cancer: Several cohort studies, including one that followed 47,000 men for eight years, have found that diets rich in lycopene—especially from tomato products—can significantly reduce the risk of prostate cancer, particularly more aggressive forms. A 2011 study

SOY

What it is: Soy is a plant in the pea family; soybeans are the seeds of the plant.

What It's Commonly Used For: Soybeans are high in protein and contain isoflavones, which are similar to estrogen. They're used to make tofu, soy milk and soy protein powders. Soy is commonly used to treat menopausal symptoms, high blood pressure, high cholesterol, osteoporosis, breast cancer and prostate cancer.

Any Proof It Works? Studies have shown that soy supplementation may lower LDL ("bad") cholesterol, and possibly reduce hot flashes; research on treatment for cardiovascular disease and cancer are inconclusive. Some studies suggest caution when taking soy isoflavones if you are at risk for hormone-sensitive cancers such as breast, uterine or ovarian. Best to get moderate levels of soy through foods such as tofu and tempeh.

on men with low-risk prostate cancer found that oxidative stress was significantly modulated with lycopene (as well as fish oil) use.

Lung Cancer: Men and women with the highest intakes of total carotenoids and lycopene have been found to be at the lowest risk of lung cancer, although not smoking is the greatest way to reduce risk.

LIMITED EVIDENCE FOR:

HPV: Most scientists who specialize in HPV research agree that the best way to battle the human papillomavirus—a major cause of cervical cancer—is to boost immunity. Lycopene is one of the supplements that, along with the herbs turmeric, echinacea and propolis, has been shown to strengthen immunity.

Breast and Other Cancers: Results from animal studies suggest that lycopene may have preventive effects against breast, ovarian, endometrial, liver and skin cancer; human studies have thus far been inconclusive. So far, the FDA recognizes this limited evidence status for lycopene (which means it probably is quite effective).

PRECAUTIONS: The only reported adverse effect of this winning antioxidant seems to be gastrointestinal, which can be managed by taking lycopene supplements with meals.

The National Cancer Institute's ongoing Prostate, Lung, Colorectal and Ovarian Cancer Screening Trial continues to seek participants; one of its main initiatives is to investigate the link between lycopene and reduced cancer risk.

17. MAGNESIUM

Magnesium is crucial to just about every organ in your body—heart, kidneys, muscles—as well as the production of teeth and bones. It also regulates calcium levels, assists in energy production and activates enzymes. So be worried: You may not be getting enough. Most American diets are sorely lacking in this essential mineral, which is found in whole grains, nuts and green vegetables, especially green leafy ones like kale.

BUT WAIT, THERE'S MORE!

Magnesium will help prevent aging, says Carolyn Dean, M.D. See how on page 23.

GOOD EVIDENCE FOR:

Osteoporosis: Magnesium is a major player in bone health; if magnesium levels in bone decrease, bone crystals become larger, making bones more brittle. A study of more than 900 elderly men and women found higher dietary magnesium intakes were associated with increased bone mineral density at the hip in both men and women, and a recent study suggests the same is true for magnesium supplementation.

Heart Health: Studies suggest that increased magnesium intake can lower the risk of cardiovascular disease, and since it helps maintain a consistent heart rhythm, magnesium is routinely given intravenously to patients in heart failure. One large observational study found that high blood levels of magnesium protected against cardiovascular disease among women (but not men). One double-blind study found magnesium supplementation to be beneficial in lowering blood pressure in individuals who were deficient, but other study findings conflict.

Anxiety Disorders: A 2011 study published in the *Journal of Neuroscience* suggests that magnesium may be a powerful tool in the treatment of anxiety disorders such as social anxiety, phobias and post-traumatic stress syndrome. According to study authors, the mineral heightens the function of the prefrontal cortex, a brain region involved in controlling fear responses.

Diabetes: Magnesium depletion has been shown to increase insulin resistance and may adversely affect blood glucose control in diabetes. One study reported that dietary magnesium supplements (400 milligrams/day) improved glucose tolerance in elderly individuals, and a 2013 study published in the journal *Nutrients* found that higher intakes of magnesium significantly reduced insulin resistance, especially for people with metabolic syndrome who had low intake of the mineral.

SOME EVIDENCE FOR:

Migraine Headaches: Two placebo-controlled trials demonstrated modest decreases in the frequency of migraine headaches after supplementation with 600 milligrams/day of magnesium. However, another placebo-controlled study found that 485 milligrams/day of magnesium did not reduce the frequency of migraine headaches.

Depression: Evidence that magnesium can benefit mental health is compelling. A 2010 study from the Clinic of Psychiatry and Psychotherapy in Malberg, Germany, found that Western diets have been depleted of dietary magnesium, that a low intake of magnesium was a major factor in depression and that supplementation of 600 to 800 milligrams/day had a significant preventative benefit.

PRECAUTIONS: Because of the potential risks of high doses of supplemental magnesium, especially if you have kidney issues, supplementation should always be under professional supervision. The most absorbable forms are magnesium citrate, glycinate taurate or aspartate, so stick to them if you can, and avoid magnesium carbonate, sulfate, gluconate and oxide, which are the cheapest and most common forms.

18. MELATONIN

If you have trouble falling and staying asleep—or want to sidestep jet lag—say hello to our little friend melatonin. Melatonin (MLT) is a hormone that maintains your body's circadian rhythm; your circadian rhythm determines when you fall asleep and wake up. When it's dark, your body produces more melatonin and so nudges you to sleep; when it's light, melatonin drops. Being exposed to bright lights in the evening or too little light during the day can disrupt your MLT cycles. Scientists believe that melatonin decreases as we age, which may be why older adults tend to struggle more with insomnia.

GOOD EVIDENCE FOR:

Insomnia and Other Sleep Disorders: MLT supplements can help people with disrupted circadian cycles—due to red-eye flights or working the graveyard shift—or those with low melatonin levels (seniors and people with schizophrenia) sleep better. Clinical studies suggest that for short-term use (days or weeks) melatonin is more effective than a placebo for reducing the time it takes to fall asleep, increasing sleep hours and boosting daytime alertness. It has been found to

SPIRULINA

What It Is: Spirulina is a blue-green algae rich in protein, minerals, vitamins and carotenoids, which are antioxidants that prevent cell damage. It also is high in GLA (an essential fatty acid).

What It's Commonly Used For: Spirulina is a high quality, non-meat protein; it's also used to treat liver damage, cancer, viral infections such as influenza, herpes and HIV; to promote immune function; and as a probiotic (to boost "good" bacteria in the intestinal tract).

Any Proof It Works? Lab studies have shown that spirulina may increase production of antibodies and other cells that fight infection, help protect against allergic reactions, and viral and bacterial infections. Experts caution that, since spirulina is harvested in the sea it could be contaminated with toxins and heavy metals, and recommend buying from a trusted source.

improve sleep for menopausal women and patients with ADHD.

SOME EVIDENCE FOR:

Schizophrenia: Fascinating ongoing research is investigating the role of melatonin as a treatment for schizophrenia. Melatonin is a hormone secreted by the pineal gland, which many consider the seat of mental health and which is light responsive. The blood of patients with schizophrenia has erratic levels of melatonin; a 2012 study in the *International Journal of Molecular Science* suggests that supplementation and monitoring can help with sleep disorders and also might be used as a treatment, but further research is required.

Breast Cancer: Women with breast cancer tend to have lower levels of the hormone, and lab experiments have shown that adding melatonin to certain types of breast cancer cells slows their growth. It also has been shown to boost the effects of medication and chemotherapy.

Huntington's Disease: Huntington's disease is a hereditary disorder characterized by movement, cognitive and psychiatric symptoms. A 2011 paper released by Stanford University found that both the antioxidant properties and the neuroprotective agents in melatonin may improve symptoms and prevent disease progression.

Fibromyalgia: A recent placebo-controlled study found that fibromyalgia patients experienced a significant reduction in their symptoms when they took a melatonin supplement either alone or in conjunction with fluoxetine (Prozac).

LIMITED EVIDENCE/MAY BE DANGEROUS:

Epilepsy: Some studies suggest melatonin may reduce the frequency

STEROLS

What It Is: Sterols, also called phytosterols, are a group of naturally occurring compounds found in plant membranes. Dietary sources include nuts, vegetable oils, whole grains, fruits and vegetables.

What It's Commonly Used For: Sterols are structurally similar to cholesterol, and compete for absorption in the digestive system. Thus, they block cholesterol absorption and are used to lower blood cholesterol levels.

Any Proof It Works? Absolutely. Studies have shown that consuming suggested levels of sterols—along with a heart-healthy eating plan—can lower cholesterol by up to 14%. The FDA has even approved a health claim for sterols, and the National Cholesterol Education Program recommends 2 grams per day to lower cholesterol.

and duration of seizures in children with epilepsy. But others have found that melatonin increases the frequency of seizures. Do not take melatonin for epilepsy or give it to a child without talking to your doctor first.

Depression: A few studies have found that melatonin can worsen depression, so always consult with a physician.

PRECAUTIONS: Don't forget that melatonin is a hormone, and while some experts suggest nightly use for consistent healthy sleep, others recommend only short-term use for insomnia or jet lag. It does cause drowsiness, so take care with that; many people report feeling a melatonin hangover the next day. MLT supplements can interact with many drugs, including antidepressants and blood pressure medications.

19. MULTIVITAMINS

Forget Allstate: The Harvard School of Public Health proclaims that a daily multivitamin is the best insurance policy. For while it's preferable to get the nutrients you need—adequate vitamins B, C, D and E, a cornucopia of antioxidants, folic acid, omega-3s and probiotics—from food, most of us just don't. Therefore, most experts agree that a standard multi, with an extra dose of vitamin D, can lower your risk for many diseases, including cancer and heart disease.

And yet the issue just got more complicated: A meta-analysis by Kaiser Permanente and the U.S. Preventive Services Task Force, published in November 2013 in the *Annals of Internal Medicine*, compared 24 studies and concluded that multivitamins alone don't help—or hurt—in preventing fatalities from cancer and heart disease, although multis with folic acid did help pregnant women have healthier babies. So where do we land? Use a multi to, as recommended by the Council of Responsible Nutrition, "fill the nutrient gaps" that most people have.

GOOD EVIDENCE FOR:

General health and disease prevention: According to the Linus Pauling Institute at Oregon State, recent research indicates that several of the nutrients found in standard multivitamin supplements do play important roles in preventing chronic diseases like heart disease, cancer and osteoporosis. A daily multivitamin supplement ensures an adequate intake of several micronutrients that are not always present

A multivitamin may also help ease anxiety. Get help on page 48.

in the diet in optimal amounts. And a good multivitamin should contain adequate daily values of folic acid; all of the alphabet vitamins, including vitamins A, C, B$_{12}$, D, E and K; biotin, iron, calcium, magnesium, selenium and zinc. The benefits from those vitamins are many and detailed here.

PRECAUTIONS: Of course, there can be too much of a good thing. It's important not to go overboard with vitamins. While a multivitamin and a vitamin D supplement can help fill some of the gaps in a less-than-optimal diet, too much can be harmful. In general, stick close to standard recommended doses in a multivitamin.

20. NIACIN

It could make you look sexier, feel stronger and last longer in bed, yet no one talks about niacin. It's a naturally occurring B vitamin whose primary duty is to convert the foods we eat into energy we can use—and in fact one sign of deficiency is fatigue. According to the University of Maryland Medical Center, niacin assists in the processes by which cells divide and regenerate, which is important for healthy skin, hair and nails. Niacin is found in meat, grains and fortified foods that include milk and orange juice.

SOME EVIDENCE FOR:

Heart Disease: Niacin often is prescribed for heart-health conditions, primarily due to its ability to raise HDL ("good" cholesterol) levels, and recent research conducted by the Linus Pauling Institute at Oregon State has confirmed its benefits; other studies have shown that high HDL levels can lower risk of heart disease by one-third. But lately there has been a question mark as to whether artificially raising HDL is enough to impart heart health, which in turn has caused Big Pharma (makers of prescription-grade niacin) to redirect efforts toward lowering the bad cholesterol, LDL. Many experts say it's back to the basics of sound diet and exercise.

Sex Drive: Niacin improves circulation, and according to the University of Maryland Medical Center, niacin works with the adrenal glands to create adequate levels of sex hormones, and boosts blood circulation to the genitals. Talk about hard evidence.

PRECAUTIONS: Too much niacin can cause skin flushing and itching, nausea and vomiting. Never take more than 35 milligrams unless told to by your doctor.

21. PROBIOTICS

This decade, probiotics enjoy rock star status in the supplement world, and probiotic supplements are considered, along with omega-3s, vitamin D and magnesium, one of the supplements every adult (and many kids) should be taking. According to the NIH National Center for Complementary and Alternative Medicine (NCCAM), probiotics are live microorganisms (in most cases, bacteria) that are similar to beneficial microorganisms found in the human gut. They are also called "friendly bacteria" or "good bacteria." Probiotics are available to consumers mainly in the form of dietary supplements and foods.

GOOD EVIDENCE FOR:

Inflammation: Ah, that word again. Many experts believe that chronic inflammation is the root of chronic disease, including heart disease, diabetes and pretty much anything with an "-itis" suffix. A study published in the journal *Gut Microbes* recently found that the mucosal immune system that lines our digestive tract offers protection against everything from colitis and chronic fatigue syndrome to psoriasis and periodontal disease. The mechanism appears to beef up the good bacteria in the intestines, which in turn strengthens the immune system so that it is better equipped to fight off disease.

IBS, Colitis and IBD: The study published in *Gut Microbes* found that the inflammatory markers related to these inflammatory conditions were significantly reduced, and patients with chronic fatigue syndrome also saw improvement in symptoms.

Allergies: Numerous studies have shown that probiotic supplementation can reduce allergy symptoms; a 2013 analysis published in *Pediatrics* found that women who took probiotics during pregnancy reduced their child's risk of developing allergies in their lifetimes. Best results were for those babies exposed to probiotics in the womb.

Vaginal Infections: A 2008 paper published by the *World Gastroenterology Organisation Practice Guidelines Probiotics and Prebiotics* found that, among other uses, probiotics were effective in fighting vaginal infections, including those brought on by antibiotic use (good-bye yeast infections!).

BUT WAIT, THERE'S MORE!

For a complete look at indigestion, uncover your eyes and see page 154.

Gastrointestinal Issues: To the relief of new parents, probiotic supplements have shown promise in the prevention and relief of colic, but a 2013 Australian review of 12 studies (and 12 different probiotics) published in *JAMA Pediatrics* found that the results were 50/50, i.e., six of the probiotics helped, six did not.

Eczema and Psoriasis: The World Gastroenterology Organisation also found strong evidence that probiotics reduced the chronic inflammation responsible for these and other skin conditions.

SOME EVIDENCE FOR:

Autism, ADHD, Dyslexia, Depression and Schizophrenia: Recent research suggests that a number of psychological conditions and learning disabilities are associated with an imbalance in the gut's bacterial "village," according to mucosal biology expert Alessio Fasano, M.D. The problem occurs when the "bad" bacteria outgrow the good.

Cancer: There is recent research that suggests probiotics may help reduce the risk of certain cancers, including colon cancer, but more studies are needed; there's good evidence that taking probiotics could minimize the side effects of chemotherapy.

PRECAUTIONS: Not all probiotics are alike, so it's best to work with someone who knows her way around the different strains. The most popular strains are acidophilus, bifidobacterium lactobacillus.

22. RESVERATROL

A powerful, naturally occurring antioxidant found in the stems, seeds and skin of red wine grapes and other plants, resveratrol often

---

TRYPTOPHAN

What It Is: Tryptophan is an essential amino acid, which means your body doesn't produce it—you must ingest it from food or supplements. Your body uses tryptophan to make niacin and serotonin; serotonin induces calm and healthy sleep. Food sources include eggs, spirulina, turkey and other poultry (famously, aka the "Thanksgiving coma"), cheese, soybean, fish, seeds and nuts, and milk.

What It's Commonly Used For: Tryptophan supplements— L-tryptophan—are commonly used as a sleep aid and to treat depression and anxiety.

Any Proof It Works? Study results have been mixed for tryptophan as a sleep inducer and antidepressant and antianxiety supplement, although they tended to be better when used as an "augmenter" of antidepressants. Proceed with caution.

pops up in the news with grabby headlines like: "Live longer by drinking wine!" It's found in peanut butter, red grapes, red grape juice, blueberries, cranberries and, yes, red and white wine. It can also be applied topically in the form of face creams.

GOOD EVIDENCE FOR:

Anti-aging: This is the big news out of 2013: A team at Harvard Medical School announced that resveratrol boosts production of SIRT1, a disease-blocking serum. "In the history of pharmaceuticals, there has never been a drug that binds to a protein to make it run faster in the way that resveratrol activates SIRT1," said the senior author. "Now that we know the exact location on SIRT1 where resveratrol works, and how it works, we can engineer even better molecules that more precisely and effectively trigger the effects of resveratrol," he says.

SOME EVIDENCE FOR:

Research also suggests that resveratrol boosts energy; inhibits the development of cancer (including breast cancer); and could be linked to a reduced risk of inflammation and blood clotting. Resveratrol also helps fight environmental toxins to keep skin supple and reduce wrinkles. But none of this research is as compelling as the Harvard study.

NO EVIDENCE FOR/POSSIBLY DANGEROUS:

A recent investigation found that researcher Dipak Das, Ph.D., falsified data suggesting that resveratrol can reduce cardiovascular disease risks. We only mention it because his work made the news; read closely.

23. SELENIUM

Selenium—maybe you remember it from the periodic table—Se?—is a chemical element found in meat, wheat germ, nuts (particularly Brazil nuts), eggs, oats, whole wheat bread and brown rice. But modern farming practices have depleted the soil, so many people don't get sufficient selenium from their diets anymore, says Tanya Edwards, M.D., medical director for the Center for Integrative Medicine at the Cleveland Clinic in Ohio. Refining and processing also reduce selenium levels, which is why eating whole, unprocessed, organic food is the best way to obtain the nutrient.

GOOD EVIDENCE FOR:

A powerful antioxidant, selenium works especially well with vitamin E to fight damaging free radicals. It's vital to the immune system, boosting the body's defenses against bacteria and viruses, and it may reduce cancer risk, particularly in the prostate, colon and lungs. Since an organic diet isn't always possible, Edwards recommends supplementing with selenium, which can be found by itself or in multivitamins. Taking selenium is particularly recommended for people with certain digestive conditions, such as Crohn's disease and ulcerative colitis.

SOME EVIDENCE FOR:

Battling Influenza: Scientists studied the selenium deficiencies in patients who had the H1N1 virus—remember that? Swine Flu?—and the "findings emphasized... the importance of Se status in infections, particularly in H1N1 influenza."

LIMITED EVIDENCE FOR:

Cancer: The National Cancer Institute is currently sponsoring a study on whether supplementing with selenium and vitamin E can help prevent or delay prostate cancer.

PRECAUTIONS: Over time, high doses (more than 900 mcg per day) may lead to depression, nervousness, vomiting and nausea. Since vitamin C can interfere with the absorption of selenium, take them at separate times.

24. VITAMIN A

Vitamin A is not a singular nutrient, but a group of organic compounds (retinol, for example, derived from eating animals, is one you'll hear a lot about). They're essential for vision and boosting immunity—hence the nickname "the anti-infective vitamin." Humans find vitamin A via two sources: in foods like fish oil, egg yolks, liver and dairy, or via pro-vitamin A carotenoids, which is a fancy word for other compounds that the body coverts into retinol. These are best found in colorful foods like squash, broccoli, greens and apricots.

Beta-carotene is the most well-known and important pro-vitamin A carotenoid—your mom was right when she said carrots, which are full of the stuff, would help your eyesight.

GOOD EVIDENCE FOR:

Acne: Topical creams with retinoid, like Isotretinoin, are the go-tos for many dermatologists, because they shrink the sebaceous glands, the microscopic organs that secrete oil and wax (when they become clogged or produce too much juice, welcome Pizza Face). Pros: The creams

BUT WAIT, THERE'S MORE!

Selenium can be a key part of detoxing. See our "Doable Detox" on page 303.

usually work. Cons: they make you prone to sunburn, and can come with side effects—most notoriously, in 2009, Accutane, then the most famous retinoid cream, was taken off the shelves after a jury found it was responsible for causing irritable bowel syndrome and other worries.

Immunity: The big research was done in the '90s, confirming what was suspected for decades, and it still stands: vitamin A boosts the immune system, party by helping develop white blood cells, which prevent disease. The essential takeaway, however, is that downing more (at the sign of a cold, say, or a cancer diagnosis) doesn't help. In fact, too much

Top Sources of Vitamin A FOOD	mcg RAE per serving	IU per serving	Percent DV*
Sweet potato, baked in skin, 1 whole	1,403	28,058	561
Beef liver, pan fried, 3 ounces	6,582	22,175	444
Spinach, frozen, boiled, ½ cup	573	11,458	229
Carrots, raw, ½ cup	459	9,189	184
Pumpkin pie, commercially prepared, 1 piece	488	3,743	249
Cantaloupe, raw, ½ cup	135	2,706	54
Peppers, sweet, red, raw, ½ cup	117	2,332	47
Mangos, raw, 1 whole	112	2,240	45
Black-eyed peas (cowpeas), boiled, 1 cup	66	1,305	26
Apricots, dried, sulfured, 10 halves	63	1,261	25

*Daily Value   Source: NIH

could lead to issues like liver problems or lower bone density. Be satisfied with the recommended dose, unless your doctor tells you otherwise.

Growth: Your baby's limbs, heart, eyes and ears grow thanks to vitamin A—though too much or too little may result in defects. If you're pregnant, talk to your doctor about any supplements before taking them.

Vision: The short story here is, retinol starts a chain of events that ultimately helps send an impulse up the optic nerve. This allows you to see—and see better in the dark. Eating foods high in beta-carotene—like sweet potatoes, kale and carrots—strengthens the eye.

LIMITED EVIDENCE FOR:

Cancer: Numerous studies have been done measuring the impact of beta-carotene on various cancers, all of them inconclusive. For example, a 2009 study from the National Cancer Institute showed participants who "took daily supplements of beta-carotene and retinyl palmitate"— a vitamin A supplement—"had a 35% lower risk of nonaggressive prostate cancer than men not taking the supplements," reports the NIH. However, the study found that baseline serum beta-carotene and retinol levels and supplemental beta-carotene had no effect on survival. More studies are to come.

NO EVIDENCE FOR/POSSIBLY DANGEROUS:

Heart Disease: A big study from Kaiser Permanente Center for Health Research (see "Multivitamins" on page 443 for more) found no consistent evidence linking vitamin A and heart disease.

Osteoporosis: Too much vitamin A, combined with a vitamin D deficiency, could "be a significant additional risk factor for osteoporosis... in postmenopausal women," according to a 2013 Spanish study published in the *Archives of Osteoporosis*.

PRECAUTIONS: Liver patients and women taking oral contraceptives are at risk for toxicity; begin at a lower dosage and have your blood levels monitored. And in general, avoid taking too much. Doctors even warn against eating paté more than once weekly, because liver is so high in vitamin A.

25. B VITAMINS

VITAMIN B$_6$

The key to metabolism: Vitamin B$_6$—also called pyridoxine—helps turn proteins and carbs into energy. It's found in fish, poultry, meats, starchy vegetables and non-citrus fruits, and is often added to other foods. All adults need 1.3 milligrams daily, unless they're over 51 years old: Then men need 1.7 milligrams and women need 1.5 milligrams. You likely get enough from your diet, unless you have kidney issues, immune disorders or bowel trouble like IBS or Crohn's disease.

Might Help: Nausea when pregnant, according to some persuasive studies. Talk to your OB-GYN.

Won't Help: Cancer. Dementia. Heart disease. No proof yet, anyway. Vitamin B$_6$ is essential to life but not a cure-all.

PRECAUTIONS: Taking more than 200 milligrams a day forever can lead to peripheral neuropathy, where you can't feel your arms and legs. So, yeah, don't do that.

VITAMIN B$_{12}$

Your brain and nervous system work because of vitamin B$_{12}$, and the vitamin also plays a key role in DNA synthesis. You'll find high levels in beef liver and clams, but it's also in staples like fish, meat, poultry and dairy, and often added to breakfast cereals.

Might Help: Dementia, because vitamin B$_{12}$ has been shown to lower homocysteine levels, but more studies must be done.

Won't Help: Heart disease. Athletic performance: Despite being touted as a booster, and reportedly used by singers like Victoria Beckham and Rita Ora, there's no solid evidence.

PRECAUTIONS: None really. A deficiency could cause permanent damage to nerve tissue. Trouble absorbing it could lead to pernicious anemia.

THE OTHER Bs

Besides B$_6$ and B$_{12}$, there are a few other B vitamins, all of which help release energy from our food: We have niacin and folate (see previous entries, arranged alphabetically); thiamin (B$_1$), which keeps your nerves and muscles strong (find it in peas, fruit and eggs); riboflavin (B$_2$), which strengthens your skin and eyes (and can be found in milk, eggs and most breakfast cereals); and pantothenic acid (B$_5$), an ingredient in some skin and hair products (found in almost all meats and vegetables). Although each of these are essential to human growth, they are not thought to cure diseases.

VANADIUM

What It Is: Vanadium is a trace mineral found in shellfish, mushrooms, parsley, dill and grains.

What It's Commonly Used For: Vanadium is popular as a sports supplement, and may improve insulin sensitivity for people with type 2 diabetes.

Any Proof It Works? No evidence exists to show that vanadium enhances performance, but some small studies suggest that it may improve blood sugar control, and possibly lower LDL levels in type 2 diabetics. High levels of vanadium can be toxic, so experts suggest a limit of 1.8 milligrams; the average diet provides six to 18 micrograms.

26. VITAMIN C

Here we go, the biggie: Vitamin C—the one we learn about first as kids, the one we pop like candy as adults, the one that supplements many diets during old age. How does this nutrient work? A few ways. First, vitamin C, also known as a L-ascorbic acid, is a bodyguard, protecting your cells from bad stuff like free radicals, the damaging compounds made when the food we eat converts into energy. (How destructive are these bad boys? They can cause everything from cancer to cardiovascular disease.) Vitamin C also helps wounds heal, and bleed less, because it's an essential ingredient in collagen, the main protein in our skin.

And, of course, it helps your immune system work better, because, well, that's common knowledge, and what the orange juice commercials claim. But is it true? And does it work when you take it after already getting a cold? Take a look at the evidence below.

But first, a note: Despite the myriad vitamin C supplements available, there's a good chance you're getting enough just by eating a diet with fruits and vegetables, and living healthily overall. Adult men need about 90 milligrams a day, and adult women need a 75-milligram daily dose,

So, Can Vitamin C Cure a Cold, or What?

The short answer is: "or what." We all want to believe vitamin C will help cure a cold, none more so than the dozens of manufacturers hawking quick relief. But here's the evidence, from the mouths of researchers: "Vitamin C may work in concert with other micronutrients rather than providing benefits alone," says a special report from Harvard Health Publications. "Controlled clinical trials of appropriate statistical power would be necessary to determine if supplemental vitamin C boosts the immune system," says the Linus Pauling Institute, the experts in micronutrients. So why have we been taught to believe it's a cure-all? As we wrote in the beginning of this section, vitamin C does help repair damage to the cells, promoting overall well-being. But once you're sick, it's too late—the vitamin doesn't target viruses, like a sharpshooter. The NIH defines the sweet spot: "Vitamin C supplements do not reduce the risk of getting the common cold," it says. "And using vitamin C supplements after cold symptoms start does not appear to be helpful. However, people who take vitamin C supplements regularly might have slightly shorter colds or somewhat milder symptoms when they do have a cold."

Top Sources of Vitamin C		
FOOD	mg per serving	Percent DV*
Red pepper, sweet, raw, ½ cup	95	158
Orange juice, ¾ cup	93	155
Orange, 1 medium	70	117
Grapefruit juice, ¾ cup	70	117
Kiwifruit, 1 medium	64	107
Green pepper, sweet, raw, ½ cup	60	100
Broccoli, cooked, ½ cup	51	85
Strawberries, fresh, sliced, ½ cup	49	82
Brussels sprouts, cooked, ½ cup	48	80
Grapefruit, ½ medium	39	65

*Daily Value   Source: NIH

according to the Office of Dietary Supplements. One orange alone has 70 milligrams, as does a glass of orange or grapefruit juice, or a kiwi. A glass of V8 has 52 milligrams. A half cup of raw red pepper has 142 milligrams. So it's easy to get there without crunching pills. (Key words above, though, were "living healthily overall." Smokers, for example, invite more free radicals, and thus require an extra 35 milligrams of vitamin C a day.)

GOOD EVIDENCE FOR:

Age-related Macular Degeneration (AMD): Older readers may recognize this one, assuming they can read this sentence: AMD affects the macula, a small part of your retina, and causes fuzzy vision or a blank patch when you look directly at something, like a book. It's not painful, very common in the elderly—and annoying as hell. The young have a chance of prevention: "In a large study, older people with AMD who took a daily dietary supplement with 500 milligrams vitamin C, 80 milligrams zinc, 400 IU vitamin E, 15 milligrams beta-carotene and 2 milligrams copper for about six years had a lower chance of developing advanced AMD," reports the NIH. "They also had less vision loss than those who did not take the dietary supplement." That said, the research doesn't indicate vitamin C will keep you from getting AMD. Same goes for cataracts—still more research to be done there.

Gout: Gout only afflicts about 2% of the population, but cases are on the rise, because it's associated with a diet high in fructose-sweetened drinks, meat and booze, three staples of the (awful) American diet. The good docs at the University of British Columbia, Vancouver, determined, over the course of a 20-year study, that "Higher vitamin C intake is independently associated with a lower risk of gout. Supplemental vitamin C intake may be beneficial in the prevention of gout."

SOME EVIDENCE FOR:

Cancer: Let's go right to the National Institutes of Health on this one: "It is not clear whether taking high doses of vitamin C is helpful as a treatment for cancer," they say, flat out. "A few studies in animals and test tubes indicate that very high blood levels of vitamin C might shrink tumors. But more research is needed to determine whether high-dose intravenous vitamin C helps treat cancer in people."

Cardiovascular Disease: The results here are muddled, too. In studies, those people who ate healthy amounts of fruits and vegetables had a lower risk for heart disease, but that may be because those foods are high in antioxidants, not because of the vitamin C. Either way, the fresh veggies had an impact: Hit up that farmer's market for your heart.

Hair: Collagen supports hair follicles and keeps blood vessels in the scalp healthy. Vitamin C also helps you absorb iron from plant proteins. Try soy yogurt with an orange; ½ cup of strawberries; or 1 cup of steamed spinach with chopped tomatoes.

Hangover: Vitamin C reduces symptoms of hangover and counteracts the effects of staying out late.

LIMITED EVIDENCE FOR:

Stroke: This is another case—as with cardiovascular disease—where vitamin C may have helped reduce the risk factors, yet can't be singled out as the sole hero. One landmark study, which followed a rural Japanese community for 20 years, showed that those who ate fruits and veggies six to seven days of the week had a 54% lower risk than those who ate zero to two days of the week. It measured the serum vitamin C concentration and found "This relationship was significant for both cerebral infarction and hemorrhagic stroke," wrote the authors, from Tokyo Medical and Dental University.

NO EVIDENCE FOR/POSSIBLY DANGEROUS:

Colds and flu: Hate to break the news, but see "So, Can Vitamin C Cure a Cold?" on page 452.

PRECAUTIONS: Pregnant women shouldn't take megadoses of C. Chewable forms can damage tooth enamel, according to some studies. Aspirin and non-esterified vitamin C taken together in large doses over time can cause stomach irritation and possibly lead to ulcers. Don't pop more than 2,000 milligrams a day. And lower your dose if diarrhea occurs—last thing you need on top of a cold or flu is more time on the throne.

27. VITAMIN D

Unlike the other vitamins on this list, your body makes one form of vitamin D—vitamin D3—when exposed to sunlight. Yet we still must consume it from outside sources, because it's so very necessary: Vitamin D aids calcium absorption and bone growth. So if you don't "got milk," get it: The U.S. has been fortifying its cow juice since the 1930s, originally to combat rickets, a softening of the bones. Also try fish and OJ.

Despite its prevalence, many people still don't get enough: Some 60% of Americans are deficient in vitamin D, according to the Centers for Disease Control and Prevention. To find out if you're at risk, ask for the 25-hydroxy test, a simple blood test. Your level for optimal health should be above 35 ng/mL. Current guidelines call for women ages 19 to 50 to get 200 IU—"international units"—daily, but experts recommend an extra

Best Sources of Vitamin D FOOD	IUs per serving	Percent DV*
Cod liver oil, 1 tablespoon	1,360	340
Swordfish, cooked, 3 ounces	566	142
Salmon (sockeye), cooked, 3 ounces	447	112
Tuna fish, canned in water, drained, 3 ounces	154	39
Orange juice fortified with vitamin D, 1 cup (check product labels, as amount of added vitamin D varies)	137	34
Milk, nonfat, reduced fat, and whole, vitamin D-fortified, 1 cup	115-124	29-31
Yogurt, fortified with 20% of the DV for vitamin D, 6 ounces (more heavily fortified yogurts provide more of the DV)	80	20
Margarine, fortified, 1 tablespoon	60	15
Sardines, canned in oil, drained, 2 sardines	46	12
Liver, beef, cooked, 3 ounces	42	11

*Daily Value   Source: NIH

2,000 IU a day if you have some sun exposure (about 20 minutes a day), or more if you have little or no sun exposure. In winter, most people need 5,000 IU daily, says John Jacob Cannell, M.D., of the Vitamin D Council.

Consider taking a supplement, but make it vitamin D3 (cholecalciferol, derived from animal products), which your body makes. Certain foods can boost your vitamin D intake. See the chart.

GOOD EVIDENCE FOR:

Arthritis: Deficient levels of the "sunshine vitamin" have been linked to higher rates of osteoarthritis (OA), as well as chronic pain and disability in OA patients, says Jason Theodosakis, M.D., author of *The Arthritis Cure.* He suggests getting a simple vitamin D blood test.

Osteoporosis: We've established that vitamin D=strong bones. And yet confusion reigns when it comes to this affliction, which weakens bone structure: Do they help or not? A 2013 study made headlines around the world: "Bad news for osteoporosis sufferers," wrote the *Independent.* "Vitamin D supplements 'do not help bone health.'" And yet other studies conclusively show otherwise. For an idea about what's what, see the "Osteoporosis" section on page 193.

SOME EVIDENCE FOR:

Cancer: A 2008 study from *Breast Journal* involving women in 107 countries found that the incidence of breast cancer was about nine times higher in women who lived in areas with the least amount of sunlight (e.g., Iceland, England, New Zealand). But results overall in cancer research are inconclusive yet tantalizing, as scientists continue to parse how geography and gender come into play. One big trial, involving 20,000 subjects and examining whether vitamin D supplements can prevent a variety of cancers, will be completed in June 2016. See the Cancer section within the "Conditions" chapter for more.

Diabetes: A 2013 study out of Almazov's Centre of Heart, Blood and Endocrinology found "Vitamin D deficiency is a potential risk factor for obesity and development of insulin resistance leading to diabetes type 2." But the jury's still out on the direct link to diabetes prevention. In 2013, the *Annals of the New York Academy of Sciences* compiled a mega-report about vitamin D. Referencing a Tufts study, they wrote: "Although the observation studies strongly suggest an important role for vitamin D in type 2 diabetes, and such a role is biologically plausible, there is lack of evidence... to support the contention that type 2 diabetes can be improved or prevented."

LIMITED EVIDENCE FOR:

Depression: With previous results showing either a positive or negative effect on depression, McMaster University out of Ontario began a systematic review in 2013 to find out once and for all. The *Journal of Clinical Endocrinology & Metabolism* did find that low dietary intake of

The Über-Antioxidant Everyone Needs

The process of keeping the body running is a dirty one. As your various internal systems fight stress and provide energy for workouts, they create harmful by-products—kind of like a car's toxic emissions. Antioxidants help get rid of this metabolic garbage.

"Glutathione is the most abundant and powerful antioxidant of all, and it's frequently depleted because of all the bad things we're exposed to," says Lauren Noel, N.D., a naturopath in private practice in San Diego. "If you're low, you're at higher risk for cancer and other diseases and you may even age faster."

Another factor working against us? We produce less glutathione as we get older. "Starting in your 30s, you lose about 10 to 20% of your glutathione production with each decade," says Michael Smith, M.D., a spokesman for the Life Extension Foundation, a nonprofit organization devoted to anti-aging research. "If you take a lot of medications, including acetaminophen, or work around chemicals like the ones you'd find in a hair salon, your glutathione production may slow down at an even faster rate."

Your doctor can check glutathione levels with a specialized blood panel or an organic acid urine test. Although some experts say you can get all the amino acids you need to make glutathione from a healthy diet, others believe supplementing is necessary. Smith suggests taking 100 to 200 milligrams of "reduced" glutathione daily on an empty stomach (aim for 200 if you're exposed to more toxins).

Best Buy: Life Extension Glutathione, Cysteine & C ($12.15 for 100; lef.org)

vitamin D may lead to depression or Alzheimer's.

PRECAUTIONS: You risk toxicity if you take too much—more than 50,000 IU daily, for example, results in a scary thing called hypercalcemia: too much calcium, resulting in an abnormal heart rhythm or ulcers. But if you're taking normal doses, there's not much to worry about—and you can't get toxicity from too much sun.

28. VITAMIN E

Like vitamin A, vitamin E is not a singular substance, but a term for a group of compounds that act as antioxidants, protecting your cells from damage. Makes sense, then, that it slows aging, keeps your hair and skin healthy and protects against coronary disease.

Vitamin E is found in nuts and seeds, cereal products and plant oils, like olive and corn oil. The recommended dose is 15 milligrams a day for men and women. As with the other vitamins on this list, there's a good chance you're getting enough already, if you eat right.

GOOD EVIDENCE FOR:

Coronary Heart Disease: Hefty research shows heart disease was lowered 30% to 40% in those with higher levels of vitamin E supplements, while a report from Brigham and Women's Hospital in Boston demonstrates "that supplementation with vitamin E may reduce the risk of VTE"—aka

Top Sources of Vitamin E FOOD	mg per serving	Percent DV*
Wheat germ oil, 1 tablespoon	20.3	100
Sunflower seeds, dry roasted, 1 ounce	7.4	37
Almonds, dry roasted, 1 ounce	6.8	34
Sunflower oil, 1 tablespoon	5.6	28
Safflower oil, 1 tablespoon	4.6	25
Hazelnuts, dry roasted, 1 ounce	4.3	22
Peanut butter, 2 tablespoons	2.9	15
Peanuts, dry roasted, 1 ounce	2.2	11
Corn oil, 1 tablespoon	1.9	10
Spinach, boiled, ½ cup	1.9	10

*Daily Value   Source: NIH

blood clots—"in women, and those with a prior history or genetic predisposition may particularly benefit." Studies from 2013 out of Tokyo, the United Arab Emirates and institutions in other countries all found something along these lines: Vitamin E may be an effective intervention strategy.

Skin and hair: Applied topically, vitamin E can boost collagen production, making you look younger (if not actually removing the wrinkles for good) and your hair look thicker. When buying creams or shampoos, choose one that mentions alpha-tocopherol instead of alpha-tocopherol acetate—the skin absorbs the former more easily, because it's alcohol-based.

SOME EVIDENCE FOR:

Diabetes: There's compelling evidence vitamin E can help counteract diabetes in animals, but additional human studies must be done.

LIMITED EVIDENCE FOR:

Cataracts: Long story short: Many reports say vitamin E prevents cataracts—an appealing conclusion, since antioxidants should prevent protein oxidation—yet other studies say there's no helpful connection.

NO EVIDENCE FOR/POSSIBLY DANGEROUS:

Cancer and cognitive decline: The logic should follow: If vitamin E protects cells, and cancer is a by-product of cell damage, vitamin E should stave off cancer. "Unfortunately, human trials and surveys that have attempted to associate vitamin E intake with cancer incidence have found that vitamin E is not beneficial in most cases," reports the NIH, and our digging through the research didn't find any definitive breakthroughs.

PRECAUTIONS: People on blood-thinning medications should talk to their doctors before supplementing with vitamin E.

29. VITAMIN K

Not as flashy as its siblings, but still essential: Vitamin K is a nutrient necessary mainly for blood clotting and to prevent abnormal bleeding. Vitamin K1 is found mostly in green leafy vegetables such as kale, cabbage, collard greens, broccoli and spinach, and some oils; vitamin K2 is found in fermented foods and some animal products such as meat and dairy. Most people get enough vitamin K from the food they eat, but a deficiency can result from extended use of antibiotics, liver damage, an intestinal disorder such as celiac or malnutrition. Newborns are usually given a supplement orally or by injection.

GOOD EVIDENCE FOR:

Blood Clotting: As we said, vitamin K is needed for normal blood clotting, and that seems to be the primary use of supplements—studies show they work.

Heart Disease: Good news here: there's growing evidence that vitamin K is a powerful inhibitor of the calcification, or hardening, of the arteries. A 2012 statement published in *Advanced Nutrition* found strong evidence from observational and clinical studies that suboptimal levels of vitamin K play an important role in vascular calcification, especially for patients who also have chronic kidney disease.

Osteoporosis: Vitamin K is involved in the formation of bone; a 2013 *Osteoporosis International* study found that supplemental vitamin K_2 taken over three years significantly improved bone density and strength in postmenopausal women; and an *American Journal of Clinical Nutrition* analysis found that low levels of vitamin K increased the risk of hip fractures in women ages 38 to 63.

SOME EVIDENCE FOR:

Cancer: A large 2008 epidemiologic study in Europe showed a higher risk of prostate cancer among men with low vitamin K intake levels. But critics say that people who get lots of vitamin K in their diets get it from fruits and vegetables, which also contain many other cancer-risk-reducing compounds.

PRECAUTIONS: The natural forms of vitamin K_1 and K_2 appear to be completely safe, although they might interfere with the action of blood thinners; but the synthetic form, vitamin K3, can interfere with the function of glutathione, one of the body's natural antioxidants.

30. ZINC

The essential mineral zinc is wildly popular as a cold remedy and cough lozenge ingredient, but it's impressively multipurpose: Besides immune function, it plays a role in DNA synthesis and cell division, and supports normal growth during pregnancy, childhood and adolescence.

Since the body doesn't store zinc, a daily dose is required. Chow down on oysters (a serving supplies 74 milligrams, or 500% of the DV), beef, seafood, poultry, nuts, beans and whole grains.

For vegetarians, beans are an important source, and allowing beans to soak until sprouts form will ensure proper absorption.

For a complete look at cold and flu remedies, visit page 88.

GOOD EVIDENCE FOR:

Colds: Zinc, when taken at the first sign of cold symptoms, has been shown in placebo-controlled, double-blind studies to significantly reduce the cough, nasal discharge and muscle aches associated with colds, says the NIH Office of Dietary Supplements. A recent Cochran review—they test the accuracy of evidence-based reports—concluded that "zinc (lozenges or syrup) is beneficial in reducing the duration and severity of the common cold in healthy people, when taken within 24 hours of onset of symptoms."

Age-related Macular Degeneration: Research has suggested that zinc, in combination with antioxidants such as vitamin C and beta-carotene, delays the progression of macular degeneration, possibly by preventing cellular damage in the retina.

Wound Healing: Zinc helps maintain the integrity of skin and mucosal membranes; deficiencies have been linked to chronic leg ulcers, and supplementation is often used to treat them.

Immunity: Zinc is essential to the production and activation of T-cells, our natural killer cells, and severe zinc deficiency depresses immune function so research is ongoing in the use of zinc supplements in the treatment and prevention of pneumonia, malaria and HIV/AIDS. A recent study found that supplementation reduced the incidence of infection and inflammation in adults ages 55 to 87.

Pregnancy Complications: A recent systematic review of 20 studies found that zinc supplements reduced premature deliveries by 14%.

PRECAUTIONS: Zinc toxicity is rare; more often gastrointestinal distress has been reported with higher doses; excessive consumption of zinc could cause a copper deficiency. In the United States, zinc deficiency is also rare; symptoms of a deficiency include weight loss, impotence, hair loss, delayed sexual maturation, delayed healing and taste abnormalities.

INDEX

A

beta carotene and, 421

breast, 73–74, 76, 78, 80–81, 439, 442

CLA and, 427–428

deep breathing and, 80

diet and, 78, 82, 83

fish oil and, 433

folate and, 434

hormone-sensitive, 413

lutein/zeaxanthin and, 437–438

lycopene and, 439

meditation and, 80–81

prevention and suppression, 390–391, 398–399, 401, 407–408

proactive attitude and, 72

probiotics and, 446

selenium and, 447–448

spirulina and, 441

supplements and, 75–76, 80–81, 85, 421, 449–451, 454, 456, 459–460

carbohydrates, 5, 67, 141

Carcinia cambogia, 239

cardio exercise, 131

cardiovascular disease. See heart disease

carnitine, 426–427

carpel tunnel syndrome, 87

cataracts, 421, 459

catuaba, 217

CBT (cognitive behavioral therapy), 8, 51–52

CFS (chronic fatigue syndrome), 112

chamomile tea, 76, 317

chaste tree berry, 404–405

CHD (coronary heart disease). See heart disease

chemical cleanse, 164

china (herbal remedy), 369

Chinese medicine. See Traditional Chinese Medicine

chiropractic medicine, 62–63, 250–253

chocolate, 388

cholesterol control, 32–33, 133–137, 401, 411, 437, 442

chromium, 105, 420

chronic fatigue syndrome (CFS), 112

cigarettes, 8–9, 53, 165

cinnamon, 103, 411–412

circulation, 406, 412

clary sage oil, 11

clay mask, natural, 4

cleanses. See detox and cleanses

coenzyme Q10, 188, 428–430

coffee, 76, 103, 116, 304–305

Coffea cruda, 369

cognitive behavioral therapy (CBT), 8, 51–52

cognitive decline, 33, 401, 427, 434, 459

cognitive therapy and weight loss, 240–243

colds and flu
food and immunity, 91–92
herbal medicine, 92, 388, 401, 411
homeopathy and, 368
remedies, 88–90, 92
selenium and, 447–448
symptoms, 89, 399–400, 461
vitamin C and, 92, 453, 454
zinc and, 92

cold water fish, 309

E

Q

R

S

sabadilla, 367

SAD (seasonal affective disorder), 204–205

sage, 408–409

salt, 66, 120–121, 196

SAM-e, 96

saw palmetto, 218

scalp massage, 340

schizophrenia, 442, 446

sciatica, 206–207

sea salt, 314

seasonal affective disorder (SAD), 204–205

season/weather, 294, 297, 299

selective serotonin reuptake inhibitors (SSRIs), 57

selenium, 240, 447–448

self-destructive tendencies, 8

self-hypnosis, 241, 373–374

sesame seeds, 424–425

sex education, 212

sex therapy, 211–212

sex toys, 212

sexual activity, 26, 28

sexual dysfunction
   antidepressant-induced, 180–181, 392
   aphrodisiacs, 165, 215–218, 219, 419
   arousal remedies, 212
   diet and, 215

herbal remedies, 211, 401
hysterectomy and, 209–210
low libido, 180–181, 209–212, 444–445
orgasmic remedies, 213
pain remedies, 214–215
psychological problems and, 210
symptoms, 208

sexual lubricants, 214

shiatsu massage, 257

SHINE fibromyalgia treatment protocol, 111–113

showering, detox and, 311

sinus congestion, 411

sinus infection, 220–221

skin health, 107, 397–398, 459

sleep
   anxiety and, 53
   detox and, 311
   diabetes risk and, 103
   longevity and, 26, 28
   melatonin and, 441–442
   pharmaceutical drug addiction and, 11–12

smoking, 8–9, 63, 165

snack foods, 35

snoring, 222–223

socialization, benefits of, 26, 339

social support, 26

soft belly breathing, 203

soy, 127, 136, 196, 438

spirulina, 441

SSRIs (selective serotonin reuptake inhibitors), 57, 93

statins, 119, 133, 136

steam, as acne treatment, 4

sterols, 442

stinging nettle, 316, 395

St. John's wort, 96, 396–397

stress
  addiction, 11
  cancer diagnosis and, 78, 80
  diet and, 237
  fertility and, 165
  heart disease and, 120
  IBS and, 145
  infertility and, 160–161
  kapha type doshas and, 299
  management, 111
  marijuana and, 400
  migraine and, 187
  milky oat seed and, 399
  negative aspects of, 226–227
  positive aspects of, 225–226, 233
  reactions, 228
  remedies
    active rest, 232
    dietary changes, 230–231
    exercise, 231–232
    meditation, 230
    prioritize, 228, 230
    sunshine, 231
    supplements, 231
  supplements and, 231
  symptoms, 224–225
  vata type doshas and, 293

stress incontinence, 149–151

strokes, 454

strontium, 35, 198

structural yoga therapy, 207

substance use, 53

sugar, 8, 23, 83

sunglasses, 41

sunshine, 231

supplements
  cancer and, 75–76, 85
  detox and, 306–307
  diabetes and, 101–105
  functions of, 10, 416–417, 419,
    420–421, 426–428
  popularity of, 415–416

support groups, 18

sweat, 311

Swedish massage, 256

T

tai chi and qigong, 19, 131, 197,
  275–278, 279–282f

TCAs (tricyclic antidepressants), 57

TCM. See Traditional Chinese
  Medicine

tea, 163, 397

tea tree oil, 4, 397–398

TENS (transcutaneous electrical
  nerve stimulation), 62

Thai massage, 257

Therapeutic Touch (TT), 321–323

thiamin, 451

thyroid health, 176–177, 238, 240,
  427

TM (transcendental meditation),
  123

tobacco, 8–9, 53, 165

toxins, 126, 340

Traditional Chinese Medicine
  (TCM)
  anxiety remedies, 55
  bloating and, 68
  diet and, 35